Vitamins as Nutraceuticals

Scrivener Publishing
100 Cummings Center, Suite 541J
Beverly, MA 01915-6106

Publishers at Scrivener
Martin Scrivener (martin@scrivenerpublishing.com)
Phillip Carmical (pcarmical@scrivenerpublishing.com)

Vitamins as Nutraceuticals

Recent Advances and Applications

Edited by
Eknath D. Ahire
Raj K. Keservani
Khemchand R. Surana
Sippy Singh
and
Rajesh K. Kesharwani

WILEY

This edition first published 2023 by John Wiley & Sons, Inc., 111 River Street, Hoboken, NJ 07030, USA
and Scrivener Publishing LLC, 100 Cummings Center, Suite 541J, Beverly, MA 01915, USA
© 2023 Scrivener Publishing LLC
For more information about Scrivener publications please visit www.scrivenerpublishing.com.

All rights reserved. No part of this publication may be reproduced, stored in a retrieval system, or transmitted, in any form or by any means, electronic, mechanical, photocopying, recording, or otherwise, except as permitted by law. Advice on how to obtain permission to reuse material from this title is available at http://www.wiley.com/go/permissions.

Wiley Global Headquarters
111 River Street, Hoboken, NJ 07030, USA

For details of our global editorial offices, customer services, and more information about Wiley products visit us at www.wiley.com.

Limit of Liability/Disclaimer of Warranty
While the publisher and authors have used their best efforts in preparing this work, they make no representations or warranties with respect to the accuracy or completeness of the contents of this work and specifically disclaim all warranties, including without limitation any implied warranties of merchantability or fitness for a particular purpose. No warranty may be created or extended by sales representatives, written sales materials, or promotional statements for this work. The fact that an organization, website, or product is referred to in this work as a citation and/or potential source of further information does not mean that the publisher and authors endorse the information or services the organization, website, or product may provide or recommendations it may make. This work is sold with the understanding that the publisher is not engaged in rendering professional services. The advice and strategies contained herein may not be suitable for your situation. You should consult with a specialist where appropriate. Neither the publisher nor authors shall be liable for any loss of profit or any other commercial damages, including but not limited to special, incidental, consequential, or other damages. Further, readers should be aware that websites listed in this work may have changed or disappeared between when this work was written and when it is read.

Library of Congress Cataloging-in-Publication Data

ISBN 978-139-417470-6

Cover image: Pixabay.Com
Cover design by Russell Richardson

Set in size of 11pt and Minion Pro by Manila Typesetting Company, Makati, Philippines

Printed in the USA

10 9 8 7 6 5 4 3 2 1

Contents

Preface		xiii
1	**Introduction to Nutraceutical Vitamins**	**1**
	Khemchand R. Surana, Eknath D. Ahire, Shital J. Patil,	
	Sunil K. Mahajan, Dhananjay M. Patil	
	and Deepak D. Sonawane	
	1.1 Introduction	2
	1.1.1 Multivitamins	4
	1.1.2 Classification of Vitamins	4
	1.2 Fat-Soluble Vitamins A, D, E, F, and K	4
	1.2.1 Vitamin A	4
	1.2.2 Vitamin D	6
	1.2.3 Vitamin E	8
	1.2.4 Vitamin F	9
	1.2.5 Vitamin K	11
	1.2.6 Water-Soluble Vitamins B1, B2, B3, B7, B9, B12 (B Complex), and C	12
	1.2.6.1 Vitamin B1	13
	1.2.6.2 Vitamin B2	15
	1.2.6.3 Vitamin B3	16
	1.2.7 Vitamin B5	17
	1.2.8 Vitamin B6	19
	1.2.9 Vitamin B9, BC, Vitamin M, or Folacin	20
	1.2.10 Vitamin B12	22
	1.2.11 Vitamin C	24
	1.3 Conclusions	26
	Acknowledgment	27
	References	27

2	Structure and Functions of Vitamins	35

*Suvarna S. Khairnar, Khemchand R. Surana,
Eknath D. Ahire, Sunil K. Mahajan, Dhananjay M. Patil
and Deepak D. Sonawane*

2.1	Introduction	36
2.2	Structural Discussion	37
	2.2.1 Vitamin A	37
	2.2.2 Vitamin D	39
	2.2.3 Vitamin E	41
	2.2.4 Vitamin K	42
	2.2.5 Vitamin B1	43
	2.2.6 Vitamin B2	44
	2.2.7 Vitamin B3	45
	2.2.8 Vitamin B7/H	46
	2.2.9 Vitamin B9/Folic Acid	47
	2.2.10 Vitamin B12	48
	2.2.11 Vitamin C	49
2.3	Conclusion	55
	References	55

3	Vitamin Intervention in Cardiac Health	61

*Shubham J. Khairnar, Eknath D. Ahire,
Madhuri D. Deshmukh, Raj K. Keservani,
Sanjay J. Kshirsagar, Amit Kumar Rajora
and Manju Amit Kumar Rajora*

3.1	Introduction	62
3.2	Vitamin Deficiency and Cardiovascular Disease	63
3.3	Vitamin Supplementation and Cardiovascular Disease	66
3.4	Clinical Research Suggesting Antioxidant Vitamins' Beneficial Effects in CVP	70
3.5	Beneficial Effects of B Vitamins in CVP	73
3.6	Role of Vitamin D in Cardiovascular Health	73
3.7	Conclusion	76
	Acknowledgment	77
	References	77

4	Impact of Vitamins on Immunity	87

*Abhijeet G. Parkhe, Khemchand R. Surana, Eknath D. Ahire,
Sunil K. Mahajan, Dhananjay M. Patil
and Deepak D. Sonawane*

4.1	Introduction	88

	4.2	Vitamin-Rich Foods for the Management of Immune System-Related Diseases	89
	4.3	Fat-Soluble Vitamins Reported in the Literature Commonly Used in the Treatment of the Immune System-Related Diseases	92
		4.3.1 Vitamin A	92
		4.3.2 Vitamin D	93
		4.3.3 Vitamin E	94
	4.4	Water Soluble Vitamins Reported in the Literature Commonly Used in the Treatment of the Immune System-Related Diseases	95
		4.4.1 Vitamin B1	95
		4.4.2 Vitamin B2	96
		4.4.3 Vitamin B3	97
		4.4.4 Vitamin B6	98
		4.4.5 Vitamin B9	98
		4.4.6 Vitamin B12	99
		4.4.7 Vitamin C	99
	4.5	Conclusion	100
		Acknowledgment	100
		References	101
5	**Nutraceuticals Potential of Fat-Soluble Vitamins**		**107**
	Jagannath Gaikwad, Shweta Jogdand, Afsar Pathan, Ashwini Mahajan, Anmol Darak, Eknath D. Ahire and Khemchand R. Surana		
	5.1	Introduction	108
		5.1.1 Categories of Nutraceuticals	109
		5.1.2 Vitamins	110
		5.1.2.1 Fat-Soluble Vitamins	111
		5.1.2.2 Fat-Soluble Vitamins in Covid-19	116
		5.1.2.3 Properties of Fat-Soluble Vitamins (Potential)	117
	5.2	Prospective Market Potential of Vitamin K2	123
	5.3	Conclusion	123
		Acknowledgment	124
		References	124

6 Marine-Derived Sources of Nutritional Vitamins 129
Neelam L. Dashputre, Rahul R. Sable, Mayur Sawant, Shubham J. Khairnar, Eknath D. Ahire, Surabhi B. Patil and Jayesh D. Kadam

- 6.1 Introduction 130
- 6.2 Marine-Based Beneficial Molecules 131
  - 6.2.1 Chitin and Chitosan 131
    - 6.2.1.1 Anti-Oxidant Properties 132
    - 6.2.1.2 Anti-Microbial Properties 133
    - 6.2.1.3 Anti-Hypertensive Activity 134
    - 6.2.1.4 Anti-Allergy and Anti-Inflammatory Activity 134
    - 6.2.1.5 Anti-Obesity and Anti-Diabetic Activity 134
    - 6.2.1.6 Anti-Cancer and Anti-Tumor Activity 135
- 6.3 Beneficial Molecules from Marine Macroalgae 136
  - 6.3.1 Pigments 136
  - 6.3.2 Polysaccharides 138
  - 6.3.3 Phenolic Compounds 140
- 6.4 Fish Oil 141
- 6.5 EAA in Protein Supplement Systems 142
- 6.6 Minerals in Seafood for Human Diet 143
- 6.7 Marine-Based Vitamin Sources 144
- 6.8 Dopamine in Seafood as Drug and Supplement 149
- 6.9 Bioactive Peptides From Marine Sources 150
- 6.10 Gelatin From Marine Sources 151
- 6.11 Health Benefit of Nano-Based Materials for Bioactive Compounds from Marine-Based Sources 153
- 6.12 Conclusions 155
- Acknowledgment 156
- References 156

7 Nutraceutical Properties of Seaweed Vitamins 167
Afsar Pathan, Mahima M. Mahajan, Pankaj G. Jain, Shital P. Zambad, Govinda S. Bhandari, Anmol D. Darak, Eknath D. Ahire, Amit Kumar Rajora and Khemchand R. Surana

- 7.1 Introduction 168
- 7.2 Bioactive Compounds from Seaweeds 170
  - 7.2.1 Vitamins 170
  - 7.2.2 Polysaccharides 170
  - 7.2.3 Lipids and Fatty Acids 170

		7.2.4 Phytochemicals	171
	7.3	Seaweed Vitamins as Nutraceuticals	171
	7.4	Types of Seaweed Vitamin	172
	7.5	Vitamin Composition in Seaweed	173
		7.5.1 Therapeutic Properties of Seaweed Vitamins	175
	7.6	Future Perspectives	178
	7.7	Conclusion	179
		Acknowledgment	180
		References	180
8	**Vitamins as Nutraceuticals for Pregnancy**		**185**

Tushar N. Lokhande, Kshitij S. Varma, Shrikant M. Gharate, Sunil K. Mahajan and Khemchand R. Surana

	8.1	Introduction	186
		8.1.1 Diet and Nourishment in Pregnancy	186
	8.2	Role of Important Vitamins in Pregnancy	188
		8.2.1 Vitamin A/Retinol	188
		8.2.2 Vitamin D/Calciferol	189
		8.2.3 Vitamin E/Tocopherol	189
		8.2.4 Vitamin B1/Thiamine	191
		8.2.5 Vitamin B7/Biotin	191
		8.2.6 Vitamin B9/Folic Acid	191
		8.2.7 Vitamin B12/Cobalamin/Cyanocobalamin	192
		8.2.8 Vitamin C/Ascorbic Acid	192
	8.3	Concept of Nutraceuticals	194
	8.4	Targeted Nutrition Foods for Pregnancy	195
	8.5	Concentrations of Vitamins During Pregnancy	196
	8.6	Role of Vitamins in the Body	197
	8.7	Herbal Sources as a Vitamin	197
	8.8	Conclusion	198
		Acknowledgment	199
		References	199
9	**Role of Vitamins in Metabolic Diseases**		**205**

Simona D'souza, Pavan Udavant, Jayesh Kadam, Shubham Khairnar, Eknath D. Ahire and Rahul Sable

		Abbreviations	206
	9.1	Introduction	207
		9.1.1 Introduction to Vitamins	207
		9.1.1.1 Fat-Soluble Vitamins	209
		9.1.1.2 Water-Soluble Vitamins	209
	9.2	Metabolic Diseases	210

		9.2.1	Role of Fat-Soluble Vitamins in Metabolic Diseases	211
			9.2.1.1 Vitamin A	211
			9.2.1.2 Vitamin D	214
			9.2.1.3 Vitamin E	217
			9.2.1.4 Vitamin K	219
		9.2.2	Role of Water-Soluble Vitamins in Metabolic Diseases	222
			9.2.2.1 Vitamin B3	222
			9.2.2.2 Vitamin B5	223
			9.2.2.3 Vitamin B6	224
			9.2.2.4 Vitamin B2	225
			9.2.2.5 Vitamin B9	225
			9.2.2.6 Vitamin B12	225
			9.2.2.7 Vitamin C	227
	9.3	Can Ascorbic Acid Lead to Cancer?		228
	9.4	Conclusion		229
		Acknowledgment		229
		References		229

10 Beneficial Effects of Water-Soluble Vitamins in Nutrition and Health Promotion — 235

Afsar S. Pathan, Pankaj G. Jain, Ashwini B. Mahajan, Vivek S. Kumawat, Eknath D. Ahire, Khemchand R. Surana, Amit K. Rajora and Manju Amit Kumar Rajora

	10.1	Introduction		236
		10.1.1	Vitamin and Its Types	237
			10.1.1.1 Water-Soluble Vitamins	237
			10.1.1.2 Fat-Soluble Vitamins	238
		10.1.2	History of Vitamins	238
			10.1.2.1 Vitamin B-Complex	239
	10.2	Beneficial Effects of Vitamins on Nutrition		244
	10.3	Beneficial Effects of Water-Soluble Vitamins in Health Promotion		247
		10.3.1	Vitamin B1	247
		10.3.2	Vitamin C	247
	10.4	Future Prospective of the Water-Soluble Vitamins		248
	10.5	Conclusion		249
		Acknowledgment		249
		References		249

11 Vitamins as Nutraceuticals for Anemia   253
Snehal D. Pawar, Shubham D. Deore, Nikita P. Bairagi, Vaishnavi B. Deshmukh, Tushar N. Lokhande and Khemchand R. Surana

    11.1 Introduction   254
         11.1.1 Classification of Nutraceuticals   255
    11.2 Anemia   255
         11.2.1 Types of Anemia   256
         11.2.2 Causes of Anemia   258
    11.3 Role of Vitamins in Nutraceuticals for Anemia   258
         11.3.1 Role of Iron in Anemia as Nutraceutical   258
         11.3.2 Vitamin A   259
         11.3.3 Vitamin C   260
         11.3.4 Vitamin E   261
         11.3.5 Folate   262
         11.3.6 Vitamin B12   263
         11.3.7 Riboflavin   263
    11.4 Structure of Vitamins   265
    11.5 Conclusion   275
    Acknowledgment   275
    References   275

12 Vitamins as Nutraceuticals for Oral Health   281
Tushar N. Lokhande, Snehal D. Pawar, Snehal S. Kolpe, Khemchand R. Surana, Smita C. Bonde and Sunil K. Mahajan

    12.1 Introduction   282
         12.1.1 Nutraceuticals Categorized Based on Food Available in Market   283
    12.2 Vitamins   285
         12.2.1 History of Vitamins   286
         12.2.2 Importance of Vitamins for Humans   287
    12.3 Role of Vitamins as Nutraceutical for Oral Health   287
         12.3.1 Vitamins Associated with the Oral Health as Nutraceuticals   287
                12.3.3.1 Vitamin C (Ascorbic Acid)   287
                12.3.3.2 Vitamin D   289
                12.3.3.3 Vitamin E   290
                12.3.3.4 Vitamin K (MKs)   291
                12.3.3.5 Vitamin A   292
                12.3.3.6 Vitamin B-Complex   293

12.4	Before Nutraceuticals	294
12.5	Conclusion	295
	Acknowledgement	295
	References	295

Index **301**

Preface

Since vitamins are widely predicted to be one of the most significant nutritional advancements over the next 25 years, the editors of this book have brought together renowned experts in the field to provide a single authoritative resource for the nutraceutical sector. This book begins by defining and classifying the field of vitamins, with a focus on legislative issues in both the United States and the European Union. The important work of vitamins as nutraceuticals in disease prevention is then summarized. Finally, a chapter on establishing vitamins as nutraceuticals is presented, which also discusses the recent advances and applications in the field.

In addition to discussing recent advances and applications, this book also includes scientific information on the importance of vitamins as nutraceuticals to human health, as well as the potential mechanisms of nutraceuticals in illness prevention, management, and control. It is being published at a time when there is a pressing need to address the rising number of cases of nutritional deficiency disorders and the high number of deaths caused by a lack of knowledge or a deviation from healthy eating habits. As such, it is intended to serve a constructive purpose as a replacement for unverifiable sources of information on the internet and within extremely outdated literature, which can be full of all kinds of promotional propaganda for profit while also leading people astray. The general population must understand what they should eat and why they should take certain nutritional supplements. This book furthers this goal by balancing the evidence in terms of the health-promoting benefits and associated hazards of vitamins as nutraceuticals. A summary of the main ideas and supporting details of the work presented in each of the 12 chapters follows:

–In Chapter 1, Introduction to Nutraceutical Vitamins, Khemchand R. Surana and his coworker present an overview of several bioactive compounds (vitamins) that operate as nutraceuticals. In addition to reviewing their health benefits, nutraceutical applications for the prevention of several diseases are also discussed.

– In Chapter 2, Structure and Functions of Vitamins, Khemchand R. Surana and his colleagues provide an extensive overview of the current evidence on the health implications of food vitamins and also include the effects of emerging technologies on vitamins.
– In Chapter 3, Vitamin Intervention in Cardiac Health, Eknath D. Ahire *et al.* analyze the pertinent research on the role of various vitamins in cardiovascular disease, taking into account both their deficiencies and their supplementation, as well as looking at a few related concerns.
– In Chapter 4, Impact of Vitamins on Immunity, Khemchand R. Surana *et al.* focus on the function of nutrients in immunity and immune-associated diseases. They present the findings of a scientific practitioner and a team of researchers, who observed the ways in which multivitamins and some micronutrients can assist in enhancing the immune system.
– In Chapter 5, Nutraceuticals Potential of Fat-Soluble Vitamins, Ashwini Mahajan *et al.* focus on fat-soluble vitamins and their potential use as nutraceuticals.
– In Chapter 6, Marine-Derived Sources of Nutritional Vitamins, Jayesh D. Kadam and his associates provide an overview of a number of recently studied beneficial compounds of marine origin that show great potential as nutraceuticals or for use in the food industry.
– In Chapter 7, Nutraceutical Properties of Seaweed Vitamins, Afsar Pathan and his coworker discuss the use of seaweeds as potential sources of seaweed-based vitamin-containing products and their potential therapeutic role in them.
– In Chapter 8, Vitamins as Nutraceuticals for Pregnancy, Tushar N. Lokhande and his colleagues discuss how vitamins aid in the development of the fetal immune system. Various herbal remedies as a source of vitamins during pregnancy are also discussed.
– In Chapter 9, Role of Vitamins in Metabolic Diseases, Eknath D. Ahire and his associates present the way in which vitamins can help avoid metabolic diseases like diabetes, obesity, cardiovascular disease, stroke, renal disease, cancer, and others, as well as how they can cause metabolic disease in some situations.
– In Chapter 10, Beneficial Effects of Water-Soluble Vitamins on Nutrition and Health Promotion, Pankaj G. Jain *et al.* discuss how vitamin deficiency causes the suffering brought on by many harsh diseases. In order to overcome this, dietary supplements are provided to maintain the proper amount of vitamins in the body for overall better body performance.
– In Chapter 11, Vitamins as Nutraceuticals for Anemia, Snehal Dilip Pawar and coworker discuss how vegetables like cabbage and cauliflower, and oil and fat like sunflower oil and soyabean oil, are rich in vitamins C and E

and various sources of folate and riboflavin that help in the prevention of anemia.

–In Chapter 12, Vitamins as Nutraceuticals for Oral Health, Snehal Dilip Pawar and his colleagues discuss the different types of vitamins which help in the prevention of oral diseases to improve oral health.

In closing, we wish to express our sincere gratitude for the outstanding efforts of the chapter contributors for their perseverance and collaboration throughout the editing process. Their dedication and hard work have greatly aided in the development of this book. Our families also deserve special recognition for their support and patience throughout the process of producing this book.

The Editors
February 2023

1

Introduction to Nutraceutical Vitamins

Khemchand R. Surana[1]*, Eknath D. Ahire[2], Shital J. Patil[3], Sunil K. Mahajan[3], Dhananjay M. Patil[4] and Deepak D. Sonawane[4]

[1]Department of Pharmaceutical Chemistry, Shreeshakti Shaikshanik Sanstha, Divine College of Pharmacy, Satana, Nashik, MH, India
[2]Department of Pharmaceutics, MET's Institute of Pharmacy, BKC, Affiliated to SPPU, Adgaon, Nashik, MH, India
[3]Department of Pharmaceutical Chemistry, MGV's Pharmacy College, Panchavati, Nashik, MH, India
[4]Department of Pharmaceutics, Shreeshakti Shaikshanik Sanstha, Divine College of Pharmacy, Satana, Nashik, MH, India

Abstract

Vitamins are low-molecular weight organic compounds that are required for life activity in trace amounts for essential metabolic reactions, with deficiency causing specific disease symptoms. Vitamins do not include other essential nutrients, such as dietary minerals, essential fatty acids, or essential amino acids, nor do they include the large number of other nutrients that promote health but do not provide cellular structural material and energy. Plants and microbes provided vitamins to animals. Vitamins are divided into two categories: fat-soluble (A, D, and E) and water-soluble (B, C, and P). Natural diets, herbal items, biofortified crops, genetically modified, and processed food products are all examples of nutraceuticals. Beyond basic diet, nutraceuticals improve health, alter immunity, and/or prevent and cure certain diseases. An overview of several bioactive compounds (vitamins) that operate as nutraceuticals has been reviewed in this chapter, as well as their involvement in health benefits. Nutraceutical applications in the prevention of several diseases have also been discussed.

Keywords: Nutraceuticals, vitamins, nutrition, dietary requirements, food

---

*Corresponding author: khemchandsurana411@gmail.com

Eknath D. Ahire, Raj K. Keservani, Khemchand R. Surana, Sippy Singh and Rajesh K. Kesharwani (eds.) *Vitamins as Nutraceuticals: Recent Advances and Applications*, (1–34) © 2023 Scrivener Publishing LLC

1.1 Introduction

Vitamins were discovered as a result of research into nutrition and their significance in the vital activities of living organisms. N. I. Lunin, a Russian physician, was the first to show in 1880 that, in addition to the recognized basic components (proteins, lipids, carbohydrates, water, and minerals), some other accessory ingredients were required for the organism's appropriate growth and maintenance [1]. While researching the causes of Beriberi in 1905, the English physician W. Fletcher noticed that eating unpolished rice instead of polished rice prevented Beriberi, and he hypothesized the existence of some specific nutrients in the rice husk. C. Funk, a Polish biochemist, coined the term "vitamin" in 1912, combining the Latin words "vita" for life and "amine" for chemicals found in the thiamine he extracted from rice bran [2]. Vitamin was eventually abbreviated to vitamin. Vitamins are chemical substances with a low molecular weight that are required in trace amounts for critical metabolic activities in the body and whose absence results in certain illness symptoms. Additional necessary nutrients, such as dietary minerals, essential fatty acids, and essential amino acids, as well as the enormous number of other nutrients that support health, are not included in the term vitamin. Vitamins, unlike other organic nutrients that give cellular structure material and energy, either engage in coenzyme formation or operate as biochemical process regulators [3]. A vitamin deficiency causes organism-specific symptoms that may or may not be alleviated by other vitamins. Plants and microbes provided vitamins to the animal world. Vitaminoids include flavonoids, inositol, carnitine, choline, lipoic acid, and essential fatty acids, which have "vitamin-like" function and are believed by some to be vitamins or to partially replace vitamins [4]. There is minimal evidence that any of these are dietary essentials, with the exception of essential fatty acids. With the exception of vitamin B6 and B12, they are easily eliminated in urine and do not store well, necessitating frequent ingestion. They are generally safe when consumed in excess of requirements, though megadoses of niacin, vitamin C, or pyridoxine may cause symptoms (B6). All of the B vitamins work as coenzymes or cofactors, helping essential enzymes in their activity and allowing energy-producing reactions to complete smoothly. Overcooking can easily destroy water-soluble vitamins. Vitamin K and several B complex vitamins are generated by bacteria in the small intestine in the human body; vitamin D is synthesized by the skin when exposed to sunshine [5].

Ascorbic acid is a vitamin for humans and guinea pigs since it is not formed in their tissues, but it is not a vitamin for rats, rabbits, or dogs because it is synthesized in their cells. Vitamins are obtained from food and gut microorganisms in humans [6].

Chronic or long-term vitamin insufficiency causes avitaminosis (beriberi, scurvy, rickets, and pellagra). Hypovitaminosis is a term used to describe a variety of disorders caused by a lack of one or more vitamins. Antivitamins are substances either degrade or inhibit a vitamin's metabolic function. Vitamin disintegrating enzymes (thiaminase and ascorbase), nonactive complexes with vitamins (avidin), and physically identical to vitamins (sulphonamides) are examples of antivitamins. Hypervitaminosis, also known as vitamin intoxication, is a disorder caused by a continuous high intake of vitamins or vitamin supplements, which can cause nausea, diarrhea, and vomiting [7]. General symptoms of hypervitaminosis, or vitamin intoxication, include lack of appetite, gastrointestinal motor function problems, severe headaches, increased nervous system excitability, hair shedding, skin desquamation, and other indicators. Hypervitaminosis has the potential to be lethal. Hypervitaminosis can be caused by consuming too much fat-soluble vitamin-rich food (for example, the liver of a polar bear or whale, which is high in vitamin A), or by taking too many vitamin pills [8].

Nutraceuticals are also said to slow the aging process, enhance life expectancy, and maintain the body's structure and function. Herbal nutraceuticals help to sustain health by fighting nutritionally induced acute and chronic diseases, as well as promoting optimal health, lifespan, and quality of life. Because of their supposed safety and possible nutritional and therapeutic advantages, nutraceuticals have sparked a lot of attention. Nutraceuticals are divided into two categories: functional foods and dietary supplements. Supplementation and the use of formulated or fortified foods can help people enhance their health [9]. Vitamin B–enriched flour helps to prevent pellagra, vitamin D-enriched milk helps to prevent rickets, and iodine-fortified salt helps to prevent goiter. Commercial nutraceuticals must pass stringent regulatory tests to ensure their quality and beneficial health effects. Functional foods are processed foods that contain nutritious elements that assist healthy body functioning and were initially developed in Japan. Beyond the fundamental nutritional content, a functional meal with novel components provides an additional function or greater benefit to human health. Medical foods and prescription medications are not the same as functional foods [10, 11].

1.1.1 Multivitamins

Multivitamins are lipid-soluble vitamins (A, D, E, and K) as well as water-soluble vitamins (thiamin (B1), riboflavin (B2), B6, B12, C, folic acid, niacin, pantothenic acid, and biotin). They are available over-the-counter (OTC) and as self-prescribed diet/nutritional supplements. Minerals such as calcium, phosphorus, iron, iodine, magnesium, manganese, copper, and zinc may be found in multivitamins [12, 13].

1.1.2 Classification of Vitamins

Vitamins are divided into two classes based on their physicochemical properties: fat-soluble vitamins and water-soluble vitamins. A letter of the Latin alphabet, as well as a chemical or physiologic name, is allocated to each vitamin in each category. Fat-soluble vitamins are absorbed and stored in bodily tissues via fat globules (chylomicrons). Excessive fat-soluble vitamin consumption can result in excessive buildup and hypervitaminosis [14, 15].

1.2 Fat-Soluble Vitamins A, D, E, F, and K

1.2.1 Vitamin A

All foods of animal origin provide vitamin A to humans. Vitamin A is abundant in fish liver particularly that of cod and banded sea perch. Pork and beef liver, egg yolk, sour cream, and whole milk are high in vitamin A. Carotenoids, which are provitamins A, are found in vegetables, such as asparagus, beet, celery, carrots, cabbage, dandelion, lettuce, endive, orange, turnip leaf, tomato, prune, parsley, spinach, and watercress. As a result, if the conversion of alimentary carotenoids to vitamin A is not impeded, vegetables give a partial supply of vitamin A to the human organism. The adult human's daily vitamin A requirement is 1.5 mg [16–18].

Chemical nature and biologically active forms
Retinol, retinal, and retinoic acid are diterpenoid alcohols (unsaturated monobasic alcohols), as are other provitamin A carotenoids such as a- and b-carotenes, b-cryptoxanthin, and others. Retinol and its derivatives are referred to as retinoids together. A typical synthetic vitamin A supplement is retinyl palmitate (vitamin A palmitate), which is an ester of retinol (vitamin A) and palmitic acid. Retinol, often known as vitamin A,

is a chemical isoprenoid generated mostly from b-carotene, which has a b-ionone ring and a side chain of two isoprene residues with a main carbinol group at the end [19]. There are at least six vitamer (vitamin with similar molecular structure) substances that qualify as "vitamin A," but each has slightly different qualities (e.g., retinol, retinal, and four carotenoids: a, b, c, and d carotenes; and b-cryptoxanthin). A vitamin's vitamer is any of several chemical molecules with comparable molecular structure and physiological activity. Plant-based foods have four vitamers (three carotenes and one xanthophyll), while animal-based foods contain retinol (alcohol) and retinal (aldehyde) forms (e.g., fish). Retinoids (retinol, retinal, retinoic acid, isotretinoin, alitretinoin, and others) are vitamin A pharmaceuticals [20]. Retinol (vitamin A alcohol) is transformed to retinal (vitamin A aldehyde) and retinoic acid in the human body (vitamin A acid). Vitamin A ester derivatives such as retinyl palmitate, retinyl acetate, and retinyl are generated in the tissues of the organism. A-, b-, and c-carotenes are three precursors or provitamins A that differ in chemical structure and biological function [21]. The most active is b-carotene, which is oxidized at the central double bond in the intestinal mucosa with the help of the enzyme carotene dihydroxygenase. Two active retinal molecules are generated. The breakdown of a- and c-carotenes, which each include only one b-ionone ring, unlike b-carotene, results in only one vitamin A molecule in both cases. Only one molecule of vitamin A is present in b-cryptoxanthin (retinol). As a result, both a- and c-carotenes, as well as b-cryptoxanthin, have lower activity than b-carotene. Retinol, retinal, retinoic acid, and their esterified counterparts are all biologically active forms of vitamin A [22, 23].

Biochemical functions
Retinoids (retinol, retinoic acid, and their derivatives) are pharmaceutical forms of vitamin A that play a variety of roles in the body, including vision, cell proliferation and differentiation in developing organisms (embryos, juvenile organisms), differentiation of rapidly proliferating tissues like cartilage and bone tissue, spermatogenic epithelium and placenta, skin epithelium, and mucosae, immune function, and immune cell activation [24, 25].

Deficiency
The dark adaption condition and night blindness are the first signs of vitamin A insufficiency. Juvenile growth retardation, follicular hyperkeratosis (excessive keratinization of the skin caused by delayed epithelial renewal), mucosal dryness (also caused by delayed epithelial renewal), xerophthalmia (dryness of the conjunctiva and cornea), keratomalacia (opacification

and softening of the cornea), and disordered reproductive function (failure of the spermatozoa [26, 27].

Uses
Natural vitamin A (which has a combination of biological forms) and its synthetic analogs (retinol acetate and retinol palmitate) are utilized in medicine. They are used to treat hypovitaminosis in people whose jobs demand them to be in front of a computer all day, as well as to stimulate growth and development in youngsters. Vitamin A formulations are also utilized as regeneration stimulants for treating poorly healable tissues, boosting infection resistance, and treating sterility prophylactically [28, 29].

1.2.2 Vitamin D

Source
Vitamin D is mostly contained in animal-derived products including liver, butter, milk, yeast, and vegetable oils, but not in vegetables, fruits, or cereals. Vitamin D is very abundant in cod liver. The daily vitamin D requirement for children ranges from 12 to 25 lg; for adults, the daily requirement is 10 times lower [30, 31].

Chemical nature and biologically active forms
Vitamin D is made up of fat-soluble secosteroids (a form of steroid with a "broken" ring) generated from cholesterol, which are chemically related to steroids. Vitamin D3 (cholecalciferol) is an example of a 9,10-secosteroid. Calcitriol is one of several vitamin D vitamers. The most active D vitamins are D2 (ergocalciferol) and D2 (cholecalciferol) (cholecalciferol). Ergocalciferol (D2) is produced from the plant sterol (provitamin D). When UV light energy is absorbed by the precursor molecule 7-dehydrocholesterol, vitamin D3 (cholecalciferol) is produced in the skin of mammals (present in the skin of humans and animals). Dihydroergocalciferol is vitamin D4. UV irradiation produces the less active vitamers D4, D5, D6, and D7 from their respective plant precursor's dihydroergosterol, 7-dehydrositosterol, 7-dehydrostig-masterol, and 7-dehydrocampesterol. Neither ergo- nor cholecalciferols, on the other hand, are physiologically active and cannot perform regulatory activities. In the course of metabolism, they produce physiologically active molecules that behave like steroid hormones [32, 33].

Biochemical functions
The biological activity of 1,25-dihydroxycalciferols is 10 times greater than parent calciferols. Vitamin D is important for calcium metabolism

and equilibrium. Vitamin D regulates the transit of calcium and phosphate ions across cell membranes and hence works as a calcium and phosphate ion regulator in the circulation. At least three vitamin D-related processes are included in this control: absorption of calcium and phosphate ions via the epithelium of the small intestine mucosa, mobilization of calcium from bone tissue, and reabsorption of calcium and phosphate in kidney tubules [34, 35].

The mechanism of action of vitamin D
Calcium is absorbed in the small intestine through facilitated diffusion, which is aided by a specific calcium-binding protein (CaBP), and active transport, which is aided by Ca^{2+} ATPase. By operating on the genetic cellular machinery of the small intestine mucosa, 1, 25-dihydroxycalciferols trigger the synthesis of CaBP and protein components of Ca^{2+} ATPase. Vitamin D-induced activation of Ca^{+} ATPase, which is found in the membranes of renal tubules, appears to result in calcium ion reabsorption in the tubules. However, the mechanisms of vitamin D's role in phosphate transmembrane transfer in the colon and kidneys, as well as calcium mobilization from bone tissue, are yet unknown. The impact of vitamin D is reflected in increased calcium and phosphate concentrations in the blood [36].

Deficiency
When vitamin D deficiency occurs in youngsters, it causes osteomalacia, often known as rickets, which is a softening of the bones. This condition is caused by a vitamin D deficient diet combined with insufficient UV irradiation (for the generation of endogenous vitamin D). A lower calciferol-responsive tissue sensitivity (presumably due to the lack of calciferol-binding receptors) could potentially be the cause. All vitamin D-controlled processes, such as the intestinal uptake of calcium ions and phosphate (even if the infant's dietary supply of these nutrients from dairy products is adequate) and their reabsorption in the kidneys, are hindered in rickets. The level of calcium and phosphorous in the blood is dropped as a result, and bone mineralization is inhibited, meaning no mineral materials are deposited on the newly produced collagen matrix of growing bones. As a result, distortion of skeletal bones of the limbs, skull, and thorax is seen in children with rickets. When the supply of vitamin D to the body is normal, a relative shortage might emerge. This could be triggered by a damaged liver or kidney, as these organs are important in the generation of active vitamin D forms [37, 38].

Uses
Natural vitamin D preparations (cod liver oil) and synthetic vitamin D preparations (ergocalciferol or cholecalciferol) are utilized in medical practice. Vitamin D preparations are employed in the prevention and treatment of rickets, as well as the treatment of other diseases (tuberculosis of the bones and joints and tuberculosis of the skin) [39].

1.2.3 Vitamin E

Sources
Wheat germ, celery, lettuce or other green leafy vegetables, parsley, spinach, turnip leaf, watercress, and vegetable oils, particularly sunflower oil, corn oil, cottonseed oil, and olive oil, are all good sources of tocopherol for humans. Wheat seedling oil has a lot of tocopherol. Tocopherol is scarce in animal-derived products, particularly dairy products. The recommended daily intake of tocopherol for adults is 20 to 50 mg [40].

Chemical nature and biologically active forms
Vitamin E is a methylated derivative chemical that comes in eight distinct forms, four of tocopherol and four of tocotrienol. The quantity and position of methyl groups on the chromanol ring dictate the a (alpha), b (beta), c (gamma), and d (delta) forms of tocopherols and tocotrienols. Tocopherols and tocotrienols are structurally similar, with the same methyl structure at the ring, the same Greek letter—methyl—notation, and an isoprenoid side chain; tocopherols have saturated isoprenoid side chains, whereas tocotrienols have unsaturated hydrophobic isoprenoid side chains with three double bonds (farnesyl isoprenoid tails) [41, 42].

Biochemical functions
Tocopherol is a biological antioxidant that controls the rate of free radical reactions in living cells by inhibiting spontaneous chain reactions of peroxide oxidation of unsaturated lipids in biomembranes. Tocopherol is a biological antioxidant that provides for the stability of cell biomembranes in the organism. Since selenium acts as a cofactor for glutathione peroxidase, which inactivates lipid hydroperoxides, a close link between tocopherol and selenium in lipid peroxide oxidation regulation has been shown. Vitamin A's biological activity is increased by tocopherol, which protects the vitamin's unsaturated side chain against peroxide oxidation. Tocopherol and its derivatives are likely engaged in other regulatory mechanisms that have yet to be found [43, 44].

Deficiency

Vitamin E hypovitaminosis in adults has never been documented. In experimental animals, tocopherol deficiency manifests as a specific membrane pathology: membrane resistance to peroxide attack is reduced, and increased permeability leads to the loss of intracellular components, such as proteins that are normally present; in premature infants, vitamin deficiency manifests as hemolytic anemia (due to a low stability of the erythrocyte membranes and their breakdown); in premature infants, tocopherol deficiency manifests as a specific membrane path. Susceptibility of erythrocytes to peroxide hemolysis; atrophy of the testes (conducive to male sterility); death of the embryo in pregnant females; muscular dystrophy and loss of intracellular nitrogenous components and muscle proteins; hepatic necrosis; and local encephalomalacia, especially cerebromalacia are all possible causes of tissue membrane pathology in E hypovitaminosis. Spinocerebellar ataxia, myopathies, peripheral neuropathy, ataxia, skeletal myopathy, retinopathy, and immune response impairment are all symptoms of vitamin E deficiency [45, 46].

Uses

Synthetic D,L-a-tocopherol acetate in vegetable oil and concentrated oil extracts of tocopherol combinations from wheat seedlings are commercially available. Tocopherolic preparations are used as antioxidants to prevent excessive lipid peroxide accumulation; they are also used in the prophylaxis (preventive measures) of sterility and impending abortion, liver diseases, muscular atrophy, and the treatment of congenital erythrocyte membrane disturbances in neonates and premature infants, among other things [47].

1.2.4 Vitamin F

Source

Vitamin F is made up of essential fatty acids (EFAs), particularly omega-3 and omega-6 fatty acids, which can only be obtained through food. Fish, canola oil, and walnut oil; raw nuts, seeds, legumes, grape seed oil, and flaxseed oil; and hemp seed, olive oil, soy oil, canola (rapeseed) oil, chia seeds, pumpkin seeds, sunflower seeds, leafy vegetables, walnuts, avocados, all kinds of sprouts; and meat, shellfish, salmon, trout, mackerel, and tuna. Vitamin F may be abundant in vegetable oils. The daily need for vitamin F in adult people is 5 to 10 g [48].

Chemical nature and biologically active
Vitamin F is a fat-soluble vitamin that contains unsaturated fatty acids, which are found in liquid vegetable oils, and saturated fatty acids, which are present in animal fat. Vitamin F is the sum of unsaturated fatty acids that cannot be produced in the tissues but are required for the organism's regular function. Only a-linoleic acid (an omega-3 fatty acid) and linoleic acid (LA) are recognized to be needed for humans (an omega-6 fatty acid). C-linoleic acid is another omega-6 fatty acid. They are polyunsaturated fatty acids (PUFA), with a-linolenic acid (ALA) having an 18-carbon chain with three cis double bonds and linoleic acid (LA) having an 18-carbon chain with two cis double bonds [49, 50].

Biochemical functions
Vitamin F is required for the formation of prostaglandins, which regulate metabolism. Vitamin F helps the tissue metabolism by preserving vitamin A reserves and facilitating vitamin A action. Vitamin F aids in the digestion of phosphorus and stimulates the conversion of carotene to vitamin A in the body, working in combination with vitamin D to make calcium available to the tissues. It is necessary for the correct functioning of the reproductive system, as well as the nutrition of skin cells and the health of mucous membranes and nerves. Vitamin F helps to minimize the risk of heart disease by lowering cholesterol levels in the blood [51, 52].

Deficiency
Unambiguous deficient symptoms have not been described in people. F hypovitaminosis is often associated with follicular hyperkeratosis, or excessive keratinization of the skin epithelium around the hair follicles. These symptoms are similar to those of vitamin A insufficiency. Vitamin F deficiency in animals can cause sterility [53].

Uses
Arachidonic acid is clearly an important fatty acid, and it is the only one that can cure all deficient symptoms. The essential fatty acid formulations xxlinetol and linol have clinical applications, primarily in the prophylaxis (preventive measures) of cholesterol deposition in arterial walls under atherosclerosis; they are also useful in the local treatment of skin problems [54].

1.2.5 Vitamin K

Source

Phylloquinomes (K1) and their derivatives are found in plants (e.g., cabbage, spinach, as well as root crops and fruits) and animal (liver) products, and are fed to the organism, whereas menaquinones (K2) are produced by the small intestinal bacterioflora or derived from naphthoquinone metabolism in the organism's tissues. The daily vitamin K requirement for adults is approximately 2 mg [55].

Chemical nature and biologically active

Vitamin K is a quinone with an isoprenoid side chain that refers to a series of substances that are 2-methyl-1, 4-naphthoquinone derivatives chemically. The "quinone" ring is shared by all K vitamins, although the length, degree of saturation, and number of side chains vary. Two naphthoquinone series, phylloquinones (K1-series) and menaquinones, are found in this fat-soluble vitamin (K2-series). Menaquinones (MQ or MK-n) are a group of related compounds that are separated into short chain (e.g., MK-4) and long chain (e.g., MK-7, MK-8, and MK-9 with 7, 8, and 9 isoprene units, respectively) menaquinones based on the length of the isoprenoid chain. Vitamin K synthetic preparations (menadione, vicasol, and synkayvite) are 2-methyl-l, 4-naphthoquinone derivatives. They are transformed into physiologically active menaquinones in the body. Menadione is a vitamin K analog with a methyl group in the second position that is occasionally used as a nutritional supplement or as a provitamin since it is metabolized by the human body into K2 [56, 57].

Biochemical functions

Vitamin K regulates blood clotting in the body by assisting in the formation of many blood clotting system components, including factor II (prothrombin), factor VII (proconvertin), factor IX (Christmas factor), and factor X. (Stewart factor). Vitamin K is required for the conversion of preprothrombin, a prothrombin precursor, to prothrombin. The liver is involved in this process. Vitamin K activates the microsomal carboxylase, which promotes the c-carboxylation of glutamic acid residues in prothrombin molecules. Prothrombin is generated and then attached to phospholipids by Ca^{2+} ions before being cleaved by enzymes to produce thrombin. The latter causes a fibrin clot to form in the blood coagulation system [58, 59].

Deficiency

A specific tendency to hemorrhagic illness, especially in traumas, is an indication of vitamin K deficiency. In adult humans, the gut flora provides the organism with a complete supply of vitamin K. K hypovitaminosis in babies (with a still-developing gut flora) could be caused by a vitamin K deficiency in the diet. Drugs that restrict the gut flora, as well as liver and gallbladder illnesses that result in decreased bile acid synthesis, are major causes of K hypovitaminosis (which are needed for the vitamin uptake). Furthermore, the liver produces active forms of vitamin K and is involved in the creation of a number of blood coagulation components as well as the conversion of preprothrombin to thrombin [60].

Uses

Vitamin K1 preparations or its synthetic counterpart vicasol are utilized in medical practice. They can be used to treat hemorrhagic illness or hemophilic hemorrhage. Human hepatocellular carcinoma, a frequent and deadly form of liver cancer, has been found to be safely suppressed by vitamin K2 (menaquinone). It has a number of impacts on these tumours, reducing the ability of growth factors and their receptor molecules to induce tumour development and progression. It stops the cell cycle from continuing, preventing further replication. It also causes apoptosis, or programmed cell death, through numerous unique ways. Three synergistic anticancer mechanisms of vitamin K have recently been discovered. DNA-building enzymes are inhibited by vitamin K3. Vitamins K2 and K3 stop new blood vessels from forming, which is necessary for tumour tissue to grow quickly. Vitamin K3 also affects microtubule-based intracellular communication networks, preventing cells from growing in a coordinated manner [61, 62].

1.2.6 Water-Soluble Vitamins B1, B2, B3, B7, B9, B12 (B Complex), and C

Vitamin B1 (thiamin), vitamin B2 (riboflavin), vitamin B3 (niacin), vitamin B5 (pantothenic acid), vitamin B6 (pyridoxine), vitamin B7 (biotin), vitamin B9 (folic acid), vitamin B12 (cobalamin), and vitamin C (ascorbic acid) are examples of water-soluble vitamins. A vitamin B complex is made up of all eight vitamins in the B group (B1, B2, B3, B5, B6, B7, B9, and B12). They are structurally diverse, and each B vitamin is either a cofactor (usually a coenzyme for critical metabolic activities) or a precursor for the production of one. Vitamin C is a cofactor in many enzymatic reactions and can help protect against oxidative stress by acting as an antioxidant (a powerful reducing agent). The l-enantiomer of ascorbate is vitamin C; the D-enantiomer has no physiological importance. The bulk of water-soluble vitamins found in food or produced by intestinal bacterial flora have biological activity when combined with metabolically generated coenzymes [63, 64].

1.2.6.1 Vitamin B1

Source
Vitamin B1 (thiamine) is a necessary nutrient for all living things, although it is only produced by bacteria, fungus, and plants. Vitamin B1 is found in a variety of foods, including coarse bread, peas, beans, pineapple, asparagus, cabbage, carrot, celery, grapefruit, coconut, lemon, parsley, pomegranate, radish, watercress, turnip leaf, and meat products, but not polished rice. It is on the WHO's List of Essential Medicines, which includes the most effective and safe medicines required in a health system. Adult people require approximately 1 to 3 mg of thiamine per day [65].

Chemical nature and biologically active
A colorless organosulfur molecule, vitamin B1 or thiamine, is made up of an aminopyrimidine and a thiazole ring joined by a methylene bridge. The thiazole's side chains are substituted with methyl and hydroxyethyl. It is soluble in water and organic solvents such as methanol and glycerol, stable at acidic pH, unstable in alkaline solutions, unstable to heat, stable during freezing storage, and unstable to UV and gamma irradiation exposure. Thiamine is an N-heterocyclic carbene that can be employed as a catalyst for benzoin condensation instead of cyanide. In Maillard reactions, thiamine reacts significantly. Food fortification is done with thiamine mononitrate rather than thiamine hydrochloride because the mononitrate is more stable and does not absorb water from natural humidity, whereas thiamine hydrochloride does. Many cellular activities rely on its phosphate derivatives, such as thiamine pyrophosphate (TPP), a coenzyme involved in sugar and amino acid catabolism. Thiamine monophosphate (ThMP), thiamine diphosphate (ThDP), also known as thiamine pyrophosphate (TPP), thiamine triphosphate (ThTP), and the recently discovered adenosine thiamine triphosphate (AThTP) and adenosine thiamine diphosphate (AThDP) are the five known natural thiamine phosphate derivatives (AThDP). While thiamine diphosphate's coenzyme role is well known and well studied, the non-coenzyme action of thiamine and derivatives may be realized by binding to a number of recently discovered proteins that do not employ thiamine diphosphate's catalytic action [66, 67].

Biochemical functions

Thiamine diphosphate (TOP), which is found in the pyruvate dehydrogenase or 2-oxoglutarate dehydrogenase complexes and transketolase, is involved in tissue metabolic control. TOP enhances the mitochondrial oxidation of pyruvate and 2-oxoglutarate, and hence the energy generation from carbs and amino acids, as a result. The nonoxidative step of the pentose phosphate cycle, which is a key source of NADP-H and the only source of ribose 5-phosphate in cells, is known to be maintained by transketolase. Thiamine is engaged in a variety of functions, including non-coenzymic ones. Thiamine triphosphate, which is found in significant concentrations in nerve cells, is implicated in the synaptic transmission of neurological impulses, either directly or indirectly [68].

Thiamine deficiency

Thiamine deficiency is widespread in areas where people consume polished rice with just trace amounts of the vitamin. Thiamine deficiency can be fatal, and symptoms include a sudden loss of appetite, decreased gastric juice and hydrochloric acid secretion, atony (lack of normal tone or strength), diarrhoea, lethargy, weight loss, irritability, and confusion. The defining symptom is skeletal muscle atrophy (distinct myasthenia or muscular debility), heart (lower cardiac contractility, dilatation of the right heart, tachycardia, sudden cardiac insufficiency), and smooth muscle contractile decrease (reduced muscular tension of intestinal smooth muscles). Beriberi, Wernicke–Korsakoff syndrome, and optic neuropathy are all well-known thiamine-deficient disorders. Beriberi causes metabolic abnormalities and poor digestive, cardiovascular, and neurological system functions. Nervous system disturbances manifest as a gradual loss of peripheral sensitivity, the loss of some peripheral reflexes, paroxysmal pain extending along nerve courses (neuralgia), decreased higher nervous activity (phobia, mental melancholy), and convulsions [69, 70].

Uses

Medicine uses a range of therapeutic formulations based on free thiamine and thiamine diphosphate (cocarboxylase). Thiamine diphosphate is susceptible to hydrolysis in the blood, and it is unknown whether this enzyme form is delivered to the cells or if it just serves as a source of free thiamine. Thiamine-based formulations are used to aid carbohydrate assimilation in diabetes, hypovitaminosis, cardiac and skeletal muscle dystrophies, peripheral nerve inflammation, and the treatment of the afflicted neurological system (including alcoholism) [71].

INTRODUCTION TO NUTRACEUTICAL VITAMINS 15

1.2.6.2 Vitamin B2

Sources
Humans get riboflavin via food and gut flora. Milk, cheese, curd, egg yolk, liver, kidney, mushrooms, almonds, grapefruit, apple, apricot, cabbage, carrot, coconut, dandelion, prune, spinach, turnip leaf, watercress, etc. contain riboflavin naturally. Animal and dairy products have more riboflavin than vegetables. Milk, milk products, and animal diets have high (free) riboflavin bioavailability. Most plant-based riboflavin is protein-bound and less bioavailable. It is on the WHO's List of Essential Medications, the most effective and safe medicines needed in a health system. Riboflavin consumption for adults is 1 to 3 mg [72, 73].

Chemical nature, biologically active forms, and biochemical functions
Cellular respiration requires it. Riboflavin is 7, 8-dimethyl-10-(1!-D-ribityl)isoalloxazine. "Flavin" comes from the Latin word for yellow, flavus. Riboflavin is a yellow-orange solid with poor water solubility. It gives vitamins colour (and bright yellow colour to the urine of persons taking a lot of it). Riboflavin is a coenzyme, meaning it helps enzymes (proteins) function normally. Active forms of riboflavin FMN and FAD function as cofactors for flavoprotein enzyme reactions. Riboflavin is photosensitive but heat stable in the dark. UV light stimulates its fluorescence. This is a detectable property. From riboflavin, FMN and FAD are derived [74, 75].

Biochemical functions
Flavin coenzymes participate in many substrate-linked oxidation reactions in cells, including electron and proton transfer in the respiratory chain, mitochondrial oxidation of pyruvate, succinate, 2-oxoglutarate, a-glycerol phosphate, fatty acids, and oxidation of biogenic amines, aldehydes, etc [76].

Deficiency
Riboflavin deficiency (ariboflavinosis) causes stomatitis, including red tongue, sore throat, chapped and fissured lips, and mouth corner inflammation (angular stomatitis). Scrotum, vulva, lip philtrum, and nasolabial folds can have oily, scaly rashes. Itchy, watery, bloodshot, light-sensitive eyes are common. Riboflavin deficiency is characterized by low tissue concentrations of coenzymic riboflavin forms, primarily FMN, and lesions of the epithelium of the cutaneous mucosa and cornea. Labial and oral mucosa are dry. Red labial mucosa, cracked lips and mouth angles. Reduced epithelium renewal makes facial skin desquamative. Dry, inflamed conjunctiva,

vascularized, keratoleucoma-prone cornea, photophobia. Since riboflavin participates in energy-generating oxidative processes, vitamin deficiency affects regenerative tissues. Vascularization increases oxygen supply to the cornea's central, nonvascular zone to compensate for a lack of flavoproteins involved in redox processes [77, 78].

Uses
Baby foods, breakfast cereals, pastas, and meal replacement products contain riboflavin. Riboflavin has poor solubility in water, so riboflavin-5′-phosphate is required. Food coloring contains riboflavin. Riboflavin, FMN, and FAD (Flavin mono- and dinucleotide) are used in medicine. Clinically, they are used to treat hyporiboflavinosis and skin and eye diseases caused by an excess of riboflavin: dermatitides, poorly healing wounds and ulcers, keratitis, and conjunctivitis (inflammation of the conjunctiva). In addition, they are used to treat respiratory poisoning (carbon monoxide CO), liver disease, and muscle soreness after exercise, etc. [79, 80].

1.2.6.3 Vitamin B3

Source
Niacin is one of 20 to 80 essential human nutrients. Niacin occurs naturally as nicotinic acid and nicotinamide, which are nutritionally equivalent. Meat (especially liver) and vegetables contain niacin. Niacin is trace in milk and egg yolk. Niacin is found in whole and processed foods, including fortified foods, meat, seafood, and spices. Fortified wheat, rice, barley, corn, and pasta have 3 to 10 mg of niacin per 100 g. Niacin can be synthesized in the human body from tryptophan, so it is not an essential food component if tryptophan isn't scarce. Milk and egg yolk, which are low in niacin but high in tryptophan, replenish a vitamin deficiency. Tryptophan consumption determines niacin needs. Niacin is found in whole and processed foods, with the most in fortified foods and meat. Adults should take 25 mg [81, 82].

Chemical nature, biologically active forms
Nicotinic acid or pyridine carboxylic acids. It is a solid, colorless, water-soluble derivative of pyridine with a 3-position carboxyl group (COOH) (pyridine-3-carboxylic acid). It is part of the vitamin B3 complex with nicotinamide, niacin, and nicotinamide riboside. Niacin and nicotinamides are precursors of NAD and NAD+ (NADP). NAD is important in fat, carbohydrate, protein, and alcohol catabolism, cell signaling, and DNA repair, and NADP in fatty acid and cholesterol synthesis [83, 84].

Biochemical functions

It is a water-soluble vitamin B with antihyperlipidemic activity found in animal and plant tissues. Niacin is used with lipid-lowering drugs. Niacin reduces cardiovascular events and deaths. Niacin coenzyme functions include hydrogen transfer in redox reactions, acting as a substrate for synthetic reactions, and acting as an allosteric effector [85, 86].

Deficiency

Niacin deficiency slows metabolism, reducing cold tolerance. Severe niacin deficiency in the diet causes pellagra, characterized by diarrhea, dermatitis, dementia, Casal's necklace lesions on the lower neck, hyperpigmentation, thickening of the skin, inflammation of the mouth and tongue, digestive disturbances, amnesia, delirium, and death, if left untreated; psychiatric symptoms of niacin deficiency include irritability, poor concentration, anxiety, Niacin deficiency reduces tryptophan absorption. Niacin hypovitaminosis is often accompanied by riboflavin and pyridoxine hypovitaminosis because they are needed to produce nicotinic acid from tryptophan [87, 88].

Uses

Nicotinic acid and nicotinamide are used in medicine. NAD and NADP's low plasmic membrane permeability makes them unsuitable as coenzymes. NAD and NADP have unknown noncoenzymic functions. Nicotinamide and nicotinic acid are used to treat pellagra and other dermatitides, peripheral nerves, cardiac muscle dystrophy, etc. Clinically, nicotinic acid has a vasodilative effect. This is unrelated to nicotinic acid's biochemical functions [89].

1.2.7 Vitamin B5

Source
Intestinal bacteria and foods like yeast, liver, hen eggs, fish, meat, milk, leguminous plants, etc. are sources of Vitamin B5 or pantothenic acid for humans. High amounts of pantothenic acid are found in fortified whole-grain cereals, egg yolks, liver, and dried mushrooms. It is a water-soluble vitamin required for coenzyme A synthesis (CoA). Adults need 10 g daily [90].

Chemical nature, biologically active forms
Vitamin B5 or pantothenic acid is a water-soluble vitamin needed to synthesize coenzyme A. (CoA). Anionic B5 is Pantothenate. Pantothenic

acid is a D-pantoic acid and b-alanine amide. $C_9H_{17}NO_5$ is a light-yellow, water-soluble, viscous beta-alanine derivative of pantoic acid. It is found as pantothenol and calcium pantothenate. It is D and L. Only the dextrorotatory (D) isomer of pantothenic acid has biologic activity, and the levorotatory (L) form may block it. Five steps synthesize coenzyme A from pantothenate, cysteine, and ATP [91, 92].

Biochemical functions
The participation of pantothenic acid's coenzyme A in biological reactions determines its relevance. In cells, CoA is a crucial enzyme. Pantothenic acid, in the form of CoA, is also required for acylation and acetylation, which are involved in signal transmission as well as enzyme activation and deactivation [93]. Pantothenic acid is necessary for glucose, protein, and lipid metabolism and synthesis. Furthermore, pantothenic acid is required for antibody creation, cholesterol conversion to stress hormones, red blood cell production, and acetylcholine production. 4-phosphopantetheine is a coenzyme for fatty acid synthetase's acyl-transporting protein; dephospho-CoA is a coenzyme for citrate lyase and plays a role in a number of acyl conversion processes [94, 95].

Deficiency
Because pantothenic acid plays so many important biological activities, it is vital to all forms of life. As a result, deficits in pantothenic acid can have a wide range of consequences. Deficiency symptoms are comparable to those of other vitamin B deficits. Due to low CoA levels, energy generation is hampered, which can lead to irritation, weariness, and apathy. Because acetylcholine synthesis is inhibited, neurological symptoms, such as numbness, paresthesia, and muscle cramping can occur in insufficiency. Hypoglycemia, or an enhanced sensitivity to insulin, can be caused by a lack of pantothenic acid. When insulin receptors refuse to bind to insulin, they are acylated with palmitic acid. As acylation reduces, more insulin binds to receptors, resulting in hypoglycemia. Restlessness, malaise, sleep problems, nausea, vomiting, and stomach cramps are all possible symptoms. More serious (but reversible) problems, such as adrenal insufficiency and hepatic encephalopathy, have been found in a few rare cases. Disorders of the neurological, gastrointestinal, and immunological systems, reduced development rate, decreased food intake, skin lesions and changes in hair coat, and abnormalities in lipid and carbohydrate metabolism are also signs of deficiency in other nonruminant species [96, 97].

Uses

Calcium pantothenate, pantetheine, and CoA preparations are utilized in a range of pharmacologic formulations in everyday medicine. They are most typically used to treat skin and hair problems, as well as to treat afflicted livers, cardiac muscle dystrophy, and other conditions. Some formulas are also utilized in the fragrance industry [98].

1.2.8 Vitamin B6

Source

Intestinal bacteria and diet are the sources of vitamin B6 (pyridoxine, pyridoxal, and pyridoxamine) for humans. Vitamin B6 is a member of the vitamin B family of nutrients. Vitamin B6 is abundant in cereals, legumes, meat, and fish. A daily dosage of 2 to 3 mg is advised for adults [99].

Chemical nature and biologically active forms

Vitamin B6 is a chemically related group of chemicals that can be interconverted in biological systems. Vitamin B6 comes in a variety of forms (vitamers), including pyridoxine (PN), pyridoxine 5′-phosphate (P5P), pyridoxal (PL), pyridoxal 5′-phosphate (PLP), the metabolically active form (sold as P-5-P vitamin supplement), pyridoxamine (PM), pyridoxamine 5′-phosphate (PMP), 4-pyridoxic acid (PA), the catabolite excretion. Except for pyridoxic acid and pyritinol, all forms can be interconverted. Pyridoxal kinase converts absorbed pyridoxamine to PMP, which is then turned to PLP by pyridoxamine phosphate transaminase or pyridoxine 5′-phosphate oxidase, which also converts PNP to PLP. Pyridoxine 5′-phosphate oxidase requires the cofactor flavin mononucleotide (FMN), which is synthesized from riboflavin (vitamin B2), implying that dietary vitamin B6 cannot be utilized in this metabolic pathway without vitamin B2. Pyridoxal 5′-phosphate, its active form, is a cofactor in over 100 enzyme processes involved in amino acid, carbohydrate, and lipid metabolism [100, 101].

Biochemical functions

PLP, the metabolically active form of vitamin B6, plays a role in macronutrient metabolism, neurotransmitter synthesis, histamine synthesis, hemoglobin synthesis and function, and gene expression, among other things. Many processes, such as decarboxylation, transamination, racemization, elimination, replacement, and beta-group interconversion, use PLP as a coenzyme (cofactor). Vitamin B6 metabolism takes place in the liver. Pyridoxal 5-phosphate is the primary coenzymic form of vitamin B6 in organism tissues. It is found in practically every type of enzyme, including oxide reductases, transferases, hydrolases, lyases, and isomerases [102, 103].

Deficiency
Children have been diagnosed with pyridoxine deficiency. It is associated with hyperexcitability of the central nervous system and repeated convulsions, which is thought to be caused by a lack of c-aminobutyric acid, the inhibitory mediator for brain neurons. Pyridoxine deficiency symptoms have been found in adult humans after long-term treatment with the tuberculostatic isoniazid, which is a pyridoxal antagonist. This condition is accompanied by nervous system hyperexcitability, polyneuritides, and skin lesions, which are all symptoms of niacin insufficiency. A seborrhoeic dermatitis-like eruption, atrophic glossitis with ulceration, angular cheilitis, conjunctivitis, intertrigo, and neurologic symptoms of somnolence, confusion, and neuropathy (due to impaired sphingosine synthesis) and sideroblastic anemia (due to impaired heme synthesis) are the classic clinical syndromes for vitamin B6 deficiency [104, 105].

Uses
Clinically, pyridoxine is applied in a variety of medicinal forms; of late, its coenzyme, pyridoxal phosphate, has gained acceptance. These agents are used in medication of B6 hypovitaminosis, in prophylaxis and therapy of isoniazid side effects, in treatment of polyneuritides, dermatitides, gestational toxicosis (assistance in biogenic amine detoxification), impaired hepatic function, congenital pyridoxine dependent anemia in children, etc. [106].

1.2.9   Vitamin B9, BC, Vitamin M, or Folacin

Source
The term "folic" is from the Latin word folium, which means leaf. Folates occur naturally in many foods especially dark green leafy vegetables and liver. Folate naturally occurs in a wide variety of foods, including vegetables (particularly dark green leafy vegetables), fruits and fruit juices, nuts, beans, peas, dairy products, poultry and meat, eggs, seafood, grains, and some beers. Avocado, beetroot, spinach, liver, yeast, asparagus, and Brussels sprouts are among the foods with the highest levels of folate. Folate naturally found in food is susceptible to high heat and ultraviolet light, and is soluble in water. It is heat labile in acidic environments and may also be subject to oxidation. Folic acid is added to grain products in many countries, and these fortified products make up a significant source

of the population's folate intake. Food is the major source of folacin (B9). Folacin is abundant in the foodstuffs of vegetable origin (lettuce, cabbage, tomato, strawberry, and spinach) and animal origin (liver, meat, and egg yolk). The recommended daily intake for the adult human is about 400 µg, and twice as large for pregnant human females [107, 108].

Chemical nature, biologically active forms
Folic acid, folinic acid, levomefolic acid, and 5-methyltetrahydrofolate are all examples of vitamin B9. Folic acid, commonly known as vitamin BC, is a B-complex vitamin that is produced by bacteria in the mammalian gut and is also necessary in the typical diet. Folic acid is required for the formation of nucleic acids and red blood cells, and a deficiency results in stunted growth and anemia. Vitamin B9 comes in two forms: folin and folate, which are found naturally in food, and folic acid, which is found in vitamin supplements. Folic acid is relatively stable in the body and is converted to folate. Folate refers to folic acid and its congeners, such as tetrahydrofolic acid, methyltetrahydrofolate, methenyltetrahydrofolate, and folinic acid. Vitamin B9, vitamin Bc, vitamin M, folacin, and pteroyl-L-glutamate are some of its other names. Tetrahydrofolate is a cofactor in a variety of processes, including all the synthesis (or anabolism) of amino acids and nucleic acids. It is water-soluble, and the majority of it is stored in the liver, which holds almost half of the body's total folate. Boiling and heating degrade the nutrition [109, 110].

Biochemical functions
Folic acid is required for cell division because it helps the body create DNA, RNA, and digest amino acids. Folate is required for the formation and maintenance of new cells, as well as for DNA and RNA synthesis via methylation, as well as for preventing DNA alterations and, thus, cancer. Folic acid is an essential vitamin because people cannot produce it and must obtain it through their food. L-5-MTHF (also known as L-methylfolate and L-5-methyltetrahydrofolate and (6S)-5-methyltetrahydrofolate and (6S)-5-MTHF) is the principal biologically active form of folate needed at the cellular level for DNA replication, the cysteine cycle, and homocysteine control. N5-formyl-THFA, N10-formyl-THFA, N5, N10-methenyl-THFA, N5, N10-methylene THFA, and N5-methyl-THFA are the coenzymes that define the functions of folacin. The active one-carbon moiety can be moved from one coenzymic form to another and employed in a number of processes to make purines, pyrimidines, and certain amino acids (glycine from serine, or methionine from homocysteine). The folacin coenzymes are involved in the biosynthesis of carbon atoms at purine ring locations

2 and 8, as well as the creation of dTMP from dUMP. As a result, folacin is essential for nucleic acid production as well as cell division [111, 112].

Deficiency in folacin
Folate deficiency in children can occur within a month of a poor diet. Adults need between 10,000 and 30,000 micrograms (g) of total body folate, with blood levels of more than 7 nmol/L (3 ng/mL). Folate deficiency can cause anemia, which is characterized by a lack of big red blood cells. Tiredness, heart palpitations, shortness of breath, open sores on the tongue, and changes in skin or hair colour are all possible symptoms. Folate deficiency can cause glossitis, diarrhea, depression, disorientation, anemia, and prenatal neural tube and brain abnormalities, among other things (during pregnancy) [113, 114]. Fatigue, grey hair, oral sores, poor growth, and a swollen tongue are some of the other symptoms. It is on the WHO's List of Essential Medicines, which includes the most effective and safe medicines required in a health system (WHO 2015). Megaloblastic anemia is caused by a lack of tetrahydrofolic acid (FH4) [115].

Uses
Folic acid formulations are used in medical practice to treat megaloblastic anemia, stimulate cell proliferation, and so on [116].

1.2.10 Vitamin B12

Source
Vitamin B12, also known as cobalamins, is only created by bacteria and archaea, which have the enzymes required for its production. No fungus, plants, people, or animals can synthesize vitamin B12. Animal items, such as meat, poultry, fish (shellfish), and to a lesser extent dairy products and eggs, contain vitamin B12. Cobalamins are abundant in the liver and kidney, while they are few in vegetable products. According to recent research, several plant-based meals, such as fermented beans and vegetables, as well as edible algae and mushrooms, contain significant amounts of functional vitamin B12. For some vegetarians, fresh pasteurized milk contains 0.9 g per cup and is an essential source of vitamin B12. Fortified food products and dietary supplements are two good sources of B12. Vitamin B12 is partially produced by gut microorganisms. For adults, a daily vitamin B12 intake of about 2 lg is suggested. These items, when combined with B vitamin fortified foods and supplements, may help to prevent vitamin B12 deficiency in vegetarians [117, 118].

Chemical nature, biologically active forms

Vitamin B12 is the largest and most complicated chemical structure; it contains the metal ion cobalt, which is why it is called cobalamin. The corrin ring, which is comparable to the porphyrin ring found in heme, chlorophyll, and cytochrome, provides the basis for B12's structure. Cobalt is the central metal ion. The corrin ring provides four of the six coordination sites, while a dimethylbenzimidazole group provides the fifth. The sixth coordination site, the centre of reactivity, can be a cyano group (–CN), a hydroxyl group (–OH), a methyl group (–CH$_3$), or a 5'-deoxyadenosyl group (here the C5' atom of the deoxyribose forms the covalent connection with cobalt), to produce the four B12 forms, respectively. For example, I Cyanocobalamin is one such form of B12, often known as a "vitamer," and (ii) Hydroxocobalamin is another type of B12 commonly seen in pharmacology but not found in the human body. The two enzymatically active cofactor forms of B12 that naturally occur in the body are (ii) hydroxocobalamin (B12a), (iii) adenosylcobalamin (adoB12), and (iv) methylcobalamin (MeB12). Vitamin B12 comes in two forms in the human body: methylcobalamin and 5-deoxyadenosylcobalamin. Most nutritional supplements and fortified meals contain cyanocobalamin, which is easily converted in the body to 5-deoxyadenosylcobalamin and methylcobalamin [119, 120].

Biochemical functions

Vitamin B12, often known as cobalamin, is one of eight B vitamins that helps the brain and nervous system operate normally by assisting in the creation of myelin (myelinogenesis) and the formation of red blood cells. It affects DNA synthesis, fatty acid and amino acid metabolism, and is involved in the metabolism of every cell in the human body. In mammals, cobalamin is required by just two enzymes: methionine synthase and L-methylmalonylcoenzyme A mutase [121].

Cofactor for methionine synthase

The folate-dependent enzyme methionine synthase requires methylcobalamin to function. This enzyme is required for the amino acid methionine to be synthesized from homocysteine. S-adenosylmethionine, a methyl group donor employed in numerous biological methylation processes, including the methylation of a variety of locations within DNA, RNA, and proteins, requires methionine [122].

Cofactor for L-methylmalonyl-coenzyme A mutase

The enzyme that catalyses the conversion of L-methylmalonyl-coenzyme A to succinyl-coenzyme A (succinyl-CoA), which subsequently enters the citric acid cycle, requires 5-deoxyadenosylcobalamin. Succinyl-CoA is essential for the synthesis of hemoglobin, the oxygen-carrying pigment in red blood cells, as well as the creation of energy from lipids and proteins [123].

Deficiency
Vitamin B12 insufficiency is frequently linked to persistent stomach inflammation, which can lead to pernicious anemia and food-bound vitamin B12 malabsorption. Megaloblastic anemia and neurologic problems can occur in people who are low in vitamin B12. Vitamin B12 shortage has the ability to harm the brain and neurological system permanently. Mild deficiency symptoms include fatigue, lethargy, sadness, poor memory, dyspnea, headaches, and pale skin, among others, especially in the elderly (age >60), owing to diminished intestinal absorption due to decreased stomach acid as people age. Mania and psychosis can both be caused by a lack of vitamin B12 [124]. Low vitamin B12 levels and excessive homocysteine levels have been linked to depression and osteoporosis. Because vitamin B12 is scarce in plant sources, vegetarians are more prone to be deficient [125].

Uses
Cyanocobalamin and, more recently, deoxyadenosylcobalamin are commonly used in medical practice. These drugs are used to treat megaloblastic anemia, spinal cord and peripheral nerve injury, and vitamin B12 metabolism disorders in children. The use of cobalamins in combination with folic acid and iron appears to be beneficial, as the latter two are required for hemoglobin formation in hemopoietic cells [126].

1.2.11 Vitamin C

Source
Vitamin C, also known as ascorbic acid, is a nutritional supplement that can be found in foods. Cabbage, cucumber, grapefruit, orange, lemon, lime, papaya, parsley, pineapple, radish, potato peels, spinach, tomato, turnip, carrot, rhubarb, and other fresh fruits and vegetables are the main sources of vitamin C for humans. Vitamin C is very high in wild-rose fruits [127]. The adult human's daily vitamin C need is 50 to 100 mg. Under certain conditions, vitamin C decomposes chemically, for example, around 60% during food cooking, possibly due to increased enzymatic destruction at sub-boiling temperatures, longer cooking times, copper food vessels (as Cu catalyzes the decomposition), length of storage time, and temperature

at which foods are stored. Leaching is another cause of vitamin C loss from cut veggies, as the water-soluble vitamin dissolves at a different rate in the boiling water, with broccoli retaining the most. When fresh fruits are stored in the refrigerator for a few days, they do not lose substantial nutrients [128].

Chemical nature, biologically active forms
Vitamin C, commonly known as ascorbic acid or L-ascorbic acid, always refers to the ascorbic acid L-enantiomer and its oxidized forms. Ascorbic acid is a sugar acid with a structure similar to glucose. Ascorbic acid is only found at low pH in biological systems, but it is mostly found in the ionized form, ascorbate, in neutral solutions above pH 5. Vitamin C activity can be found in all of these compounds. Ascorbic acid contains no coenzyme forms, thus ascorbate acid is the active form of vitamin C. Vitamin C (ascorbic acid), L-ascorbic acid (reduced form), Vitamin C, dehydroascorbic acid (oxidized form), calcium ascorbate, calcium salt of ascorbic acid, and sodium L-ascorbate [129].

Biochemical functions
Vitamin C (ascorbate) is primarily used as a reducing agent in a variety of reactions, and it has the ability to reduce respiratory chain cytochromes a and c, as well as molecular oxygen. In enzymic redox processes, ascorbic acid works as a hydrogen donor. With dehydroascorbic acid, it forms a redox pair. Ascorbate reductase, with the help of the reductant glutathione, converts dehydroascorbic acid to ascorbic acid in the tissues. The most important reaction in which ascorbate acts as a cofactor appears to be the hydroxylation of proline and lysine residues in collagen production. As a result, vitamin C is necessary for wound healing as well as the preservation of normal connective tissue. It also participates in the hydroxylation of tryptophan to 5-hydroxytryptophan (in serotonin biosynthesis), the conversion of 3, 4-dihydroxyphenylethylamine to noradrenalin, the hydroxylation of p-hydroxyphenylpyruvate to homogentisic acid, the hydroxylation of steroids during the biosynthesis of adrenocortical hormones from cholesterol, the hydroxylation of 5-biityrobetain Scurvy is a condition caused by a lack of vitamin C, and vitamin C plays a critical role in treating it [130].

Ascorbic acid deficiency
Scurvy, also known as scorbutus, is a condition caused by a lack of ascorbic acid. Scurvy is an avitaminosis caused by a shortage of vitamin C, because

the body's collagen is too unstable to perform its role without it. This causes the blood capillaries to become more permeabile and fragile, resulting in subcutaneous hemorrhages. Brown stains on the skin, spongy gums, and bleeding from the mucous membranes are all symptoms of scurvy. Acute variants of this condition show evidence of ascorbic acid biochemical processes being disrupted, such as the ability to use stored iron for marrow cell hemoglobin synthesis and folic acid participation in hemopoietic cell proliferation being diminished, resulting in anemia. Outward scorbutic signs include loosening and loss of teeth (dedentition), gingivae bleeding, dolorous and edemic joints, skin pallor (anemia), hemorrhages, damaged bones, and impaired wound healing [131].

Uses
Ascorbic acid is used in medicine to treat hypovitaminosis, to stimulate hemopoiesis (along with folic acid, vitamin B12, and iron), to strengthen the inner wall of blood capillaries that have ruptured, to stimulate regenerative processes, and to treat afflicted connective tissues and acutely diseased respiratory ducts [132–134].

1.3 Conclusions

Nutraceuticals have been shown to offer health advantages, and when consumed in moderation (within acceptable Recommended Dietary Intakes), they can help people stay healthy. Although nutraceuticals show great promise in the promotion of human health and disease prevention, health professionals, nutritionists, and regulatory toxicologists should collaborate strategically to plan appropriate regulation that will provide mankind with the greatest health and therapeutic benefit. As a result, the establishment of a regulating agency is required to standardize the nutraceutical industry. It is especially important to revisit this topic because the nutraceutical industry is outpacing the food and pharmaceutical industries in terms of growth. Vitamins, as a nutraceutical, are an effective tool for sustaining health and fighting nutritionally induced acute and chronic disorders, supporting optimal health, lifespan, and quality of life.

Acknowledgment

The authors thank MET's Institute of Pharmacy, BKC, which is affiliated with Savitribai Phule Pune University, Nashik. EDA wishes to express gratitude to the NFST/RGNF/UGC, Government of India, for providing financial assistance in the form of a fellowship (Award No - 202021-NFST-MAH-01235).

References

1. Chauhan, B., Kumar, G., Kalam, N., Ansari, S.H., Current concepts and prospects of herbal nutraceutical: A review. *J. Adv. Pharm. Technol. Res.*, 4, 1, 4, 2013.
2. McClements, D.J., Enhancing nutraceutical bioavailability through food matrix design. *Curr. Opin. Food Sci.*, 4, 1–6, 2015.
3. Goggs, R., Vaughan-Thomas, A., Clegg, P.D., Carter, S.D., Innes, J.F., Mobasheri, A., Shakibaei, M., Schwab, W., Bondy, C.A., Nutraceutical therapies for degenerative joint diseases: A critical review. *Crit. Rev. Food Sci. Nutr.*, 45, 3, 145–164, 2005.
4. Murugesan, R. and Orsat, V., Spray drying for the production of nutraceutical ingredients—A review. *Food Bioprocess Technol.*, 5, 1, 3–14, 2012.
5. Haar, C.V., Peterson, T.C., Martens, K.M., Hoane, M.R., Vitamins and nutrients as primary treatments in experimental brain injury: Clinical implications for nutraceutical therapies. *Brain Res.*, 1640, 114–129, 2016.
6. Bernal, J., Mendiola, J.A., Ibáñez, E., Cifuentes, A., Advanced analysis of nutraceuticals. *J. Pharm. Biomed. Anal.*, 55, 4, 758–774, 2011.
7. Houston, M., The role of nutrition and nutraceutical supplements in the treatment of hypertension. *World J. Cardiol.*, 6, 2, 38, 2014.
8. Ajjawi, I. and Shintani, D., Engineered plants with elevated vitamin E: A nutraceutical success story. *Trends Biotechnol.*, 22, 3, 104–107, 2004.
9. Chen, L., Remondetto, G.E., Subirade, M., Food protein-based materials as nutraceutical delivery systems. *Trends Food Sci. Technol.*, 17, 5, 272–283, 2006.
10. Houston, M.C., Nutrition and nutraceutical supplements in the treatment of hypertension. *Expert Rev. Cardiovasc. Ther.*, 8, 6, 821–833, 2010.
11. Shinde, N., Bangar, B., Deshmukh, S., Kumbhar, P., Nutraceuticals: A review on current status. *Res. J. Pharm. Technol.*, 7, 1, 110–113, 2014.
12. Grima, N.A., Pase, M.P., Macpherson, H., Pipingas, A., The effects of multivitamins on cognitive performance: A systematic review and meta-analysis. *J. Alzheimer's Dis.*, 29, 3, 561–569, 2012.

13. Hoover, N., Aguiniga, A., Hornecker, J., In the adult population, does daily multivitamin intake reduce the risk of mortality compared with those who do not take daily multivitamins? *Evid.-Based Pract.*, 22, 3, 15, 2019.
14. Ugli, B.S.U. and Bekchanovich, K.Y., Classification of vitamins and disease syndrome. *Sci. Educ.*, 1, 1, 54–57, 2020.
15. Lorenzini, J., Classification of vitamins. *Presse Medicale*, 35, 166–7, 1927.
16. Grune, T., Lietz, G., Palou, A., Ross, A.C., Stahl, W., Tang, G., Thurnham, D., Yin, S.A., Biesalski, H.K., β-carotene is an important vitamin A source for humans. *J. Nutr.*, 140, 12, 2268S–2285S, 2010.
17. Cortese, M., Riise, T., Bjørnevik, K., Holmøy, T., Kampman, M.T., Magalhaes, S., Pugliatti, M., Wolfson, C., Myhr, K.M., Timing of use of cod liver oil, a vitamin D source, and multiple sclerosis risk: The EnvIMS study. *Mult. Scler. J.*, 21, 14, 1856–1864, 2015.
18. Bikle, D. and Christakos, S., New aspects of vitamin D metabolism and action—Addressing the skin as source and target. *Nat. Rev. Endocrinol.*, 16, 4, 234–252, 2020.
19. Barua, A.B., Retinoyl β-glucuronide: A biologically active form of vitamin A. *Nutr. Rev.*, 55, 7, 259–267, 1997.
20. Blunt, J.W., DeLuca, H.F., Schnoes, H.K., 1,25-hydroxycholecalciferol. A biologically active metabolite of vitamin D3. *Biochemistry*, 7, 10, 3317–3322, 1968.
21. Szterk, A., Roszko, M., Małek, K., Czerwonka, M., Waszkiewicz-Robak, B., Application of the SPE reversed phase HPLC/MS technique to determine vitamin B12 bio-active forms in beef. *Meat Sci.*, 91, 4, 408–413, 2012.
22. Fraser, D. and Kodicek, E., Unique biosynthesis by kidney of a biologically active vitamin D metabolite. *Nature*, 228, 5273, 764–766, 1970.
23. Singh, A. and Sharma, S., Bioactive components and functional properties of biologically activated cereal grains: A bibliographic review. *Crit. Rev. Food Sci. Nutr.*, 57, 14, 3051–3071, 2017.
24. Napoli, J.L., Biochemical pathways of retinoid transport, metabolism, and signal transduction. *Clin. Immunol. Immunopathol.*, 80, 3, S52–S62, 1996.
25. Nau, H. and Blaner, W.S. (Eds.), *Retinoids: The biochemical and molecular basis of vitamin A and retinoid action*, Springer Science & Business Media, 2012.
26. Rice, A.L., West Jr., K.P., Black, R.E., Vitamin A deficiency, in: *Comparative Quantification of Health Risks: Global and Regional Burden of Disease Attributable to Selected Major Risk Factors*, vol. 1, pp. 0211–0256, 2004.
27. West, K.P. and Darnton-Hill, I., Vitamin A deficiency, in: *Nutrition and Health in Developing Countries*, pp. 377–433, Humana Press, Totowa, New Jersey, United States, 2008.
28. Chapman, M.S., Vitamin A: History, current uses, and controversies. *Semin. Cutan. Med. Surg.*, 31, 1, 11–16, 2012, March. WB Saunders.
29. Sommer, A., Uses and misuses of vitamin A. *Curr. Issues Public Health*, 2, 4, 161–164, 1996.

30. Cardwell, G., Bornman, J.F., James, A.P., Black, L.J., A review of mushrooms as a potential source of dietary vitamin D. *Nutrients*, *10*, 10, 1498, 2018.
31. Lund, J. and DeLuca, H.F., Biologically active metabolite of vitamin D3 from bone, liver, and blood serum. *J. Lipid Res.*, *7*, 6, 739–744, 1966.
32. Reeve, L.E., Chesney, R.W., DeLuca, H.F., Vitamin D of human milk: Identification of biologically active forms. *Am. J. Clin. Nutr.*, *36*, 1, 122–126, 1982.
33. Norman, A.W., Lund, J., Deluca, H.F., Biologically active forms of vitamin D3 in kidney and intestine. *Arch. Biochem. Biophys.*, *108*, 1, 12–21, 1964.
34. Hewison, M., Bouillon, R., Giovannucci, E., Goltzman, D. (Eds.), *Vitamin D: Volume 1: Biochemistry, physiology and diagnostics*, Elsevier Academic Press 2017.
35. Haussler, M.R., Vitamin D receptors: Nature and function. *Annu. Rev. Nutr.*, *6*, 1, 527–562, 1986.
36. DeLuca, H.F. and Schnoes, H.K., Metabolism and mechanism of action of vitamin D. *Annu. Rev. Biochem.*, *45*, 1, 631–666, 1976.
37. Holick, M.F., Vitamin D deficiency. *N. Engl. J. Med.*, *357*, 3, 266–281, 2007.
38. Prentice, A., Vitamin D deficiency: A global perspective. *Nutr. Rev.*, *66*, suppl_2, S153–S164, 2008.
39. Deluca, H.F. and Cantorna, M.T., Vitamin D: Its role and uses in immunology 1. *FASEB J.*, *15*, 14, 2579–2585, 2001.
40. Murphy, S.P., Subar, A.F., Block, G., Vitamin E intakes and sources in the United States. *Am. J. Clin. Nutr.*, *52*, 2, 361–367, 1990.
41. Hajibabaei, K., Antioxidant properties of vitamin E. *Ann. Res. Antioxid.*, *1*, 2, 1–7, 2016.
42. Traber, M.G. and Atkinson, J., Vitamin E, antioxidant and nothing more. *Free Radical Boil. Med.*, *43*, 1, 4–15, 2007.
43. Qian, J., Atkinson, J., Manor, D., Biochemical consequences of heritable mutations in the α-tocopherol transfer protein. *Biochemistry*, *45*, 27, 8236–8242, 2006.
44. Cornwell, D.G. and Ma, J., Studies in vitamin E: Biochemistry and molecular biology of tocopherol quinones. *Vitam. Horm.*, *76*, 99–134, 2007.
45. Binder, H.J., Herting, D.C., Hurst, V., Finch, S.C., Spiro, H.M., Tocopherol deficiency in man. *N. Engl. J. Med.*, *273*, 24, 1289–1297, 1965.
46. Witting, L.A. and Horwitt, M.K., Effect of degree of fatty acid unsaturation in tocopherol deficiency-induced creatinuria. *J. Nutr.*, *82*, 1, 19–33, 1964.
47. Mergens, W.J., Kamm, J.J., Newmark, H.L., Fiddler, W., Pensabene, J., Alpha-tocopherol: Uses in preventing nitrosamine formation. *IARC Sci. Publ.*, *19*, 199–212, 1978.
48. Grandel, F., Vitamin F. *Fette Seifen*, *46*, 150–152, 1939.
49. Watanabe, F., Yabuta, Y., Tanioka, Y., Bito, T., Biologically active vitamin B12 compounds in foods for preventing deficiency among vegetarians and elderly subjects. *J. Agric. Food Chem.*, *61*, 28, 6769–6775, 2013.

50. Lund, J. and DeLuca, H.F., Biologically active metabolite of vitamin D3 from bone, liver, and blood serum. *J. Lipid Res.*, 7, 6, 739–744, 1966.
51. Shimizu, S. and Yamada, H., Microbial production of polyunsaturated fatty acids (vitamin-F group), in: *Biotechnology of Vitamins, Pigments and Growth Factors*, pp. 105–121, Springer, Dordrecht, 1989.
52. Lecoq, R., Chauchard, P., Mazoue, H., Disturbances of neuromuscular excitability in nutritional imbalance and vitamin deficiencies. 22. Vitamin F deficiency in the rat and pigeon. *Bull. Soc. Chim. Biol.*, 29, 724–727, 1947.
53. Perlenfein, H.H., A survey of vitamin F. *A survey of vitamin F., Lee Found. Nutrit. Res.*, 1, 21–36, 1942.
54. Suttie, J.W., Vitamin K and human nutrition. *J. Am. Diet. Assoc.*, 92, 5, 585–590, 1992.
55. Stenflo, J. and Suttie, J.W., Vitamin K-dependent formation of γ-carboxyglutamic acid. *Annu. Rev. Biochem.*, 46, 1, 157–172, 1977.
56. Gröber, U., Reichrath, J., Holick, M.F., Kisters, K., Vitamin K: An old vitamin in a new perspective. *Dermatoendocrinol.*, 6, 1, e968490, 2014.
57. Booth, S.L., Roles for vitamin K beyond coagulation. *Annu. Rev. Nutr.*, 29, 89–110, 2009.
58. Gröber, U., Reichrath, J., Holick, M.F., Kisters, K., Vitamin K: An old vitamin in a new perspective. *Dermatoendocrinol.*, 6, 1, e968490, 2014.
59. Anastasi, E., Ialongo, C., Labriola, R., Ferraguti, G., Lucarelli, M., Angeloni, A., Vitamin K deficiency and COVID-19. *Scand. J. Clin. Lab. Invest.*, 80, 7, 525–527, 2020.
60. Jin, D.Y., Tie, J.K., Stafford, D.W., The conversion of vitamin K epoxide to vitamin K quinone and vitamin K quinone to vitamin K hydroquinone uses the same active site cysteines. *Biochemistry*, 46, 24, 7279–7283, 2007.
61. Berkner, K.L. and Runge, K.W., The physiology of vitamin K nutriture and vitamin K-dependent protein function in atherosclerosis. *J. Thromb. Haemost.*, 2, 12, 2118–2132, 2004.
62. Martin, F., Giménez, E.C., Konings, E., New methods for the analysis of water-soluble vitamins in infant formula and adult/pediatric nutritionals. *J. AOAC Int.*, 99, 1, 19–25, 2016.
63. Szczuko, M., Migrała, R., Drozd, A., Banaszczak, M., Maciejewska, D., Chlubek, D., Stachowska, E., Role of water soluble vitamins in the reduction diet of an amateur sportsman. *Open Life Sci.*, 13, 1, 163–173, 2018.
64. Du, Q., Wang, H., Xie, J., Thiamin (vitamin B1) biosynthesis and regulation: A rich source of antimicrobial drug targets? *Int. J. Boil. Sci.*, 7, 1, 41, 2011.
65. Knight, B.C.J.G., The nutrition of Staphylococcus aureus; Nicotinic acid and vitamin B1. *Biochem. J.*, 31, 5, 731, 1937.
66. Bauer-Petrovska, B. and Petrushevska-Tozi, L., Mineral and water soluble vitamin content in the Kombucha drink. *Int. J. Food Sci. Technol.*, 35, 2, 201–205, 2000.
67. Peters, E.A., The biochemical lesion in vitamin B1 deficiency. Application of modern biochemical analysis in its diagnosis. *Lancet*, 230, 1161–1165, 1936.

68. Martin, P.R., Singleton, C.K., Hiller-Sturmhöfel, S., The role of thiamine deficiency in alcoholic brain disease. *Alcohol Res. Health*, 27, 2, 134, 2003.
69. Abdou, E. and Hazell, A.S., Thiamine deficiency: An update of pathophysiologic mechanisms and future therapeutic considerations. *Neurochem. Res.*, 40, 2, 353–361, 2015.
70. Gibson, G.E., Hirsch, J.A., Fonzetti, P., Jordan, B.D., Cirio, R.T., Elder, J., Vitamin B1 (thiamine) and dementia. *Ann. N. Y. Acad. Sci.*, 1367, 1, 21–30, 2016.
71. Aykroyd, W.R. and Roscoe, M.H., The distribution of vitamin B2 in certain foods. *Biochem. J.*, 23, 3, 483, 1929.
72. Northrop-Clewes, C.A. and Thurnham, D.I., The discovery and characterization of riboflavin. *Ann. Nutr. Metab.*, 61, 3, 224–230, 2012.
73. Massey, V., The chemical and biological versatility of riboflavin. *Biochem. Soc. Trans.*, 28, 4, 283–296, 2000.
74. Bacher, A., Eberhardt, S., Fischer, M., Kis, K., Richter, G., Biosynthesis of vitamin B2 (riboflavin). *Annu. Rev. Nutr.*, 20, 1, 153–167, 2000.
75. Ashoori, M. and Saedisomeolia, A., Riboflavin (vitamin B2) and oxidative stress: A review. *Br. J. Nutr.*, 111, 11, 1985–1991, 2014.
76. Schramm, M., Wiegmann, K., Schramm, S., Gluschko, A., Herb, M., Utermöhlen, O., Krönke, M., Riboflavin (vitamin B2) deficiency impairs NADPH oxidase 2 (Nox2) priming and defense against Listeria monocytogenes. *Eur. J. Immunol.*, 44, 3, 728–741, 2014.
77. Buehler, B.A., Vitamin B2: Riboflavin. *J. Evid.-Based Complementary Altern. Med.*, 16, 2, 88–90, 2011.
78. Bacher, A., Eberhardt, S., Fischer, M., Kis, K., Richter, G., Biosynthesis of vitamin b2 (riboflavin). *Annu. Rev. Nutr.*, 20, 1, 153–167, 2000.
79. Chi, Y. and Sauve, A.A., Nicotinamide riboside, a trace nutrient in foods, is a vitamin B3 with effects on energy metabolism and neuroprotection. *Curr. Opin. Clin. Nutr. Metab. Care*, 16, 6, 657–661, 2013.
80. Sauve, A.A., NAD+ and vitamin B3: From metabolism to therapies. *J. Pharmacol. Exp. Ther.*, 324, 3, 883–893, 2008.
81. Tewari, K.S. and Monk, B.J., Chemotherapy drugs and regimens, in: *The 21st Century Handbook of Clinical Ovarian Cancer*, p. 165, 2015.
82. Svedäng, H., Hammer, M., Heiskanen, A.S., Häggblom, M., Ilvessalo-Lax, H., Kvarnström, M., Tunon, H., Vihervaara, P., *Nature's contributions to people and human well-being in a nordic coastal context*, Publishers Nordic Council of Ministers, 2018.
83. Yawata, Y., Kanzaki, A., Yawata, A., Nakanishi, H., Kaku, M., Hereditary red cell membrane disorders in Japan: Their genotypic and phenotypic features in 1014 cases studied. *Hematology*, 6, 6, 399–422, 2001.
84. Lopez-Guerrero, J.A. and Alonso, M.A., Nitric oxide production induced by herpes simplex virus type 1 does not alter the course of the infection in human monocytic cells. *J. Gen. Virol.*, 78, 8, 1977–1980, 1997.

85. Zimmermann, M.B., Jooste, P.L., Mabapa, N.S., Schoeman, S., Biebinger, R., Mushaphi, L.F., Mbhenyane, X., Vitamin A supplementation in iodine-deficient African children decreases thyrotropin stimulation of the thyroid and reduces the goiter rate. *Am. J. Clin. Nutr.*, 86, 4, 1040–1044, 2007.
86. Darnton-Hill, I., Public health aspects in the prevention and control of vitamin deficiencies. *Curr. Dev. Nutr.*, 3, 9, nzz075, 2019.
87. Prousky, J., Vitamin B3 for depression: Case report and review of the literature. *J. Orthomol. Med.*, 25, 3, 137–147, 2010.
88. Sheppard, S.K., Didelot, X., Meric, G., Torralbo, A., Jolley, K.A., Kelly, D.J., Bentley, S.D., Maiden, M.C., Parkhill, J., Falush, D., Genome-wide association study identifies vitamin B5 biosynthesis as a host specificity factor in Campylobacter. *Proc. Natl. Acad. Sci.*, 110, 29, 11923–11927, 2013.
89. Shibata, K. and Fukuwatari, T., The chemistry of pantothenic acid (vitamin B5), in: *B Vitamins and Folate*, pp. 127–134, 2012.
90. Mittermayr, R., Kalman, A., Trisconi, M.J., Heudi, O., Determination of vitamin B5 in a range of fortified food products by reversed-phase liquid chromatography–mass spectrometry with electrospray ionisation. *J. Chromatogr. A*, 1032, 1-2, 1–6, 2004.
91. Vergeres, G. and Waskell, L., Cytochrome b5, its functions, structure and membrane topology. *Biochimie*, 77, 7-8, 604–620, 1995.
92. Dürr, U.H., Waskell, L., Ramamoorthy, A., The cytochromes P450 and b5 and their reductases—Promising targets for structural studies by advanced solid-state NMR spectroscopy. *Biochim. Biophys. Acta (BBA)-Biomembr.*, 1768, 12, 3235–3259, 2007.
93. Hodges, R.E., Ohlson, M.A., Bean, W.B., Pantothenic acid deficiency in man. *J. Clin. Investig.*, 37, 11, 1642–1657, 1958.
94. Smith, C.M. and Song, W.O., Comparative nutrition of pantothenic acid. *J. Nutr. Biochem.*, 7, 6, 312–321, 1996.
95. Wittwer, C.T., Schweitzer, C., Pearson, J., Song, W.O., Windham, C.T., Wyse, B.W., Hansen, R.G., Enzymes for liberation of pantothenic acid in blood: Use of plasma pantetheinase. *Am. J. Clin. Nutr.*, 50, 5, 1072–1078, 1989.
96. Selhub, J., Folate, vitamin B12 and vitamin B6 and one carbon metabolism. *J. Nutr. Health Aging*, 6, 1, 39–42, 2002.
97. Tully, D.B., Allgood, V.E., Cidlowski, J.A., Modulation of steroid receptor-mediated gene expression by vitamin B6. *FASEB J.*, 8, 3, 343–349, 1994.
98. Schneider, G., Käck, H., Lindqvist, Y., The manifold of vitamin B6 dependent enzymes. *Structure*, 8, 1, R1–R6, 2000.
99. Bender, D.A., Novel functions of vitamin B6. *Proc. Nutr. Soc.*, 53, 3, 625–630, 1994.
100. Shideler, C.E., Vitamin B6: An overview. *Am. J. Med. Technol.*, 49, 1, 17–22, 1983.
101. Malouf, R. and Evans, J.G., Vitamin B6 for cognition. *Cochrane Database Syst. Rev.*, 4, 1–22, 2003.

102. Rail, L.C. and Meydani, S.N., Vitamin B6 and immune competence. *Nutr. Rev.*, *51*, 8, 217–225, 1993.
103. Bender, D.A., Non-nutritional uses of vitamin B6. *Br. J. Nutr.*, *81*, 1, 7–20, 1999.
104. Simmons, S., Folic acid vitamin B9: Friend or foe? *Nursing2020*, *43*, 3, 55–60, 2013.
105. Rawalpally, T.R., Folic acid, in: *Kirk-Othmer Encyclopedia of Chemical Technology*, pp. 1–18, 2000.
106. Naderi, N. and House, J.D., Recent developments in folate nutrition. *Adv. Food Nutr. Res.*, *83*, 195–213, 2018.
107. Chango, A., The chemistry of folate, in: *B Vitamins and Folate*, pp. 158–163, 2012.
108. Fenech, M., Folate (vitamin B9) and vitamin B12 and their function in the maintenance of nuclear and mitochondrial genome integrity. *Mutat. Res./Fundam. Mol. Mech. Mutagen.*, *733*, 1-2, 21–33, 2012.
109. Abbasi, I.H.R., Abbasi, F., Wang, L., Abd El Hack, M.E., Swelum, A.A., Hao, R., Yao, J., Cao, Y., Folate promotes S-adenosyl methionine reactions and the microbial methylation cycle and boosts ruminants production and reproduction. *AMB Express*, *8*, 1, 1–10, 2018.
110. Zamierowski, M.M. and Wagner, C., Effect of folacin deficiency on folacin-binding proteins in the rat. *J. Nutr.*, *107*, 10, 1937–1945, 1977.
111. Lee, C.D., Belcher, L.V., Miller, D.L., Field observation of folacin deficiency in poults. *Avian Dis.*, *9*, 4, 504–512, 1965.
112. Bailey, L.B., Mahan, C.S., Dimperio, D., Folacin and iron status in low-income pregnant adolescents and mature women. *Am. J. Clin. Nutr.*, *33*, 9, 1997–2001, 1980.
113. Watanabe, F., Vitamin B12 sources and bioavailability. *Exp. Biol. Med.*, *232*, 10, 1266–1274, 2007.
114. Watanabe, F., Yabuta, Y., Bito, T., Teng, F., Vitamin B12-containing plant food sources for vegetarians. *Nutrients*, *6*, 5, 1861–1873, 2014.
115. Szterk, A., Roszko, M., Małek, K., Czerwonka, M., Waszkiewicz-Robak, B., Application of the SPE reversed phase HPLC/MS technique to determine vitamin B12 bio-active forms in beef. *Meat Sci.*, *91*, 4, 408–413, 2012.
116. Watanabe, F., Yabuta, Y., Tanioka, Y., Bito, T., Biologically active vitamin B12 compounds in foods for preventing deficiency among vegetarians and elderly subjects. *J. Agric. Food Chem.*, *61*, 28, 6769–6775, 2013.
117. Scott, J.M., Folate and vitamin B12. *Proc. Nutr. Soc.*, *58*, 2, 441–448, 1999.
118. Banerjee, R.V. and Matthews, R.G., Cobalamin-dependent methionine synthase. *FASEB J.*, *4*, 5, 1450–1459, 1990.
119. Gaire, D., Sponne, I., Droesch, S., Charlier, A., Nicolas, J.P., Lambert, D., Comparison of two methods for the measurement of rat liver methylmalonyl-coenzyme A mutase activity: HPLC and radioisotopic assays. *J. Nutr. Biochem.*, *10*, 1, 56–62, 1999.
120. Stabler, S.P., Vitamin B12 deficiency. *N. Engl. J. Med.*, *368*, 2, 149–160, 2013.

121. Oh, R.C. and Brown, D.L., Vitamin B12 deficiency. *Am. Fam. Physician*, 67, 5, 979–986, 2003.
122. Romain, M., Sviri, S., Linton, D.M., Stav, I., van Heerden, P.V., The role of Vitamin B12 in the critically ill—A review. *Anaesth. Intensive Care*, 44, 4, 447–452, 2016.
123. Devaki, S.J. and Raveendran, R.L., Vitamin C: Sources, functions, sensing and analysis, in: *Vitamin C*, IntechOpen, London, 2017.
124. Doseděl, M., Jirkovský, E., Macáková, K., Krčmová, L.K., Javorská, L., Pourová, J., Mercolini, L., Remião, F., Nováková, L., Mladěnka, P., OEMONOM, Vitamin C—Sources, physiological role, kinetics, deficiency, use, toxicity, and determination. *Nutrients*, 13, 2, 615, 2021.
125. Telang, P.S., Vitamin C in dermatology. *Indian Dermatol. Online J.*, 4, 2, 143, 2013.
126. Rock, C.L., Jacob, R.A., Bowen, P.E., Update on the biological characteristics of the antioxidant micronutrients: Vitamin C, vitamin E, and the carotenoids. *J. Am. Diet. Assoc.*, 96, 7, 693–702, 1996.
127. Padh, H., Vitamin C: Newer insights into its biochemical functions. *Nutr. Rev.*, 49, 3, 65–70, 1991.
128. Schlueter, A.K. and Johnston, C.S., Vitamin C: Overview and update. *J. Evid.-Based Complementary Altern. Med.*, 16, 1, 49–57, 2011.
129. Bendich, A., Machlin, L.J., Scandurra, O., Burton, G.W., Wayner, D.D.M., The antioxidant role of vitamin C. *Adv. Free Radic. Biol. Med.*, 2, 2, 419–444, 1986.
130. Ahire, E.D., Sonawane, V.N., Surana, K.R., Talele, G.S., Drug discovery, drug-likeness screening, and bioavailability: Development of drug-likeness rule for natural products, in: *Applied Pharmaceutical Practice and Nutraceuticals*, pp. 191–208, Apple Academic Press, New Jersey and Canada, 2021.
131. Robertson, W.V.B. and Schwartz, B., Ascorbic acid and the formation of collagen. *J. Biol. Chem.*, 201, 689, 1953.
132. Hodges, R.E., Hood, J., Canham, J.E., Sauberlich, H.E., Baker, E.M., Clinical manifestations of ascorbic acid deficiency in man. *Am. J. Clin. Nutr.*, 24, 4, 432–443, 1971.
133. Vilter, R.W., Nutritional aspects of ascorbic acid: Uses and abuses. *West. J. Med.*, 133, 6, 485, 1980.
134. Keservani, R.K., Kesharwani, R.K., Sharma, A.K., Pulmonary and respiratory health: Antioxidants and nutraceuticals, in: *Nutraceutical and Functional Foods in Human Life and Disease Prevention*, D. Bagchi, H.G. Preuss, A. Swaroop (Eds.), pp. 279–295, CRC Press, Taylor and Francis, Boca Raton, Fl, 2015.

2
Structure and Functions of Vitamins

Suvarna S. Khairnar[1], Khemchand R. Surana[2*], Eknath D. Ahire[3], Sunil K. Mahajan[4], Dhananjay M. Patil[5] and Deepak D. Sonawane[5]

[1]Department of Pharmacology, Shreeshakti Shaikshanik Sanstha, Divine College of Pharmacy, Satana, Nashik, India
[2]Department of Pharmaceutical Chemistry, Shreeshakti Shaikshanik Sanstha, Divine College of Pharmacy, Satana, Nashik, India
[3]Department of Pharmaceutics, MET's Institute of Pharmacy, Adgaon, Nashik, India
[4]Department of Pharmaceutical Chemistry, MGV's Pharmacy College, Panchvati, Nashik, India
[5]Department of Pharmaceutics, Shreeshakti Shaikshanik Sanstha, Divine College of Pharmacy, Satana, Nashik, India

Abstract

Vitamins are wide a group of organic compounds that are required for normal body function. There are 13 nutrients classified as vitamins: four "fat-soluble" and nine "water-soluble." All are essential to maintain healthy homeostasis and metabolic function. Today, there is increased interest in nutritionally rich foods that are either natural or minimally processed. The use of emerging technologies aimed at improving the stability and bioaccessibility of vitamins in foods to maintain their functionality through their bioavailability, metabolism, and health-promoting activity has also increased. This chapter discusses these emerging technologies, as well as the challenges and opportunities for vitamins as food additives. An extensive overview of current evidence on the health implications of food vitamins, as well as the effects of emerging technologies on vitamins, is included in this chapter.

Keywords: Vitamins, structure and functions of vitamins, fat-soluble, water-soluble

---

*Corresponding author: khemchandsurana411@gmail.com

2.1 Introduction

Vitamins are wide a group of organic compounds, generally unable to be synthesized by the human body but necessary for the correct maintenance of its normal functions. Under normal circumstances, we can receive various vitamins via food and proper nutrition, but minimum nutritional requirements are frequently not satisfied, necessitating supplementation. Vitamins are necessary for metabolism, growth, and normal physiological function [1]. Only vitamin D is produced by the body; all other vitamins are obtained from food. The key essential nutrients, vitamins were equally important for the body [2]. Vitamins were derived from the Latin term viva, which meant "life," and were discovered to be chemically an amine. Once it was discovered that not all vitamins were amines, the "e" was eliminated, and the term was shortened to "vitamins." Vitamin A was the first vitamin identified by Cashmir, followed by the vital nutrients. Vitamins are equally crucial for the body. Vitamins were derived from the Latin term viva, which meant "life," and were discovered to be chemically an amine. Once it was discovered that not all vitamins were amines, the "e" was eliminated and the term was shortened to "vitamins." Vitamins are little organic chemicals that the body need in minute amounts (micrograms to milligrams per day) to carry out metabolic processes. Because the chemical nature of vitamins was unknown at the time, letter designations, such as a, b, and c, were used in their name. Today, aldehydes, alcohols, organic acids, their derivatives, and even nucleotide compounds, such as vitamin B1, are discovered to have various chemical natures. Vitamins include 13 essential

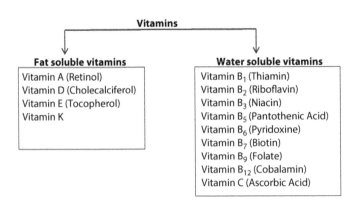

Figure 2.1 Classification of vitamins.

compounds that cannot be synthesized or produced in sufficient quantities by the body and hence requires to be supplied in diet [3, 4].

There are two major classifications (Figure 2.1) of vitamins.

2.2 Structural Discussion

2.2.1 Vitamin A

Vitamin A is an essential nutrient in mammals that occurs in several forms known as retinoids. Each form is characterized by a common skeleton known as the retinyl group. The vitamin A family includes vitamin A1 (retinol) and vitamin A2 (dehydroretinol) (Figure 2.2). These vitamins and their biologically active metabolites are known as retinoids. Two main preforms of vitamin A are usually found in human diet, namely retinol and beta carotenoid. Mammals do not synthesize retinoids de novo, so they depend on the dietary intake of retinol, derivatives, and precursors (provitamins A). Provitamin A is widely dispersed in the body. Carrots, tomatoes, peaches, sweet potatoes, beef, dark green, yellow, and orange

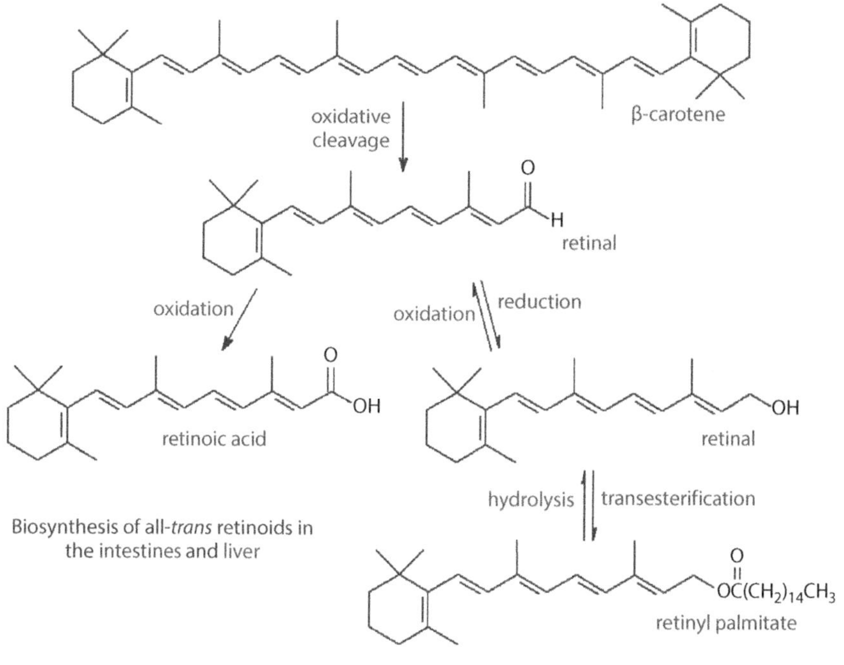

Figure 2.2 The chemical structure of vitamin A.

fruits and vegetables, such as oranges, broccoli, spinach, carrots, squash, pumpkins, and cod liver, are all good providers of these nutrients. It is a fat-soluble vitamin made up of a six-membered ring with an 11-carbon side chain. Retinol, retinal, and retinoic acid are the three active biological components generated from beta carotene that make up vitamin A [5, 6].

Vitamin A in humans consists of a group of molecules with a common retinyl group. The functional molecules are retinal and retinoic acid. Dietary sources are principally retinyl esters from meat and dairy products and provitamin A (PVA) carotenoids from plants. The synthesis of vitamin A takes place in the intestine, where beta carotene deoxygenated acts on beta carotene in the presence of NADPH to reduce retinal to retinol. The retinol is further esterified with palmitic acid in chylomicrons along with dietary lipid for absorption [7, 8].

Functional Roles of Vitamin A: Implications for Public Health

Anemia: Vitamin A deficiency negatively affects hemoglobin concentrations. Vitamin A plus iron supplementation increased hemoglobin concentrations more than either nutrient alone [9].

Cancer: Meta-analyses of human studies have found an adverse relationship between vitamin A intake and a variety of malignancies, including bladder, breast, cervical, and stomach cancers. Clinical trials have used both synthetic and naturally occurring retinoids (e.g., all-trans retinoic acid, 9-cis retinoic acid, 13-cis retinoic acid) (Institute of Medicine, 1999). Certain retinoid inhibit the growth of various tumors (e.g., lung, gastrointestinal, breast) and may have chemopreventive and/or chemotherapeutic properties, d all-trans retinoic acid is used as a chemotherapeutic agent to treat acute promyelocytic leukemia, and in the vast majority of these patients, this treatment leads to a complete remission [10].

Diabetes: Patients with type 1 diabetes have reduced quantities of serum retinol and its carrier proteins (RBP and transthyretin). The relationship between serum retinol and carrier proteins and type 2 diabetes is less obvious, with some studies indicating no change and others reporting reductions in type 2 diabetes. Vitamin A shortage and excess have different impacts on macronutrient metabolism in different tissues and cells [11].

RBP secreted by adipose tissue has been linked to obesity and insulin resistance by interfering with insulin signaling in muscle and increasing hepatic glucose output [12].

Structure and Functions of Vitamins 39

HIV and pregnancy: Because there is currently no solid evidence of vitamin A supplementation reducing the risk of vertical HIV transmission in HIV-positive pregnant women, the WHO does not suggest supplementation to minimize the risk of mother-to-child transmission. Vitamin A supplementation to mothers at delivery was linked to a lower risk of HIV transmission in newborns with mannose-binding lectin-2 variations [13].

Measles: The WHO recommends that age-appropriate doses of vitamin A be given twice 24 hours apart to infants and children with measles in populations where vitamin A deficiency may be present to reduce the risk of death from measles, based on a randomized, placebo-controlled clinical trial in children with measles and other clinical research.

In places where vitamin A deficiency is a public health problem, preventing vitamin A deficiency with periodic, high-dose supplements reduces the risk of measles in children aged 6 to 59 months [14].

For an adult man and woman, the recommended daily average (RDA) vitamin A intake is roughly 900 mcg and 700 mcg, respectively. It is vital to remember not to consume too much vitamin A because it can cause toxicity and hypervitaminosis A, which can cause bone discomfort, eyesight changes, and even death, as well as birth problems in pregnant women. Night blindness, xerophthalmia, skin illnesses, nerve lesions, reduced lipid absorption and chylomicron production, and some enzymatic abnormalities are also symptoms of vitamin A insufficiency. As a result, it is critical to get enough vitamin A every day. As a medicinal supplements vitamin A megadoses appear effective in reducing mortality from measles in children under two years old and have few associated adverse events [15].

2.2.2 Vitamin D

Vitamin D deficiency affects about half of the world population. There are around 1 billion individuals in the world, representing all races and age categories. Vitamin D is unique in that it can be produced in the skin as a result of sun exposure. Sunlight has also been discovered to be a source of vitamin D for humans, as the UV light in sun rays allows skin to produce its own vitamin D. In spring, summer, and fall, exposure to the skin normally ranges between 1000 and 1500 hours [16].

There are two types of vitamin D. Vitamin D2 is produced by irradiating the yeast sterol ergosterol with ultraviolet light, and it is found naturally in sun-exposed mushrooms. The most "natural" form is vitamin D3, which is produced by humans when UVB radiation contacts the skin. Vitamin D2 is not produced by humans, although it is found in most oily fish, such as

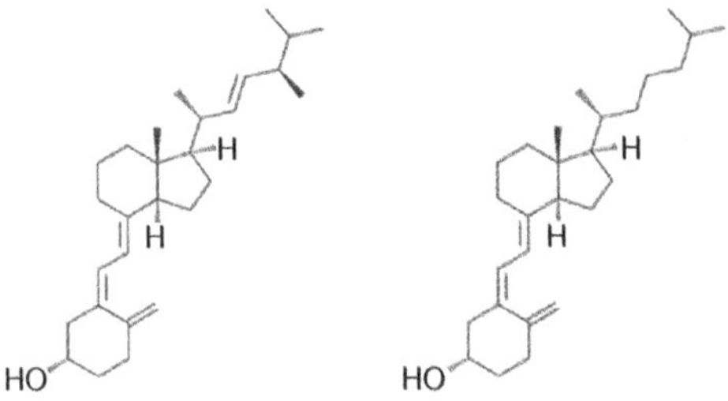

Figure 2.3 The chemical structure of vitamin D.

salmon, mackerel, and herring. Ingested vitamin D (Figure 2.3) (D stands for D2, D3, or both) is combined into chylomicrons, which are absorbed into the lymphatic system and enter the venous bloodstream. Vitamin D obtained through the skin or the diet is physiologically inactive and must be converted to 25(OH) D in the liver by the enzyme vitamin D-25-hydroxylase (25-OHase) [17, 18].

Functional Roles of Vitamin D: Implications for Public Health

Bone health and muscle strength: Vitamin D supplementation may prevent such fractures as long as it is taken in high enough higher intakes of vitamin D supplements about 500 to 800 IU per day reduced hip and non-spine fractures by about 20%, while lower intakes (400 IU or less) failed to offer any fracture prevention benefit [19, 20].

Heart disease: The coronary heart is largely a massive muscle and prefers skeletal muscle, it has receptors for nutrition D. Immune and inflammatory cells that play a function in cardiovascular ailment situations, like atherosclerosis, are regulated via way of means of nutrition D [21].

Type 2 diabetes: Vitamin D deficiency can also additionally negatively have an effect on the biochemical pathways that cause the improvement of type 2 diabetes (T2DM), consisting of impairment of beta cellular feature within the pancreas, insulin resistance, and inflammation. Prospective observational research has proven that better nutrition D blood tiers are related to decrease quotes of T2DM [22].

Immune function: Vitamin D function in regulating the immune device has led scientists to discover parallel studies paths: Does nutrition D deficiency make a contribution to the improvement of a couple of sclerosis, type 1 diabetes, and different so-called autoimmune diseases, in which the body's immune device assaults its personal organs and tissues? And should nutrition D dietary supplements assist increase our body's defenses to combat infectious ailment [23]?

Flu and the Common Cold: The flu virus causes the most devastation during the winter months and then fades away during the summer months. Because of this periodicity, a British medical specialist hypothesized that influenza outbreaks were caused by a sunlight-related "seasonal stimulus." Many scientists published an article more than two decades after this preliminary theory, claiming that vitamin D is a seasonal stimulant. Vitamin D levels are lowest during the winter months. The active form of vitamin D reduces the detrimental inflammatory response of some white blood cells while also increasing immune cell production of antimicrobial proteins [24].

2.2.3 Vitamin E

Vitamin E includes eight clearly happening lipophilic compounds along with four tocopherols (α-, β-, γ-, and δ-) and four tocotrienols (α-, β-, γ-, and δ-) that range their aspect chain saturation and diploma of methylation in their chromanol heads (Figure 2.4). Vitamin E is well known for its

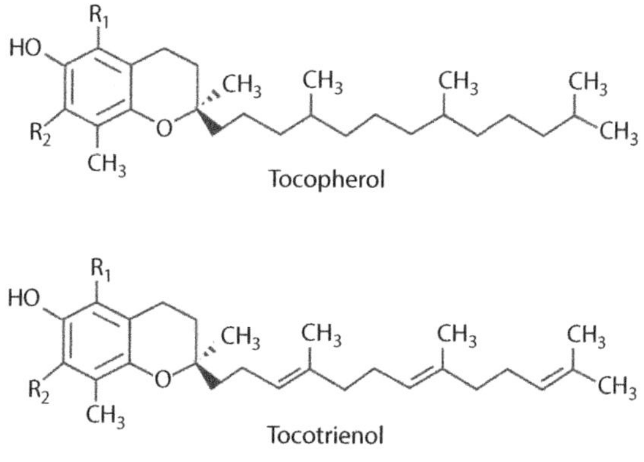

Figure 2.4 The chemical structure of vitamin E.

antioxidant properties, which help to break the self-perpetuating cycle of lipid peroxidation. Vitamin E is an important component that also serves as an antioxidant. The phrase "nutrition E" is generic, and it refers to everything that displays the organic activity of tocopherol [25, 26].

2.2.4 Vitamin K

Vitamin K1 and vitamin K2 are fat-soluble vitamins that are found and function in the membranes of living organisms. The chemical backbone of both forms (menadione and vitamin K3) is 2-methyl-1, 4-naphtoquinone, although their lipophilic side chains are different. Vitamin K2 has unsaturated isoprenyl side chains with numbers ranging from MK-4 to MK-13 depending on their length, whereas vitamin K1 has a phytyl substituted chain [27]. Vitamin K1 is found mostly in green leafy vegetables, vegetable oils, and some fruits, and is the most common source of vitamin K in the diet (Figure 2.5). Vitamin K2 is created by bacteria in the human gut or found in animal-based and fermented meals. MK-4 is an example because it is not a typical bacterial product and is therefore thought to be of animal origin because of its tissue-specific conversion

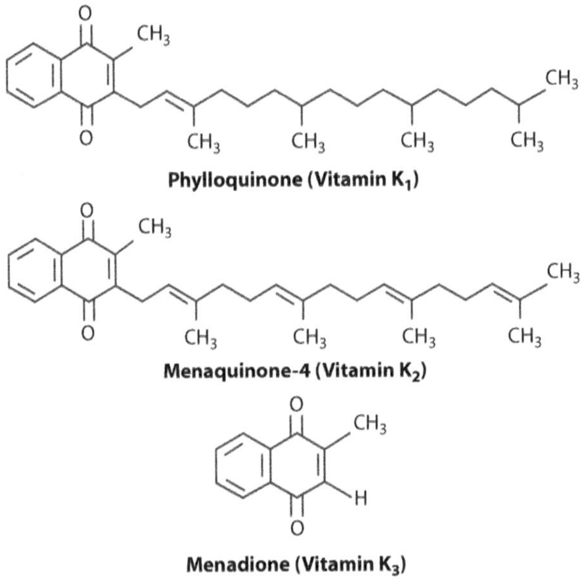

Figure 2.5 The chemical structure of vitamin K.

from vitamin K1. Menadione, on the other hand, is a result of vitamin K1 catabolism and a circulating precursor of tissue MK-4 despite being referred to as vitamin K3. As a result, it is more appropriately characterized as a provitamin [28, 29].

Functional Roles of Vitamin K: Implications for Public Health

Blood clotting action: Vitamin K enables to make four of the thirteen proteins needed for blood clotting, which stops wounds from constantly bleeding so one can heal. People who are prescribed anticoagulants (additionally known as blood thinners) to save you blood clots from forming within the coronary heart, lung, or legs are regularly knowledgeable approximately nutrition K. Nutrition K has the ability to counteract the effects of blood thinning drugs due to its blood clotting function. A common technique that estimates blood tiers of nutrition K is measuring prothrombin time (PT), or how lengthy it takes for blood to clot [30, 31].

Bone: Vitamin K is involved in the production of proteins in bone, including osteocalcin, which is needed to prevent bone deterioration. Some research has proven that better nutrition K intakes are related to a decrease occurrence of hip fractures and low bone density. In addition, low blood levels of nutrition K had been related with low bone density [32].

Heart disease: A few research have researched the position of nutrition K for coronary heart health. Vitamin K is worried with the manufacturing of matrix Gla proteins (MGP), which assist to save you calcification or hardening of coronary heart arteries, a contributor to coronary heart disease. Because studies on this region may be very limited, extra research are wanted earlier than a selected quantity of nutrition K past the usual advice is proposed for this condition [33].

2.2.5 Vitamin B1

Thiamin (thiamine), or vitamin B1 (Figure 2.6), is a water-soluble vitamin found naturally in some foods, added to foods, and sold as a supplement. Thiamin plays a vital role in the growth and function of various cells [34].

Thiamine consists of a pyrimidine ring structure bonded to a thiazole ring via a methylene bridge. Hence, synthesis of thiamine requires an independent formation of the two ring structures and their subsequent condensation. When phosphorylated, thiamine forms an activated coenzyme, thiamine pyrophosphate (TPP), upon the addition of pyrophosphate from ATP [35].

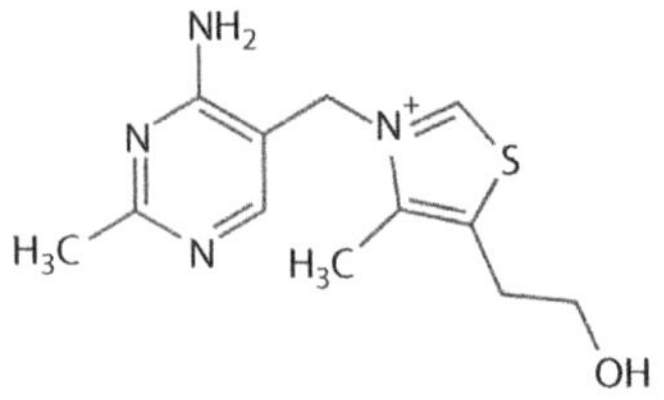

Figure 2.6 The chemical structure of vitamin B1.

Thiamine consists of a pyrimidine ring structure bonded to a thiazole ring via a methylene bridge. Hence, synthesis of thiamine requires an independent formation of the two ring structures and their subsequent condensation. When phosphorylated, thiamine forms an activated coenzyme, thiamine pyrophosphate (TPP), upon the addition of pyrophosphate from ATP. The active coenzyme form of thiamine serves several functions [36].

1. TPP is the coenzyme for all alpha ketos decarboxylation and alpha-oxoglutaric acid decarboxylation in the citric acid cycle.
2. Alanine is converted to pyruvic acid and then to acetyl coenzyme A.
3. TPP functions as a phosphate donor for phosphorylation of the Na+ nerve membrane transporter, making it essential for brain function.
4. Necessary for ATP, ribose, NAD, and DNA production (Vitamin B1).

The recommended daily average requirement of thiamine is approximately 1.2 to 1.4 mg in men and 1 mg in women (more for pregnant and lactating women). For infants, the suggested daily intake is between 0.2 and 0.5mg. It is vital that the diet includes proper amounts of vitamin B1 to avoid deficiency symptoms, such as lactic acidosis, Wernicke's encephalopathy with Korsakoff's psychosis, which is associated with alcohol and drug abuse, with extended cases of heart failure and edema [37, 38].

2.2.6 Vitamin B2

Egg, dark meat, kidneys, liver, milk, and green vegetables all contain vitamin B2 (Figure 2.7) or riboflavin. It is a yellow compound with an isoalloxazine ring and a ribitol side chain that is extensively used as food colouring [39].

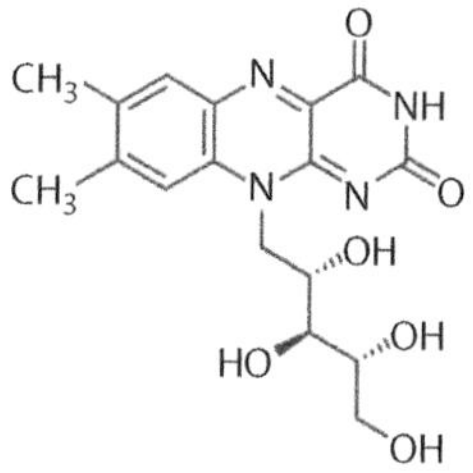

Figure 2.7 The chemical structure of vitamin B2.

Flavinmononucleotide (FMN) and flavin adenine dinucleotide (FAD) are the two active forms of riboflavin (Figure 2.7). These riboflavin-derived flavocoenzymes are among the most chemically flexible cofactors [40].

2.2.7 Vitamin B3

Vitamin B3 is the name given to the third water-soluble vitamin found. Mushrooms, liver, almonds, green vegetables, eggs, yeasts, chicken, pork, and pumpkins are all good sources of vitamin B3 (Figure 2.8). Niacin is a derivative of pyridine, technically known as pyridine-3-carboxylic acid and is named after nicotine acid and nicotinamide ($C_6H_5NO_2$). Vitamin B3, often known as niacin, is the only other known vitamin that the body can produce. The liver produces niacin from the necessary amino acid tryptophan in the diet, which goes through a sequence of reactions to produce niacin [41].

Function of Niacin

1. Used in the formation of NAD+ and NADP+ which are active coenzymes of dehydrogenases for various oxidation reduction reactions, primarily in citric acid cycle and glycolysis.
2. NAD has been linked to DNA repair.

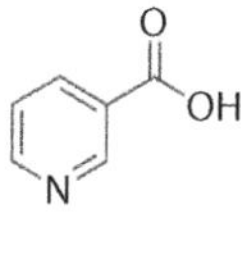

Figure 2.8 The chemical structure of vitamin B3.

3. Plays role in cholesterol and fatty acid synthesis and pentose phosphate pathways.
4. High doses of nicotinic acid are known to reduce risks of cardiovascular diseases, hence used as an additional supplement to lipid lowering medications.

However, over dosage/high intake of niacin may lead to liver damage and vasodilation resulting adverse effects. Hence, the RDA for Vitamin B3 is around 15 to 20 mg, where tryptophan alone provides 10% of the total daily requirement [42]. Deficiency of niacin can lead to pellagra, a disease that can result dermatitis, diarrhoea, dementia, and even death. However, a deficiency of vitamin B6 can also lead to niacin deficiency due to vitamin B6' conezymatic activity in niacin synthesis pathway [43].

2.2.8 Vitamin B7/H

Egg yolk, liver, kidneys, and veggies are a number of the critical sources of biotin or nutrition H. It also can be synthesized through the intestine microbiome present within the small intestine. Biotin is located in nature acts as a precursor of biotin. Biotin includes a fused imidazole and thiophene ring with a valeric acid side chain (consisting amino institution of lysine residue and carboxylase bonded collectively readily absorbed by the liver and muscle tissues [44]. Figure 2.9 indicates the chemical structure of vitamin B7.

Functions: The significant organic roles of biotin are:

1. Required in the conversion of acetyl CoA to malonyl CoA via acetyl CoA carboxylase.
2. Helps in fatty acid synthesis.
3. Helps within the conversion of pyruvate to oxaloacetate.
4. Catabolizes branched chain amino acids

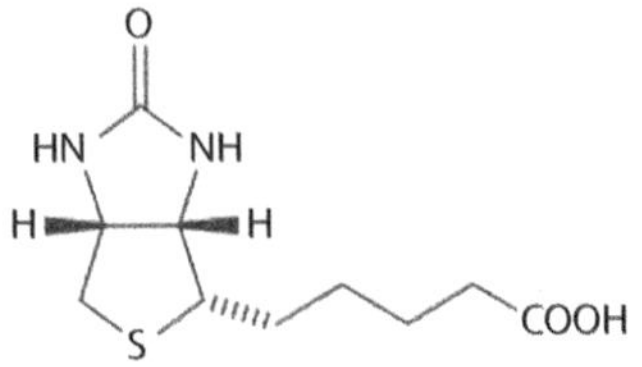

Figure 2.9 The chemical structure of vitamin B7.

5. Converts propionate to succinate.
6. Helps to keep right hair cell, pores and skin.

There is no unique RDA set for biotin since it is miles synthesized through the intestinal flora. Deficiency of biotin causing nausea, depression, hair loss is consequently uncommon and might arise if diet includes excessive antibiotic intake (effecting the intestine microbiome) and ingestion of raw egg (that is composed avidin which reacts with imidazole of biotin) [45, 46].

2.2.9 Vitamin B9/Folic Acid

A pteridine ring and a para-aminobenzoic acid residue (PABA), consisting variable glutamyl units joined through amide linkages, together form folic acid. Leafy veggies, legumes, asparagus, beets, broccoli, citrus fruits, and rice are a few significant sources of folic acid. Folic acid calls for to be activated to tetrahydrofolate (THF), with the help of nutrition C, to perform positive organic functions. First, folate is decreased and methylated and then carried in the plasma once bound to unique proteins [47, 48].

The activation of folic acid (Figure 2.10) to THF is proven below.

Functions of THF

1. A provider of 1 carbon fragment by accepting carbon units from degradation sites through N5, N10, and donating to synthesis reactions, such as in the conversion of serine to glycine, synthesis of thymidylate, methionine, purine, homocysteine, catabolism of histidine.
2. Prevents changes in the DNA that can cause cancer.
3. Helps to save you anemia.
4. Associated with boom and development.
5. Aids nutrition B12 at some stage in methyl institution transfer.

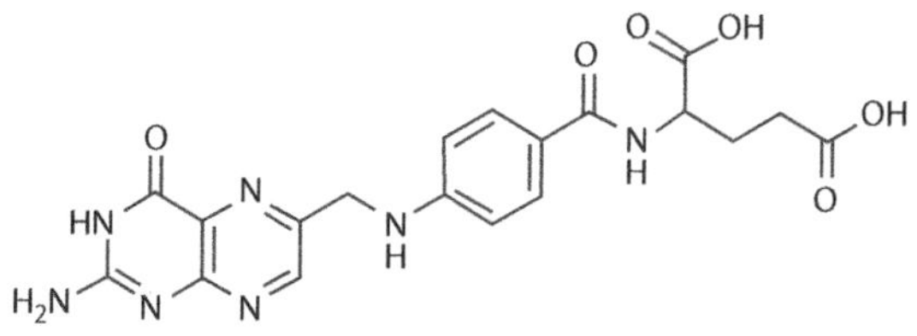

Folic acid

Figure 2.10 The chemical structure of vitamin B9.

The RDA of folic acid is around 200 mg, which is possibly to boom at some stage in being pregnant and lactation. Folic acid is an important requirement for the frame and deficiency can cause start defects in pregnant women, neural. tube defects, sensory loss, megaloblastic anemia (when you consider that DNA synthesis is impaired) and excretion of formiminoglutamic acid (FIGLU) through urine. Folic acid may be taken as a nutritional complement; however, for human beings with kidney diseases; hemolytic anemia is counseled to have unique dosage changes below clinical supervision because of certain facet consequences of the supplement consisting of shortness of breath, pores and skin irritability, dizziness, etc. Hence, its miles continually recommended making sure folic acid is obtained from the nutrients infood via a balanced diet [49, 50].

2.2.10 Vitamin B12

Vitamin B12, known as cobalamin is commonly of animal origin, found in eggs, milks, fishes, meat, sardines, with small quantities made to be had from the intestine microbiome. Having a coring ring, Cobalamin is a complicated, consisting a cobalt atom in a co-ordinate bond with nitrogen of pyrol groups, dimethylbenzimidiazolenulcetotide. Commercially, cyanocobalamin acts as diet B12 supplement. The energetic types of vitamin B12 are methycobalamin and deoxyadenosylcobalamin. Given that cobalamin is a complicated compound, for the absorption of diet B12, it first calls for to be observed with the aid of using salivary proteins known as haptocorin to the stomach, in which it is far damaged down while certain to intrinsic elements, which can be secreted with the aid of using the patrialc cells of the stomach. From the stomach, v12-IF complicated (damaged shape of vitamin B12) is then transported thru hepatic portal vein with the aid of using the hepatocytes and transported in plasma with the aid of using transcobalamin I (haptocorrin) and transcobalamin II, earlier than being saved in liver, bone marrow, and tissues in big quantities. Hence, vitamin B12 (Figure 2.11) deficiency is commonly now no longer evident [51, 52].

Function:

1. Deoxyadenosylcobalamin (a coenzyme, an activated vitamin B12 shape), coverts methylmalonic acid to succinic acid.
2. Maintains the metabolism of fatty acids and aliphatic amino acids.

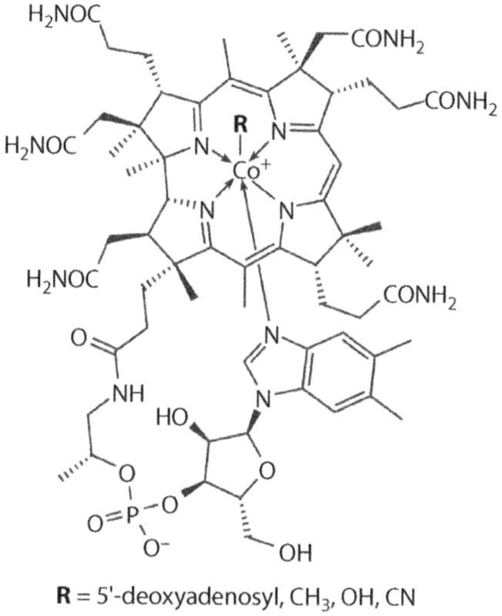

Structure and Functions of Vitamins 49

R = 5'-deoxyadenosyl, CH_3, OH, CN

Figure 2.11 The chemical structure of vitamin B12.

3. Methylcobalamin converts homocysteine to methionine appearing as a transferase, helping in metabolic procedure of folic acid and vitamin B12 itself.
4. Helps un neuronal metabolism, mind function.
5. Helps within the manufacturing of crimson blood cells.

The RDA for a grownup is four hundred micrograms, with better requirement in the course of being pregnant and lactation. High consumption of vitamin B12 is not always acknowledged to be toxic; however, a deficiency can end result irreversible neurological disorders, megaloblastic anemia, or even folate deficiency. Furthermore, conditions such as pernicious anemia and altrophic gastritis, can promote vitamin B12 malabsorption, resulting in a deficit. In addition, a lack of vitamin B12 might lead to an accumulation of methyl malonyl CoA in the blood and urine. As a result, vegetarians and vegans are frequently advised to ensure that vitamin B12 is included in their diet to avoid the repercussions of such deficiency conditions [53, 54].

2.2.11 Vitamin C

Vitamin C, or ascorbic acid, is a water-soluble diet (Figure 2.12). This approach that dissolves in water and is added to the body's tissues, however,

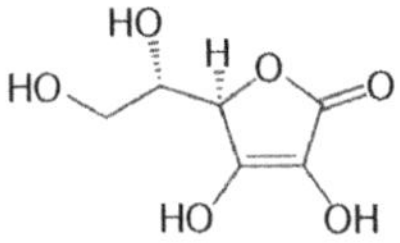

Figure 2.12 Ascorbic acid.

is not always properly stored, so it ought to be taken each day via meals or supplements is rich in citrus culmination inclusive of oranges, strawberries, potatoes, lemons, grapes, tomatoes, broccoli, cauliflower, and spinach. Humans are not able to synthesize diet C and are consequently a crucial nutritional requirement. Sensitive to oxygen, metallic ions, alkali, heat, diet C is more often than not a lowering agent and an antioxidant [55].

Ascorbic acid is a by-product of hexose D-glucose. However, in addition oxidation can cause the inactive form, 2, 3- Diketo-L-gulonic acid [56].

Function:

1. Hydroxides proline and lysin at some point of collagen biosynthesis.
2. Involved within the hydroxylation technique of steroid hormones.
3. Plays position in hydroxylation reactions at some point of adrenaline synthesis.
4. During carnitine synthesis, converts gamma-butyrobetaine to carnitine.
5. Helps at some point of bile acid (cholic acid) formation.
6. Enhances enzymatic pastime at some point of tyrosine degradation.
7. Metabolizes folic acid to THF.
8. Facilitates the absorption of iron.
9. Prevents coronary coronary heart ailment with the aid of using impairing LDL oxidation.
10. Its antioxidant belongings scavenge unfastened radicals, stopping most cancers with the aid of using inhibiting nitrosamine formation.

Readily absorbed with the aid of using the frame from the stomach, the RDA of diet C is 60 mg for adults and 70 mg and 95 mg for pregnant and lactating girls respectively. For humans who have greater fried substances, a junk meal, etc., of their diet, the RDA is generally better to fight the unfastened radicals produced [57]. See Table 2.1 for a summary of vitamins.

Table 2.1 Summary of vitamins [59–74].

Vitamin	Chemical name	Food source	Solubility	Consequence of deficiency	Recommended dietary allowance	Overdose disease
Vitamin A	Retinal, retinol and four carotenoids including beta carotene	Cod liver oil	Fat-soluble	Night blindness, nyctalopia, xerophthalmia, keratomalacia	900 μg	Hyper-vitaminosis A
Vitamin D	Cholecalciferol	Cod Liver Oil	Fat-soluble	Rickets (in children) and osteomalacia (in adult)	5.0–10 μg	Hypervitaminosis D
Vitamin E	Tocopherol forms—alpha, beta, gamma, delta, tocotrienols	Wheat germ oil, unrefined vegetable oil	Fat-soluble	Occurrence of lipid peroxidation, hemolytic anemia in new born	15 mg	Increased congestive heart failure seen in one large randomized study

(Continued)

Table 2.1 Summary of vitamins [59–74]. (Continued)

Vitamin	Chemical name	Food source	Solubility	Consequence of deficiency	Recommended dietary allowance	Overdose disease
Vitamin K	Phylloquinone, menaquinones	Leafy green vegetables	Fat-soluble	Increased clotting time, hemorrhage in children	120 µg	Increased Coagulation in warfarin
Vitamin B_1	Thiamine	Rice bran	Water-soluble	Causes Beriberi, Wernicke Korsakoff syndrome	1.2 mg	Drowsiness or muscle relation when overdose
Vitamin B_2	Riboflavin	Meat, eggs	Water-soluble	Dermatitis photophobia, angular stomatitis.	1.3 mg	Liver damage with doses >2g/day
Vitamin B_3	Niacin, niacin amide	Meat, eggs, grains	Water-soluble	Pellagra	16.0 mg	Diarrhea, possibility of nausea and heartburn

(Continued)

Table 2.1 Summary of vitamins [59–74]. (Continued)

Vitamin	Chemical name	Food source	Solubility	Consequence of deficiency	Recommended dietary allowance	Overdose disease
Vitamin B_5	Panthoehic acid	Meat, whole grains, in many foods	Water-soluble	Burning feet syndrome	5.0 mg	Diarrhea; possibly nausea and heartburn
Vitamin B_6	Pyridoxine, pyridoxamine, pyridoxal	Meat, dairy products	Water-soluble	Epileptiform convulsions, dermatitis, hypochromic anemia	13– 1.7 mg	Impairment of proprioception, nerve damage (doses > 100 mg/day)
Vitamin B_7	Biotin	Meat, dairy products, eggs	Water-soluble	Biotin inhibition	30.0 μg	Not known
Vitamin B_9	Folic acid, folinic acid	Leafy vegetables	Water-soluble	Megaloblastic anemia	400 μg	May mask symptoms of vitamin B12 deficiency; other effects

(Continued)

Table 2.1 Summary of vitamins [59–74]. (*Continued*)

Vitamin	Chemical name	Food source	Solubility	Consequence of deficiency	Recommended dietary allowance	Overdose disease
Vitamin B_{12}	Cyanocobalamin, cobalamin, hydroxocobalamin, methylcobalamin	Liver, eggs, animal product	Water-soluble	Pernicious anemia, dementia	2.4 µg	Acne like rash (not conclusively established)
Vitamin C	Ascorbic acid	Citrus, most fresh fruits and vegetables	Water-soluble	Scurvy	90.0 mg	Vitamin C mega dosage

Deficiency of diet c ends in scurvy, gum diseases, ache in joints, extended capillary fragility main to clean bruising of skin, osteoporosis, anemia, not on time wound healing, susceptible immunity and cell regeneration capability. Although diet C is understood to be an antioxidant that enhances immunity and regarded to assist with not unusual place cold, excessive consumption of diet C cannot be absorbed from the gut causing diarrhea and oxalate stones in kidneys [58, 64–66].

2.3 Conclusion

Vitamins and their possible chemical compounds have played a significant role in enhancing health and illness outcomes. Thus, functional food may represent a powerful tool for combating a very important known name need in very small quantities and group of complex organic compounds present in natural food stuffs, which play a key role in normal metabolism and whose lack in the diet causes deficiency in a number of critical diseases. Vitamins are distinguished from trace elements, which are likewise present in minute amounts in the diet for health, growth, reproduction, and other critical metabolic processes. Vitamins are not produced in the body and must be obtained from natural sources; however, some vitamins, such as A and K (fat-soluble vitamins), are stored in the body. Water-soluble vitamins B complex and C (water-soluble vitamin) do not store in the body and are easily excreted. Deficiency signs and symptoms will appear if a single vitamin is missing from the diet of a species that requires it. Vitamin deficiency and excesses can have a negative impact on the body and cause a variety of symptoms.

References

1. Velić, D., Klarić, D.A., Velić, N., Klarić, I., Tominac, V.P., Mornar, A., Chemical constituents of fruit wines as descriptors of their nutritional, sensorial and health-related properties, in: *Descriptive Food Science*, pp. 59–91.2, 2018.
2. Drewke, C. and Leistner, E., Biosynthesis of vitamin B6 and structurally related derivatives. *Vitam. Horm.*, 61, 121–155, 2001.
3. Bai, C., Twyman, R.M., Farré, G., Sanahuja, G., Christou, P., Capell, T., Zhu, C., A golden era—Pro-vitamin A enhancement in diverse crops. *In Vitro Cell. Dev. Biol.-Plant*, 47, 2, 205–221, 2011.

4. Farré, G., Sanahuja, G., Naqvi, S., Bai, C., Capell, T., Zhu, C., Christou, P., Travel advice on the road to carotenoids in plants. *Plant Sci., 179*, 1-2, 28–48, 2010.
5. Farré Martinez, G., Sanahuja Solsona, G., Naqvi, S., Bai, C., Capell Capell, T., Zhu, C., Christou, P., Travel advice on the road to carotenoids in plants. *Plant Sci., 179*, 28–48, 2010.
6. Zhu, C., Bai, C., Sanahuja, G., Yuan, D., Farré, G., Naqvi, S., Shi, L., Capell, T., Christou, P., The regulation of carotenoid pigmentation in flowers. *Arch. Biochem. Biophys., 504*, 1, 132–141, 2010.
7. Harrison, E.H., Mechanisms of digestion and absorption of dietary vitamin A. *Annu. Rev. Nutr., 25*, 87–103, 2005.
8. Holick, M.F., Vitamin D deficiency. *N. Engl. J. Med., 357*, 3, 266–281, 2007.
9. Lips, P., Hosking, D., Lippuner, K., Norquist, J.M., Wehren, L., Maalouf, G., Ragi-Eis, S., Chandler, J., The prevalence of vitamin D inadequacy amongst women with osteoporosis: An international epidemiological investigation. *J. Intern. Med., 260*, 3, 245–254, 2006.
10. Institute of Medicine, Food and nutrition board. *Dietary reference intakes: Calcium, phosphorus, magnesium, vitamin D and fluoride*, Phys. Rev. J., United State, 1999.
11. Moan, J., Porojnicu, A.C., Dahlback, A., Setlow, R.B., Addressing the health benefits and risks, involving vitamin D or skin cancer, of increased sun exposure. *Proc. Natl. Acad. Sci., 105*, 2, 668–673, 2008.
12. Boonen, S., Lips, P., Bouillon, R., Bischoff-Ferrari, H.A., Vanderschueren, D., Haentjens, P., Need for additional calcium to reduce the risk of hip fracture with vitamin D supplementation: Evidence from a comparative metaanalysis of randomized controlled trials. *J. Clin. Endocrinol. Metab., 92*, 4, 1415–1423, 2007.
13. Cauley, J.A., LaCroix, A.Z., Wu, L., Horwitz, M., Danielson, M.E., Bauer, D.C., Lee, J.S., Jackson, R.D., Robbins, J.A., Wu, C., Stanczyk, F.Z., Serum 25-hydroxyvitamin D concentrations and risk for hip fractures. *Ann. Intern. Med., 149*, 4, 242–250, 2008.
14. Sanders, K.M., Stuart, A.L., Williamson, E.J., Simpson, J.A., Kotowicz, M.A., Young, D., Nicholson, G.C., Annual high-dose oral vitamin D and falls and fractures in older women: A randomized controlled trial. *JAMA, 303*, 18, 1815–1822, 2010.
15. Norman, P.E. and Powell, J.T., Vitamin D and cardiovascular disease. *Circ. Res., 114*, 2, 379–393, 2014.
16. Holick, M.F., The vitamin D deficiency pandemic and consequences for nonskeletal health: Mechanisms of action. *Mol. Aspects Med., 29*, 6, 361–368, 2008.
17. Pilz, S., März, W., Wellnitz, B., Seelhorst, U., Fahrleitner-Pammer, A., Dimai, H.P., Boehm, B.O., Dobnig, H., Association of vitamin D deficiency with heart failure and sudden cardiac death in a large cross-sectional study of

patients referred for coronary angiography. *J. Clin. Endocrinol. Metab., 93,* 10, 3927–3935, 2008.
18. Wang, T.J., Pencina, M.J., Booth, S.L., Jacques, P.F., Ingelsson, E., Lanier, K., Benjamin, E.J., D'Agostino, R.B., Wolf, M., Vasan, R.S., Vitamin D deficiency and risk of cardiovascular disease. *Circulation, 117,* 4, 503–511, 2008.
19. Wang, T.J., Pencina, M.J., Booth, S.L., Jacques, P.F., Ingelsson, E., Lanier, K., Benjamin, E.J., D'Agostino, R.B., Wolf, M., Vasan, R.S., Vitamin D deficiency and risk of cardiovascular disease. *Circulation, 117,* 4, 503–511, 2008.
20. Ascherio, A. and Munger, K.L., Epidemiology of multiple sclerosis: From risk factors to prevention—An update. *Semin. Neurol.,* 36, 02, 103–114, 2016, April, Thieme Medical Publishers.
21. Cannell, J.J., Vieth, R., Umhau, J.C., Holick, M.F., Grant, W.B., Madronich, S., Garland, C.F., Giovannucci, E., Epidemic influenza and vitamin D. *Epidemiol. Infect., 134,* 6, 1129–1140, 2006.
22. Hope-Simpson, R.E., The role of season in the epidemiology of influenza. *Epidemiol. Infect., 86,* 1, 35–47, 1981.
23. Astley, S.B., ANTIOXIDANTS| role of antioxidant nutrients, in: *Defense Systems, Encyclopedia of Food Sciences and Nutrition,* pp. 282–289, 2003.
24. Glynn, R.J., Ridker, P.M., Goldhaber, S.Z., Zee, R.Y., Buring, J.E., Effects of random allocation to vitamin E supplementation on the occurrence of venous thromboembolism: Report from the Women's Health Study. *Circulation, 116,* 13, 1497–1503, 2007.
25. Nesaretnam, K., Yew, W.W., Wahid, M.B., Tocotrienols and cancer: Beyond antioxidant activity. *Eur. J. Lipid Sci. Technol., 109,* 4, 445–452, 2007.
26. Sesso, H.D., Buring, J.E., Christen, W.G., Kurth, T., Belanger, C., MacFadyen, J., Bubes, V., Manson, J.E., Glynn, R.J., Gaziano, J.M., Vitamins E and C in the prevention of cardiovascular disease in men: The Physicians' Health Study II randomized controlled trial. *JAMA,* 300, 18, 2123–2133, 2008.
27. Christen, S., Woodall, A.A., Shigenaga, M.K., Southwell-Keely, P.T., Duncan, M.W., Ames, B.N., γ-Tocopherol traps mutagenic electrophiles such as NOx and complements α-tocopherol: Physiological implications. *Proc. Natl. Acad. Sci., 94,* 7, 3217–3222, 1997.
28. Kryscio, R.J., Abner, E.L., Schmitt, F.A., Goodman, P.J., Mendiondo, M., Caban-Holt, A., Dennis, B.C., Mathews, M., Klein, E.A., Crowley, J.J., A randomized controlled Alzheimer's disease prevention trial's evolution into an exposure trial: The PREADViSE Trial. *J. Nutr. Health Aging, 17,* 1, 72–75, 2013.
29. Jo Harris, P., Caceres, C.A., Bell, B., Ganser, A., Greher, J., Völkers, B., Staszewski, S., Hoelzer, D., Richman, D.D., Fischl, M.A., Nusinoff-Lehrman, S., Azidothymidine in the treatment of AIDS. *N. Engl. J. Med., 318,* 4, 250–251, 1988.
30. Feskanich, D., Weber, P., Willett, W.C., Rockett, H., Booth, S.L., Colditz, G.A., Vitamin K intake and hip fractures in women: A prospective study. *Am. J. Clin. Nutr., 69,* 1, 74–79, 1999.

31. Doseděl, M., Jirkovský, E., Macáková, K., Krčmová, L.K., Javorská, L., Pourová, J., Mercolini, L., Remião, F., Nováková, L., Mladěnka, P., OEMONOM, Vitamin C—Sources, physiological role, kinetics, deficiency, use, toxicity, and determination. *Nutrients*, *13*, 2, 615, 2021.
32. Nivina, A., Escudero, J.A., Vit, C., Mazel, D., Loot, C., Efficiency of integron cassette insertion in correct orientation is ensured by the interplay of the three unpaired features of attC recombination sites. *Nucleic Acids Res.*, 44, 16, 7792–7803, 2016.
33. Yakovlev, G., Vít, Č., Polyanskikh, I., Gordina, A., Pudov, I., Gumenyuk, A., Smirnova, O., The effect of complex modification on the impedance of cement matrices. *Materials*, 14, 3, 557, 2021.
34. Mameesh, M.S. and Johnson, B.C., Production of dietary vit. K deficiency in the rat. *Proc. Soc. Exp. Biol. Med.*, 101, 3, 467–468, 1959.
35. Booth, S.L., Tucker, K.L., Chen, H., Hannan, M.T., Gagnon, D.R., Cupples, L.A., Wilson, P.W., Ordovas, J., Schaefer, E.J., Dawson-Hughes, B., Kiel, D.P., Dietary vitamin K intakes are associated with hip fracture but not with bone mineral density in elderly men and women. *Am. J. Clin. Nutr.*, 71, 5, 1201–1208, 2000.
36. Booth, S.L., Roles for vitamin K beyond coagulation. *Annu. Rev. Nutr.*, 29, 89–110, 2009.
37. Vermeer, C., Jie, K.S., Knapen, M.H.J., Role of vitamin K in bone metabolism. *Annu. Rev. Nutr.*, 15, 1, 1–21, 1995.
38. Harshman, S.G. and Shea, M., The role of vitamin K in chronic aging diseases: Inflammation, cardiovascular disease, and osteoarthritis. *Curr. Nutr. Rep.*, 5, 2, 90–98, 2016.
39. Hartley, L., Clar, C., Ghannam, O., Flowers, N., Stranges, S., Rees, K., Vitamin K for the primary prevention of cardiovascular disease. *Cochrane Database Syst. Rev.*, 9, 1–28, 2015.
40. Chu, A.S., Mataga, M.A., Krueger, L., Barr, P.A., Nutrient deficiency-related dermatoses after bariatric surgery. *Adv. Skin Wound Care*, 32, 10, 443–455, 2019.
41. Vandamme, E.J. (Ed.), *Biotechnology of vitamins, pigments and growth factors*, Springer Science & Business Media, Berlin, Germany, 1989.
42. Fischer, M. and Bacher, A., Biosynthesis of vitamin B2: Structure and mechanism of riboflavin synthase. *Arch. Biochem. Biophys.*, 474, 2, 252–265, 2008.
43. Bacher, A., Eberhardt, S., Fischer, M., Kis, K., Richter, G., Biosynthesis of vitamin b2 (riboflavin). *Annu. Rev. Nutr.*, 20, 1, 153–167, 2000.
44. Jacobson, M.K. and Jacobson, E.L., Vitamin B3 in health and disease: Toward the second century of discovery, in: *ADP-Ribosylation and NAD+ Utilizing Enzymes*, pp. 3–8, 2018.
45. Amanullah, S. and Seeber, C., Niacin deficiency resulting in neuropsychiatric symptoms: A case study and review of literature. *Clin. Neuropsychiatry*, 7, 1, 10–4, 2010.

46. Gao, L., Zhou, F., Wang, K.X., Zhou, Y.Z., Du, G.H., Qin, X.M., Baicalein protects PC12 cells from Aβ25–35-induced cytotoxicity via inhibition of apoptosis and metabolic disorders. *Life Sci.*, *248*, 117471, 2020.
47. Zeman, M., Vecka, M., Perlík, F., Hromádka, R., Staňková, B., Tvrzická, E., Žák, A., Niacin in the treatment of hyperlipidemias in light of new clinical trials: Has niacin lost its place? *Med. Sci. Monit.: Int. Med. J. Exp. Clin. Res.*, *21*, 2156, 2015.
48. Ismail, N., Kureishy, N., Church, S.J., Scholefield, M., Unwin, R.D., Xu, J., Patassini, S., Cooper, G.J., Vitamin B5 (d-pantothenic acid) localizes in myelinated structures of the rat brain: Potential role for cerebral vitamin B5 stores in local myelin homeostasis. *Biochem. Biophys. Res. Commun.*, *522*, 1, 220–225, 2020.
49. Demirci, B., Demir, O., Dost, T., Birincioglu, M., Protective effect of vitamin B5 (dexpanthenol) on cardiovascular damage induced by streptozocin in rats. *Bratisl. Lek. Listy*, *115*, 4, 190–196, 2014.
50. Malouf, R. and Evans, J.G., Vitamin B6 for cognition. *Cochrane Database Syst. Rev.*, 4, 1–24, 2003.
51. B., Kris-Etherton, P., Harris, W.S., Howard, B., Karanja, N., Diet and lifestyle recommendations revision 2006: A scientific statement from the American Heart Association Nutrition Committee. *Circulation*, *114*, 1, 82–96, 2006.
52. Heinivaara, O. and Palva, I.P., Malabsorption of vitamin B7 during treatment with para-aminosalicylic acid. A preliminary report. *Acta Med. Scand.*, 175, 469–471, 1964.
53. Bhardwaj, R. and Choudhary, S., Weighted goal programming for vitamin, structure and control of diet. *Mater. Today: Proc.*, 29, 651–660, 2020.
54. Guilland, J.C. and Aimone-Gastin, I., Vitamin B9. *Rev. Prat.*, 63, 8, 1079–1081, 2013.
55. Bourre, J.M., The role of nutritional factors on the structure and function of the brain: An update on dietary requirements. *Rev. Neurol.*, 160, 8-9, 767–792, 2004.
56. Knyazev, A.V., Smirnova, N.N., Plesovskikh, A.S., Shushunov, A.N., Knyazeva, S.S., Low-temperature heat capacity and thermodynamic functions of vitamin B12. *Thermochim. Acta*, 582, 35–39, 2014.
57. Murakami, Y., Hisaeda, Y., Fan, S.D., Matsuda, Y., Redox behavior of simple vitamin B12 model complexes and electrochemical catalysis of carbon-skeleton rearrangements. *Bull. Chem. Soc. Jpn.*, 62, 7, 2219–2228, 1989.
58. Johnson, L.J., Meacham, S.L., Kruskall, L.J., The antioxidants-vitamin C, vitamin E, selenium, and carotenoids. *J. Agromedicine*, 9, 1, 65–82, 2003.
59. Helliwell, K.E., The roles of B vitamins in phytoplankton nutrition: New perspectives and prospects. *New Phytol.*, 216, 1, 62–68, 2017.
60. Revuelta, J.L., Buey, R.M., Ledesma-Amaro, R., Vandamme, E.J., Microbial biotechnology for the synthesis of (pro) vitamins, biopigments and antioxidants: Challenges and opportunities. *Microb. Biotechnol.*, 9, 5, 564–567, 2016.

61. Volpe, S.L. and Nguyen, H., Vitamins, minerals, and sport performance, in: *The Encyclopaedia of Sports Medicine: An IOC Medical Commission Publication*, vol. 19, pp. 215–228, 2013.
62. Driskell, J.A., Summary—Vitamins and trace elements in sports nutrition, in: *Sports Nutrition*, pp. 323–331, CRC Press, London, 2005.
63. Kutsky, R.J., *Handbook of vitamins, minerals, and hormones*, Van Nostrand Reinhold Co., London, 1981.
64. Ahire, E.D., Sonawane, V.N., Surana, K.R., Talele, G.S., Drug discovery, drug-likeness screening, and bioavailability: Development of drug-likeness rule for natural products, in: *Applied Pharmaceutical Practice and Nutraceuticals*, pp. 191–208, Apple Academic Press, London, 2021.
65. Surana, K.R., Ahire, E.D., Sonawane, V.N., Talele, S.G., Talele, G.S., Molecular modeling: Novel techniques in food and nutrition development, in: *Natural Food Products and Waste Recovery*, pp. 17–31, Apple Academic Press, London, 2021.
66. Surana, K.R., Ahire, E.D., Sonawane, V.N., Talele, S.G., Biomolecular and molecular docking: A modern tool in drug discovery and virtual screening of natural products, in: *Applied Pharmaceutical Practice and Nutraceuticals*, pp. 209–223, Apple Academic Press, London, 2021.
67. Keservani, R.K., Kesharwani, R.K., Vyas, N., Jain, S., Raghuvanshi, R., Sharma, A.K., Nutraceutical and functional food as future food: A review. *Der Pharm. Lett.*, 2, 1, 106–116, 2010a.
68. Keservani, R.K., Kesharwani, R.K., Sharma, A.K., Vyas, N., Chadoker, A., Nutritional supplements: An overview. *Int. J. Curr. Pharm. Rev. Res.*, 1, 1, 59–75, 2010b.
69. Keservani, R.K. and Sharma, A.K., Flavonoids: Emerging trends and potential health benefits. *J. Chin. Pharm. Sci.*, 23, 12, 815, 2014.
70. Keservani, R.K., Sharma, A.K., Kesharwani, R.K., Nutraceutical and functional foods for cardiovascular health, in: *Food Process Engineering*, pp. 291–312, Apple Academic Press, CRC Press, 2016a, pp. 257–278.
71. Keservani, R.K., Sharma, A.K., Kesharwani, R.K., Medicinal effect of nutraceutical fruits for the cognition and brain health. *Scientifica*, Article ID 3109254, 1–10, 2016b.
72. Keservani, R.K., Sharma, A.K., Kesharwani, R.K., An overview and therapeutic applications of nutraceutical and functional foods, in: *Recent Advances in Drug Delivery Technology*, pp. 160–201, 2017.
73. Keservani, R.K., Sharma, A.K., Kesharwani, R.K. (Eds.), *Nutraceuticals and dietary supplements: Applications in health improvement and disease management*, CRC Press, 2020.
74. Singh, P., Kesharwani, R.K., Keservani, R.K., Antioxidants and vitamins: Roles in cellular function and metabolism, in: *Sustained Energy for Enhanced Human Functions and Activity*, pp. 385–407, Academic Press, 2017.

3
Vitamin Intervention in Cardiac Health

Shubham J. Khairnar[1], Eknath D. Ahire[1*], Madhuri D. Deshmukh[1], Raj K. Keservani[2], Sanjay J. Kshirsagar[1], Amit Kumar Rajora[3] and Manju Amit Kumar Rajora[4]

[1]METs, Institute of Pharmacy, Bhujbal Knowledge City, SPPU, Adgaon, Nashik, Maharashtra, India
[2]CSM Group of Institutions, Prayagraj, Uttar Pradesh, India
[3]NanoBiotechnology Lab, School of Biotechnology, Jawaharlal Nehru University, New Mehrauli Road, New Delhi, India
[4]College of Nursing, All India Institute of Medical Sciences, New Delhi, India

Abstract

Both hydrosoluble and liposoluble vitamins are thought to be crucial in sustaining cardiovascular function in both health and sickness because of their regulatory roles in numerous metabolic and biosynthetic pathways for energy status and cellular integrity. Vitamin deficiencies, such as those in vitamin A, B6, folic acid, C, D, and E, have been linked to cardiovascular abnormalities, whereas vitamin supplements have been proven to lower the risk of heart failure, hypertension, atherosclerosis, myocardial ischemia, and arrhythmias. However, there is disagreement in the evidence from numerous experimental and clinical investigations about the pathophysiology of cardiovascular disease caused by vitamin deficiency, as well as the therapeutic effects of certain vitamins. In this article, we have made an effort to analyze the pertinent research on the role of various vitamins in cardiovascular disease, taking into account both their deficiencies and their supplementation, as well as looking at a few related concerns. The use of several antioxidant vitamins for the treatment of cardiovascular problems has shown some promise in both epidemiological and observational research, but the findings are not definitive.

Keywords: Cardiovascular diseases, vitamin deficiency, vitamin supplements, cardiac dysfunction

---

*Corresponding author: eknathahire05@gmail.com; eknatha_iop@bkc.met.edu

Eknath D. Ahire, Raj K. Keservani, Khemchand R. Surana, Sippy Singh and Rajesh K. Kesharwani (eds.) *Vitamins as Nutraceuticals: Recent Advances and Applications,* (61–86) © 2023 Scrivener Publishing LLC

3.1 Introduction

A balanced diet, with respect to proteins, carbohydrates, and lipids is crucial for maintaining cardiovascular health as it is now well known that malnutrition over an extended period is one of the major factors linked to the development of heart disease [1–3]. It is also recognized that different proteins, carbohydrates, and lipids are digested by the body through various but connected metabolic pathways in order to preserve the structural and functional integrity of every component of the circulatory system.

Vitamin changes are thought to cause circulatory irregularities since both liposoluble and hydrosoluble vitamins have been shown to be crucial in the control of several metabolic pathways for cellular biosynthesis and energy production. It is noted that several liposoluble vitamins, including A, D, and E, as well as hydrosoluble vitamins, including B6 (pyridoxine), B9 (folic acid), and C, have been shown to play a significant role in modifying cardiovascular function [4–6]. Although the majority of vitamins are present in plasma concentrations that are within normal ranges in healthy animals and human beings, patients with various forms of heart disease have been found to lack both liposoluble and hydrosoluble vitamins [7–10]. In order to promote, a variety of vitamins are frequently advised. Different vitamins are effective in treating cardiovascular disease, according to a number of experimental and observational research [11–15]. The effects of several vitamins on alterations in the levels of oxidative stress, inflammation, homocysteine, lipoproteins, and nitric oxide have been used to establish links between these conditions [16–18]. Although neither liposoluble nor hydrosoluble vitamins directly alter cardiovascular function, they are thought to have an impact on certain cardiovascular illnesses through modifying the associated risk factors. However, there is conflicting evidence on their beneficial effects, and in particular, the outcomes of several clinical trials for the use of various vitamins in the treatment of heart disease have been disappointing [19–24].

The American Heart Association has advised eating of vitamin-rich fresh fruits and vegetables rather than vitamin pills due to the uncertainty around the shown beneficial cardiovascular effects of various vitamins. It is noted that the molecular targets of individual vitamins may differ for their efficiency in health and disease, and that the pathophysiology of various forms of cardiovascular diseases is a complex issue. In order to determine whether there is a connection between a certain vitamin and a particular type of heart disease under circumstances of vitamin deficiency or vitamin supplementation, this article will review the body of available research.

Additionally, by detailing the pathophysiology of heart disease as a result of vitamin insufficiency, the function of several vitamins will be studied.

Evidence will also be offered to highlight the potential role that different vitamin may have in the prevention of cardiovascular problems. Due to the fact that oxidative stress is a significant factor in the emergence of cardiovascular disease and that several vitamins are known to have antioxidant potential [25–29]. The positive benefits of several vitamins will be assessed in relation to some oxidative stress markers.

3.2 Vitamin Deficiency and Cardiovascular Disease

Vitamin shortage is typically rarely seen in healthy persons due to the availability of the majority of vitamins in food, including fruits, vegetables, dairy products, and meat preparations. The development of many cardiovascular abnormalities, such as hypertension, atherosclerosis, diabetes, ischemic heart disease, heart failure, and stroke, however, has been linked to low levels of several vitamins in both men and women. Vitamin shortage is typically rarely seen in healthy persons because the majority of vitamins are readily available in foods, such as fruits, vegetables, dairy products, and meat preparations. While developing several sorts of cardiovascular irregularities, such as hypertension, atherosclerosis, diabetes, ischemic heart disease, heart failure, and stroke, however, men and women have been found to have low levels of some vitamins.

Deficiency in Hydrosoluble Vitamins Patients with heart failure have been found to have deficiencies in a variety of vitamins, including vitamins B1, B2, and B6 [30]. Additionally, cardiovascular disease risk factors, such as diabetes, dyslipidemia, obesity, and vascular inflammation, have been linked to vitamin B1 deficiency [31]. Anemia and higher homocysteine levels are linked to vitamin B2 deficiency in cardiovascular disease [32, 33].

Additionally, elevated homocysteine levels have been linked to vitamin B6 and B12 insufficiency in patients with peripheral and coronary artery disorders [34, 35]. Diabetes, atherosclerosis, myocardial infarction, and stroke patients all had low levels of vitamin B12 and endothelial dysfunction [36–38]. Along with congenital heart disease, vascular diseases have been linked to folic acid deficiency [39–41]. A lack of vitamin B6 has also been linked to coronary artery disease, atherosclerosis, and hypertension [42–44]. Atherosclerosis, coronary artery disease, hypertension, and increased sympathetic activity were all observed in rats fed a diet lacking in vitamin B6 [45–48]. Cardiomyocytes from B6-deficient rats displayed a substantial amplification of the KCl-induced increase in [Ca2C]i without any alterations in the basal level of [Ca2C]i [49].

On the other hand, vitamin B6 deficiency inhibited the ATP-induced increase in [Ca2C]i in cardiomyocytes, and this alteration was connected to a reduction in sarcolemmal (SL) ATP binding. These changes in the cardiomyocytes of B6-deficient animals can be used as evidence in favor of the theory that vitamin B6 deficiency may increase the chance of developing certain cardiovascular diseases. Although low plasma levels of vitamin C, which are a result of its lower intake, have been linked to a higher risk of cardiovascular disease [50, 51], the connection between these two variables is still unclear.

Vitamin C deficiency was observed to increase the incidence of coronary artery disease in women [52], likely as a result of increased low-density lipoprotein oxidation and the development of atherosclerosis [53, 54]. On the other hand, elderly adults who were vitamin C deficient had a higher probability of dying from a stroke than from coronary artery disease [55]. However, some researchers found a substantial link between vitamin C deficiency and risk of acute myocardial infarction in a population study of males [56]. It should be noted that adult heart failure was shown to be accompanied by high sensitivity of C-reactive proteins and vitamin C insufficiency [57]. Additionally, it has been observed that the plasma level of vitamin C can predict the likelihood of developing heart failure due to its antioxidant function [58, 59].

Deficiency in Liposoluble Vitamins
Since vitamin D deficiency is the most prevalent nutritional issue, significant research has been done to understand how it affects cardiovascular health and the processes by which it does so. Numerous researchers have stressed that a lack of vitamin D is a major factor in the development of cardiovascular illness, such as hypertension, heart failure, and ischemic heart disease [60–63]. It is interesting that peripheral vascular disease, hypertension, and poor systolic and diastolic functions were all linked to congestive heart failure in vitamin D insufficiency [64]. Because of inflammation, autoimmune, endothelial dysfunction, the creation of foam cells, and the proliferation of smooth muscle cells, low levels of vitamin D have been found to favor the development of atherosclerosis and myocardial infarction [65, 66]. Additionally, diabetes, obesity, dyslipidemia, metabolic syndrome, and hypertension have all been linked to vitamin D insufficiency [67, 68]. The development of insulin resistance, increased parathyroid hormone levels, activation of the renin-angiotensin system, aberrant nitric oxide regulation, increased oxidative stress, and inflammatory pathway

were all linked to both diabetes and hypertension caused by vitamin D deficiency [69, 70]. Experimental findings revealing cardiac hypertrophy, arterial hypertension, and enhanced activity of the renin-angiotensin system in vitamin D receptor knockout mice provide evidence that vitamin D deficiency plays a role in cardiovascular disease [71]. Contrary to other dietary deficiencies, vitamin E insufficiency in humans is uncommon due to adequate ingestion of widely accessible food [72, 73]. However, vitamin E insufficiency has been identified in infants, those who have a problem absorbing fat, and those who have certain genetic disorders [74, 75]. On the other hand, many animal species have shown varying degrees of anemia, cardiac cell damage, and cardiomyopathy as a result of vitamin E insufficiency [75–78]. Numerous electrocardiographic abnormalities were observed in the hearts of rabbits fed a diet lacking in vitamin E, and these heart changes were accompanied by lower levels of high-energy phosphate and glycogen reserves. Animals kept on a diet lacking in vitamin E also developed heart failure and noticeable metabolic abnormalities [78]. Additionally, the activity of the sarcoplasmic reticular (SR) Ca2C-pump ATPase, SL NaC-KC ATPase, and SR Ca2C uptake and Ca2C release were

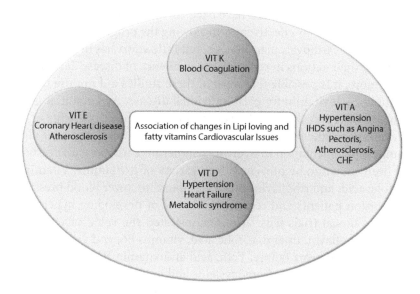

Figure 3.1 Associations between variations in the plasma concentration of several liposoluble vitamins and distinct cardiovascular disease risk factors.

markedly altered in vitamin E-deficient rat heart tissue. Muscular dystrophy coexisted with cardiac problems brought on by vitamin E insufficiency, it should be noted. It is likely that the cardiac problems observed in experimental animals owing to vitamin E shortage are caused by the formation of higher levels of oxidative stress given the antioxidant activity of vitamin E [79]. Figure 3.1 indicates the associations between variations in the plasma concentration of several liposoluble vitamins and distinct cardiovascular disease risk factors.

3.3 Vitamin Supplementation and Cardiovascular Disease

Excellent evaluations on how different vitamins can treat cardiovascular disease are accessible in the literature [80]. The outcomes of adding these nutrients to diets for both animal and human subjects with heart disease, however, are inconclusive. The use of several vitamins in treating various cardiovascular problems is supported by a number of epidemiological, observational, and animal experiments, but well-controlled clinical investigations have not been able to detect their therapeutic benefits in any of the cardiovascular diseases. It should be noted that the majority of vitamin randomized clinical trials have been conducted to ascertain the therapeutic aspect of their effectiveness in slowing the progression or reducing the severity of cardiovascular diseases, but little effort has been devoted to examining their actions in reducing the incidence of disease development. Furthermore, it is possible that most of these studies did not use the right amount of each vitamin for each individual disease. As a result, it is challenging to interpret these findings in terms of the health benefits of various vitamins for the prevention or treatment of any cardiovascular illness. Vitamin supplementation in hydrosols numerous cardiovascular disorders have been shown to be prevented by a variety of B vitamins. Vitamin B6, B12, folic acid, and riboflavin intake was found to lower blood pressure in hypertension patients and reduce the chance of developing hypertension [81, 82]. Clinical trials have also demonstrated the value of vitamins B, including riboflavin, thiamine, folic acid, vitamin B6, and vitamin B12, in the treatment of heart failure. Folic acid and vitamin B12 administration has been shown to reduce homocysteine and oxidative stress levels, as well as the damage to cardiac cells caused by isoproterenol in hyperhomocysteinemic rats. Folic acid also restored tetrahydrobiopterin-induced endothelial dysfunction in rabbit aortic rings. In fact, it has been demonstrated that folic acid supplementation helps individuals with cardiovascular disease with endothelial dysfunction [83]. Niacin was found to lower total cholesterol and triglycerides, suggesting that it may be used to treat hypertriglyceridemia, as well as prevent cardiovascular illnesses [84]. By acting as an anti-inflammatory, the vitamin B complex, which includes vitamins B1, B2, and B6, as well as vitamin B12 and folic acid, has been shown to lessen atherosclerosis and ischemic heart disease. By lowering plasma homocysteine levels, vitamin B12 and folic acid have both been shown to postpone the early start of coronary artery disease. Furthermore, patients with coronary artery disease who took antioxidant vitamins and folic acid saw a decreased incidence of endothelial dysfunction. Folic acid, vitamin B6, and vitamin B12 administration corrected endothelial impairment in patients with hyperhomocysteinemia caused by methionine loading, In fact, it is thought that using these vitamins is the mainstay therapy for treating hyperhomocysteinemia. It should be noted, nonetheless, that a meta-analysis of data from multiple clinical trials using folic acid, vitamin B12, and vitamin B6 did not provide any proof of their preventative effects against the development of atherosclerosis. The active vitamin B6 metabolite pyridoxal 50-phosphate (PLP), which should be noted, has been demonstrated to have outstanding potentials for the treatment of ischemic heart disease [85]. In this regard, it is interesting that PLP was discovered to inhibit oxyradical production and lipid peroxidation brought on by. Additionally, it was discovered that this substance inhibited the ATP-induced rise in [Ca2Cl] in cardiomyocytes as well as SL ATP-binding. PLP not only decreased the cardiac dysfunction brought on by I/R, but it was also seen to decrease infarct size. It has been demonstrated that giving PLP to patients after coronary angioplasty and coronary bypass surgery reduces ischemic injury. However, significant clinical research including high-risk patients undergoing coronary artery bypass graft surgery found no evidence of the therapeutic effects of PLP. Although the precise causes of PLP's ineffectiveness in preventing various cardiovascular events in advanced ischemic heart disease are unknown, pretreatment of animals with PLP has been shown to attenuate arrhythmias, incidence of ventricular tachycardia, and mortality from myocardial infarction (MI). Additionally, pretreatment of rats with PLP reduced I/R-induced cardiac dysfunction as well as modifications in SR Ca2C uptake and Ca2C-release activities [86].

Given these findings, it is clear that PLP may be more effective in preventing ischemic heart disease than in treating it. In patients with ischemic heart disease, vitamin C inhibits the oxidation of low-density lipoproteins while also enhancing endothelial function and lipid profile, according to epidemiologic research. A higher intake of vitamin C has also been proven to lower the risk of ischemic heart disease in people who smoke heavily. In individuals with ischemic heart disease, vitamin C treatment was seen to improve coronary flow and stop the re-induction of coronary constriction. In human individuals, this vitamin also offered defense against I/R-mediated oxidative stress. Vitamin C's advantageous effects on high-density lipoprotein remodeling and attenuating ischemic heart disease in mice were also seen. Numerous researches on the benefits of vitamin C on various cardiovascular disorders are debatable, in contrast to its beneficial effects in the domain of ischemic heart disease. Some researchers have found that vitamin C administration lowers blood pressure in patients with hypertension [21]; however, others have found no decrease in the rate of bad outcomes associated with pregnancy-related hypertension. Although vitamin C has been found to lessen the heart's susceptibility to postoperative atrial fibrillation brought on by oxidative damage, this treatment had no effect on dogs' tendency to develop atrial fibrillation as a result of atrial-tachycardia remodeling. The effects of vitamin C on endothelial dysfunction and atherosclerosis linked to oxidative stress were also found to be detrimental. Due to its antioxidant action, it appears that vitamin C may be helpful for the treatment of ischemic heart disease; however, its value for the therapy of other cardiovascular disorders cannot currently be determined with certainty.

Supplementing with Liposoluble Vitamins
It was suggested that vitamin A and its precursors, a-carotene or b-carotene, could prevent the onset of many cardiovascular illnesses. Patients with hypertension who received treatment to raise their serum vitamin A levels saw a reduction in both their systolic and diastolic blood pressure. Because of its antioxidant and anti-inflammatory properties, vitamin A was also found to reduce atherosclerosis in both animals and humans when used consistently. Vitamin A supplementation has reportedly been shown to reduce oxidative stress in diabetic patients with ischemic heart disease. B-carotene reduced the extent of the Ischemia-Reperfusion (I/R)-induced infract and increased the recovery of post-ischemic heart function in Zucker diabetic rats, Additionally, taking b-carotene protected the heart from SR stress, apoptosis, and autophagy brought on by advanced glycation end products [87]. B-carotene, however, had no positive impact on the metabolic syndrome in rats fed a high-fat diet. It has been demonstrated that giving vitamin D (calcitriol) to people with hypertension and heart failure has positive effects by preventing the release of parathyroid hormone and the renin-angiotensin system as well as by directly interacting with the vitamin D receptors found in vascular smooth muscle cells,

endothelial cells, and cardiomyocytes. Another recent research states that the evidence is "mixed and inconclusive at this time" regarding a link between low vitamin D level and CVD. Although it is not known for sure if supplementing improves cardiovascular outcomes (a precursor of calcitriol) and decreases risk of cardiovascular disease such as myocardial infarction, heart failure, and aortic stenosis, it is possible to draw the conclusion that a lack of vitamin D is a risk factor for cardiovascular disease (CVD). Vitamin D supplementation has been shown to slow the development of acute myocardial infarction and the progression of coronary artery disease by inhibiting the intracellular NF-kB pathway. By reducing serum levels of total cholesterol, triglycerides, and low-density lipoproteins and raising levels of high-density lipoproteins and endothelial nitric oxide, 25-hydroxyvitamin D supplementation has been shown to delay the onset of atherosclerosis. Additionally, it has been discovered that giving vitamin D to obese rats fed a high-fat diet reduces various oxidative stress and inflammation indicators. On the other hand, numerous clinical investigations have been unable to demonstrate any positive effects of vitamin D medication in ischemic heart disease prevention or mortality reduction. Additionally, certain randomized controlled trials in the treatment of chronic heart failure and other cardiovascular diseases did not yield conflicting and equivocal findings when using vitamin D. Vitamin E (a-tocopherol) is the most popular dietary supplement due to its antioxidant and anti-inflammatory qualities, capacity to boost immunological function, and low risk of any negative effects on human health. In reality, the use of vitamin E for the treatment of cardiovascular disease has been backed by several observational and experimental investigations. According to Rodrigo et al. (2008), supplementing with vitamin E can lower blood pressure in people with essential hypertension and shield them from pregnancy-related hypertension's consequences. According to certain research, vitamin E therapy prevented the development of atherosclerosis and reduced the severity of endothelial dysfunction. In fact, a-tocopherol was found to reduce oxidative stress and inflammation, which in turn prevented ischemia-reperfusion-induced heart dysfunction and damage. Additionally, vitamin E supplementation had positive benefits on animals with ischemic heart disease and decreased the incidence of coronary artery disease in men. Vitamin E's protective impact in myocardial infarction was linked to the modification of several processes. Vitamin E pretreatment of rats has also been demonstrated to stop ventricular arrhythmias and alterations in heart function brought on by MI [88].

Additionally, pretreatment of mice with vitamin E reduced the severity of arrhythmias, cardiac cell damage, lipid peroxidation, and subcellular abnormalities brought on by catecholamines. These findings imply that supplementing with vitamin E can help protect the heart against a variety of pathogenic stressors. Despite substantial evidence pointing to vitamin E's health benefits, a number of clinical studies have produced contradictory and equivocal findings. According to one study, large doses of vitamin E reduced myocardial infarction and cardiovascular death whereas modest levels of vitamin E supplementation reduced angina risk in patients without a history of coronary artery disease. Vitamin E's beneficial benefits depended not only on the right dosage but also on the a- or b-tocopherol forms for preventing the production of proinflammatory cytokines and the activity of the enzymes 5-lipoxygenase, cyclooxygenase, and tyrosine kinase. On the other hand, excessive doses of vitamin E were also found to raise the risk of myocardial infarction and coronary artery disease. The literature has shown contrasting findings regarding the protective effects of vitamin E treatment for atherosclerosis and coronary artery calcification. The primary and secondary cardiovascular events were unaffected despite evidence that vitamin E use lowers the risk of coronary heart disease in middle-aged to older men and women. Furthermore, vitamin E supplementation had little effect on postmenopausal women's coronary heart disease. In actuality, chronic vitamin E administration to high-risk individuals had no impact on any type of cardiovascular event. It is interesting to note that while vitamin E therapy has been demonstrated to reduce the risk of heart disease, some populations and subjects who consume a nutritious diet may not experience additional protection from vitamin E supplementation. Additionally, when patients without a history of cardiovascular illness were evaluated, it was clear that vitamin E plays a preventive effect in coronary heart disease. As a result, in light of the aforementioned data, it would seem that vitamin E administration may be more important for preventing cardiovascular disease than for treating it [89].

3.4 Clinical Research Suggesting Antioxidant Vitamins' Beneficial Effects in CVP

Clinical trials and studies using dietary supplements of vitamin C, vitamin E, and carotenoids have examined the benefits of antioxidant vitamins. The results of these trials and studies on the function of antioxidant vitamins in the treatment and prevention of CVD are inconclusive. There are "successful" trials and research that show antioxidant vitamins have positive benefits in the prevention of CVD in addition to the trials and studies that are regarded as "negative." Twenty years ago, cohort studies were done that hinted at the function of vitamins in CVP. A study found that vitamin E intake lowered the risk of coronary heart disease (CHD) by 34%. The study involved female nurses who were free from CVD and were monitored for 8 years. An inverse relationship between vitamin C intake and risk of CHD was shown in a cohort research involving 16 years of follow-up on female nurses, with a 27% risk decrease. In the European Prospective Investigation into Cancer and Nutrition trial, the patients' chance of developing heart failure was inversely correlated with their plasma vitamin C content. This study suggests that the prevalence of heart failure may be predicted by plasma vitamin C levels. Additionally, there was a significant correlation between participants' plasma vitamin C levels and blood pressure. Higher plasma vitamin C levels in subjects were associated with decreased blood pressure. Short-term vitamin C treatment decreased both the systolic and diastolic blood pressure in a meta-analysis of 29 trials (-4.85 mmHg and -1.67 mmHg, respectively). The typical length of the test was 8 weeks, and the median vitamin C dose was 500 mg/day [90].

The combination of vitamin C, vitamin E, -carotene, selenium, and zinc decreased the incidence of ischemic CVD by 11% in the Supplementation in Vitamins and Mineral Antioxidants Study (SU.VI.MAX). Eight years of supplementation also resulted in a 36% reduction in total mortality among men. In a different study14, vitamin E supplementation (60 IU/day) reduced the risk of CHD by 36% in those who did not have the disease. Men who consumed 100 IU of vitamin E per day for two years had a lower risk of CHD. Supplementing with vitamin E decreased the risk of cardiovascular death and nonfatal myocardial infarction (MI) by 47% in the Cambridge Heart Antioxidant Study (CHAOS) (41 versus 64 events). Vitamin C and vitamin E supplements slowed the advancement of carotid atherosclerosis in males by 74% in the Antioxidant Supplementation in Atherosclerosis Prevention study (ASAP), a randomized experiment. In the ASAP research, treatment with a mix of vitamins C and E during a 6-year follow-up period in hypercholesterolemic individuals reduced the progression of carotid intima-media thickness (CIMT) [91].

Vitamin E supplementation (800 IU/day) decreased the incidence of CVD endpoints and MI in the Secondary Prevention with Antioxidants of Cardiovascular disease in Endstage Renal Disease research (SPACE), a randomized placebo-controlled trial in hemodialysis patients with pre-existing CVD. After a 16.5-year follow-up, the Japan Collaborative Cohort Study for Evaluation of Cancer Risk (JACC) looked at the impact of vitamin C intake on cardiovascular morbidity and mortality. For women, there was an inverse relationship between vitamin C intake and morbidity and death from CVD, CHD, and stroke. Nine prospective studies investigating the effects of vitamin C, vitamin E, and carotenoids on CHD risk were examined by Knekt *et al.* Subjects who were CHD-free at the beginning of the vitamin supplementation and who were monitored for 10 years were included in the study. According to the findings, those who consumed 700 mg of vitamin C per day had a 25% lower risk of CHD and mortality than those who did not take any supplements [92].

The Women's Antioxidant Cardiovascular Study (WACS) was designed to examine the impact of vitamins C, E, and -carotene on the combined outcome of MI, stroke, coronary revascularization, and CVD death in female health professionals who were at increased risk for developing CVD and had a history of the disease or risk factors for developing it. The participants were monitored for a median of 9.4 years. Despite the fact that 26–27% of participants in all groups used multivitamins, which may have been biased, vitamin E administration resulted with a 21% reduction in ischemic stroke risk and a 20% reduction in nonfatal stroke risk. The primary endpoints were significantly reduced by 23% as a result of participant noncompliance, while the secondary endpoints showed reductions in MI, stroke, CVD mortality, and the sum of MI, stroke, and CVD fatalities of 22%, 27%, 9%, and 23%, respectively [93, 94].

There is a link between supplemental vitamin E use and a slowed progression of coronary artery lesions as seen on angiograms. Subjects with supplemental vitamin E consumption of at least 100 IU/day showed slower progression of coronary artery lesions than those with intake of less than 100 IU/day. During the three years of follow-up, an increase in vitamin C intake was negatively correlated with the advancement of CIMT [95].

It has been amply proven that oxidative stress plays a critical role in the pathophysiology of atrial fibrillation following cardiac surgery. Following coronary artery bypass grafting, oxidative stress contributes to the early postoperative emergence of rhythm abnormalities. Vitamin C administration within the first 24 hours following surgery was successful in reducing heart rhythm abnormalities. In comparison to the treatment of -blockers alone, vitamin C with -blockers dramatically decreased the incidence of postoperative atrial fibrillation in patients undergoing bypass grafting surgery. Vitamin C supplementation decreased the frequency of post-coronary artery bypass grafting atrial fibrillation, as well as the amount of time needed to restore rhythm and the length of hospital stay [96].

3.5 Beneficial Effects of B Vitamins in CVP

In atherosclerotic subjects, kidney disease subjects, including recipients of renal transplants, chronic hemodialysis patients, and cases of elevated levels of HCY, FA supplementation slowed the progression of CIMT. Dietary FA consumption and the likelihood of acute coronary events have been demonstrated to be negatively correlated. High blood FA concentrations are linked to a decreased incidence of acute coronary events, whereas low dietary FA intake is linked to an elevated incidence of acute coronary events and stroke. A higher intake of FA has been linked to a lower risk of MI, while low FA serum levels may be a risk factor for CVD and stroke. In North America, the incidence of CVD, notably the occurrences of MI68 and stroke mortality, dropped after the FA food fortification programme was implemented. In 80,082 women without a history of CVD. The effect of FA and vitamin B6 intake on the incidence of fatal CHD and nonfatal MI has been looked at. After 14 years of follow-up, women who regularly took multiple vitamins saw a reduction in their risk of CHD of 24% (median consumption of FA 0.696 mg/day, vitamin B6 4.6 mg/day). The results of this study suggest that taking low-dose multivitamin supplements may help to prevent MI. More research indicates that consuming FA may help with MI's primary prevention. The risk of MI was found to be negatively correlated with the daily usage of multivitamin supplements (including 400 g FA) in a Swedish study called the Stockholm Heart Epidemiology Program (SHEEP). In a cohort of Swedish women drawn from the general population, the SHEEP results have been verified. In this investigation, multivitamin consumption (particularly long-term use among women without a history of CVD) was found to be negatively correlated with MI. These multivitamins contained 400 g of FA (31,671 cases) [96].

3.6 Role of Vitamin D in Cardiovascular Health

Although vitamin D (25-hydroxyvitamin D) is crucial for bone metabolism, there is mounting evidence that it is also crucial for preserving cardiovascular function. Vascular and cardiac cells exhibit the vitamin D receptor 92 and enzymes for vitamin D metabolism, suggesting that vitamin D exerts effects in the cardiovascular system. By decreasing the activity of the renin-angiotensin system and inflammation, lowering blood pressure, and lowering the risk of type II diabetes mellitus, vitamin

D causes its cardiovascular effects. Vitamin D insufficiency has been linked to CVD, all-cause premature death, heart failure, coronary artery disease, hypertension, and diabetes mellitus, according to research. Low serum vitamin D levels, which are present in between 30% and 50% of the general population, are also thought to be a risk factor for CVD and PAD. In the Framingham Offspring Study, patients with low vitamin D levels had a 53% to 80% increased chance of major CVD events. Mortality was inversely correlated with vitamin D levels, according to the National Health and Nutrition Examination Survey (NHANES) III study, which had a follow-up of 8.7 years. The analysis of the individuals, a meta-analysis of 73 cohort studies and 22 RCTs, and a recent study that demonstrated an inverse relationship between the level of circulating 25-hydroxyvitamin D and death from CVD and other causes all lend credence to this conclusion. Additionally, a number of experimental investigations on vitamin D's impact contend that it possesses cardioprotective properties. For instance, vitamin D3 supplementation dramatically decreased mortality in older persons, and vitamin D supplementation increased survival. A review of

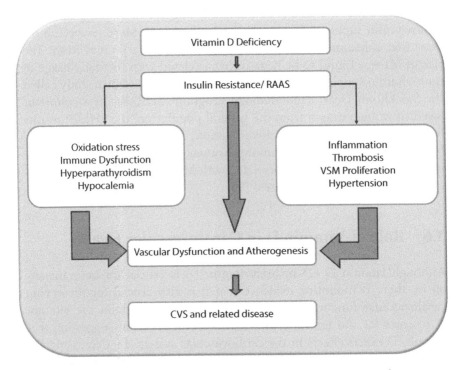

Figure 3.2 Conceptual diagram illustrating the main routes that a vitamin D shortage may take to cause cardiovascular disease.

17 prospective studies and RCTs indicates that taking vitamin D supplements may lower the risk of developing CVD [97]. Figure 3.2 showing the conceptual diagram illustrating the main routes that a vitamin D shortage may take to cause cardiovascular disease.

The meta-analysis of 51 studies on the impact of vitamin D on cardiovascular outcomes was completed. While there was no impact on MI or stroke, the risk of death decreased by a non-significant (4%) amount. However, if we look at the combined mortality results, we can see that the RR for death ranged from 0.28 to 0.94 in 16 out of 30 trials. Significant variability was evident in the calcium and vitamin D intake dosages across the trials that were analysed. Only stratified analysis in this situation may produce a more impartial assessment; otherwise, the data can be deceptive. Furthermore, diseases, ageing, drug use, and other factors could skew the results. The fact that vitamin D trials may be impacted by calcium intake is another issue with these studies, as oral calcium may raise the risk of CVD. 113 According to a summary of vitamin D's pleiotropic effects on cardiac function and dysfunction, as well as its effects on cardiac physiology, vitamin D supplementation is recommended for people who are vitamin D deficient, as well as for people who are at a high risk of developing myocardial diseases [98–102].

Vitamin D3 reduced mortality by roughly 6%, according to a Cochrane Review of 50 trials (94,148 individuals) on the topic. However, vitamin D2 (ergocalciferol), alfacalcidol, and calcitriol had no discernible impact. The authors of a review116 update also came to the conclusion that vitamin D3 reduced senior mortality. Despite these encouraging findings, a recent "umbrella" review (which looked at 107 systematic reviews, 74 meta-analyses of observational studies, and 87 meta-analyses of RCTs on vitamin D and multiple health outcomes) revealed that there is only "suggestive" evidence linking high D vitamin levels to a lower risk of CVD and stroke (i.e., the association is possible, but not convincing or probable). According to different recent research, "the evidence suggesting a causal relationship between low vitamin D status and CVD is now equivocal and confusing." While it is possible to conclude that a lack of vitamin D is an independent risk factor for cardiovascular disease (CVD), Kienreich *et al.* stress that it is uncertain whether supplementation has any positive effects on cardiovascular outcomes. There are now two RCTs looking at the effects of vitamin D supplementation on the cardiovascular system. One study focuses on primary prevention, the vitamin D and Omega 3 Trial (VITAL), and the other study examines secondary prevention of cardiovascular events [103–114].

3.7 Conclusion

The merits and downsides of both liposoluble and hydrosoluble vitamins in treating various cardiovascular disorders, including hypertension, atherosclerosis, ischemic heart disease, and heart failure, have been discussed in this article. We have looked at the concerns surrounding the link between vitamin deficiencies and the onset of cardiovascular illness, as well as the advantages of vitamin supplements for enhancing circulatory function in both people and animals. Results from well-controlled clinical investigations are inconsistent, inconclusive, and conflicting, despite the fact that numerous epidemiological, observational, and experimental studies have shown the beneficial effects of some vitamins showing antioxidant, anti-inflammatory, and autoimmune activities in attenuating cardiovascular disorders. A valid conclusion on the use of various vitamins in the treatment of cardiovascular disease cannot be drawn in light of these disparities between experimental and clinical observations. It appears that prior to starting treatment, the majority of clinical trials using vitamins for cardiovascular disease were conducted without first determining their plasma levels. One reason why reasonably big double blind clinical trials with various vitamins failed could have been because the positive benefits of these nutrients might only be observed in individuals with low levels of plasma vitamins prior to treatment. Antioxidant vitamin consumption may also be advantageous for the prevention of cardiovascular irregularities brought on by various pathogenic stressors. This opinion is supported by observations that pretreatment with vitamin B6 and vitamin E reduced the severity of I/R-induced injury and the changes in cardiac function, myocardial metabolism, Ca2C-handling by cardiomyocytes, and ventricular arrhythmias brought on by coronary occlusion. Vitamins A, C, B6, and E pretreatment of rats was also found to suppress catecholamine-induced ventricular arrhythmias.

These encouraging findings serve as an excellent impetus for conducting in-depth investigations into the dose-response and cause-and-effect interactions of different vitamins to determine their specificity in avoiding various cardiovascular illnesses. It should be understood that in healthy people, vitamins have no effect, and that a specific vitamin deficit is what causes a certain cardiovascular abnormality to occur. Therefore, it would be wise to investigate vitamin efficacy in individuals under circumstances where their plasma levels are low. The role of various vitamins as a specific adjunct therapy for a specific condition may be established using novel approaches to the treatment of cardiovascular patients.

Acknowledgment

The authors thank the MET's Institute of Pharmacy, BKC, which is affiliated with Savitribai Phule Pune University, Nashik. EDA wishes to express gratitude to the NFST/RGNF/UGC, Government of India, for providing financial assistance in the form of a fellowship (award no 202021-NFST-MAH-01235).

References

1. Adameova, A., Shah, A.K., Dhalla, N.S., Role of oxidative stress in the genesis of ventricular arrhythmias. *Int. J. Mol. Sci.*, 21, 4200, 2020.
2. Agarwal, M., Phan, A., Willix, R., Jr, Barber, M., Schwarz, E.R., Is vitamin D deficiency associated with heart failure? A review of current evidence. *J. Cardiovasc. Pharmacol. Ther.*, 16, 354–363, 2011.
3. Alpers, D.H., Clouse, R.E., Stenson, W.F., *Manual of nutritional therapeutics*, p. 457, Little, Brown and Company, Boston, 1983.
4. Altoum, A.E.A., Osman, A.L., Babker, A., Comparative study of levels of selective oxidative stress markers (malondialdehyde, zinc, and antioxidant vitamins A, E, and C) in ischemic and non-ischemic heart disease patients suffering from type-2 diabetes. *Asian J. Pharm. Clin. Res.*, 11, 508–510, 2018.
5. Antoniades, C., Tousoulis, D., Tentolouris, C., Toutouzas, P., Stefanadis, C., Oxidative stress, antioxidant vitamins, and atherosclerosis. From basic research to clinical practice. *Herz*, 28, 628–638, 2003.
6. Azizi-Namini, P., Ahmed, M., Yan, A.T., Keith, M., The role of B vitamins in the management of heart failure. *Nutr. Clin. Pract.*, 27, 363–374, 2012.
7. Balasubramanian, S., Christodoulou, J., Rahman, S., Disorders of riboflavin metabolism. *J. Inherit. Metab. Dis.*, 42, 608–619, 2019.
8. Bartekova, M., Adamcova, A., Gorbe, A., Ferenczyova, K., Pechanova, O., Lazou, A. *et al.*, Natural and synthetic antioxidants targeting cardiac oxidative stress and redox signaling in cardiometabolic diseases. *Free Radic. Biol. Med.*, 169, 446–477, 2021.
9. Bilagi, U., Vitamin D and heart disease. *J. Assoc. Physicians India*, 66, 78–83, 2018.
10. Bleys, J., Edgar, R., Pastor-Barriuso, R., Appel, L.J., Guallar, E., Vitamin-mineral supplementation and the progression of atherosclerosis: A meta-analysis of randomized controlled trials. *Am. J. Clin. Nutr.*, 84, 880–887, 2006.
11. Bostick, R.M., Kushi, L.H., Wu, Y., Meyer, K.A., Sellers, T.A., Folsom, A.R., Relation of calcium, vitamin D, and dairy food intake to ischemic heart disease mortality among postmenopausal women. *Am. J. Epidemiol.*, 149, 151–161, 1999.

12. Brinkley, D.M., Ali, O.M., Zalawadiya, S.K., Wang, T.J., Vitamin D and heart failure. *Curr. Heart Fail. Rep.*, 14, 410–420, 2017.
13. Carrier, M., Emery, R., Kandzari, D.E., Harringtion, R., Guertin, M.C., Tardif, J.C., Protective effect of pyridoxal-50-phosphate (MC-1) on perioperative myocardial infarction is independent of aortic cross clamp time: Results from the MEND-CABG trial. *J. Cardiovasc. Surg.*, 49, 249–253, 2008.
14. Chasan-Taber, L., Selhub, J., Rosenberg, I.H., Malinow, M.R., Terry, P., Tishler, P.V. et al., A prospective study of folate and vitamin B6 and risk of myocardial infarction in US physicians. *J. Am. Coll. Nutr.*, 15, 136–43, 1996.
15. Chen, J., He, J., Hamm, L., Batuman, V., Whelton, P.K., Serum antioxidant vitamins and blood pressure in the United States population. *Hypertension*, 40, 810–816, 2002.
16. Chow, C.K., Vitamin E and oxidative stress. *Free Radic. Biol. Med.*, 11, 215–232, 1991, doi: 10.1016/0891-5849(91)90174-2.
17. Contreras-Duarte, S., Chen, P., Andía, M., Uribe, S., Irarrázaval, P., Kopp, S. et al., Attenuation of atherogenic apo B-48-dependent hyperlipidemia and high density lipoprotein remodeling induced by vitamin C and E combination and their beneficial effect on lethal ischemic heart disease in mice. *Biol. Res.*, 51, 34–36, 2018.
18. Csepanyi, E., Czompa, A., Szabados-Furjesi, P., Lekli, I., Balla, J., Balla, G. et al., The effects of long-term, low- and high-dose beta-carotene treatment in zucker diabetic fatty rats: The role of HO-1. *Int. J. Mol. Sci.*, 19, 1132, 2018.
19. Czeizel, A.E., Dudas, I., Vereczkey, A., Banhidy, F., Folate deficiency and folic acid supplementation: The prevention of neural-tube defects and congenital heart defects. *Nutrients*, 5, 4760–4775, 2013.
20. Dakshinamurti, S., Wang, X., Musat, S., Dandekar, M., Dhalla, N.S., Alterations of KCl- and ATP-induced increase in [Ca2C]i in cardiomyocytes from vitamin B6 deficient rats. *Can. J. Physiol. Pharmacol.*, 76, 837–842, 1998.
21. Das, U.N., Vitamin C for type 2 diabetes mellitus and hypertension. *Arch. Med. Res.*, 50, 11–14, 2019.
22. Davis, J.L., Paris, H.L., Beals, J.W., Binns, S.E., Giordano, G.R., Scalzo, R.L. et al., Liposomal-encapsulated ascorbic acid: Influence on vitamin C bioavailability and capacity to protect against ischemia-reperfusion injury. *Nutr. Metab. Insights*, 9, 25–30, 2016.
23. de la Guia-Galipienso, F., Martinez-Ferran, M., Vallecillo, N., Lavie, C.J., Sanchis- Gomar, F., Pareja-Galeano, H., VitaminDand cardiovascular health. *Clin. Nutr.*, 40, 2946–2957, 2021.
24. Dhalla, K.S., Rupp, H., Beamish, R.E., Dhalla, N.S., Mechanisms of alterations in cardiac membrane Ca2C transport due to excess catecholamines. *Cardiovasc. Drugs Ther.*, 10, 231–238, 1996.
25. N.S. Dhalla, R. Sethi, K. Dakshinamurti, Treatment of cardiovascular and related pathologies. US Patent 6, 2000b.

26. Dhalla, N.S., Fedelesova, M., Toffler, I., Biochemical alterations in the skeletal muscle of vitamin E deficient rats. *Can. J. Physiol.*, 49, 1202–1208, 1971.
27. Dhalla, N.S., Takeda, S., Elimban, V., Mechanisms of the beneficial effects of vitamin B6 and pyridoxal 5-phosphate on cardiac performance in ischemic heart disease. *Clin. Chem. Lab. Med.*, 51, 535–543, 2013.
28. Dosedel, M., Jirkovsky, E., Macakova, K., Krcmova, L.K., Javorska, L., Pourova, J. et al., Vitamin C-sources, physiological role, kinetics, deficiency, use, toxicity, and determination. *Nutrients*, 13, 615, 2021.
29. Draper, H.H., James, M.F., Johnson, B.C., Tri-o-cresyl phosphate as a vitamin E antagonist for the rat and lamb. *J. Nutr.*, 47, 583–599, 1952.
30. Ellis, J.M. and McCully, K.S., Prevention of myocardial infarction by vitamin B6. *Res. Commun. Mol. Pathol. Pharmacol.*, 89, 208–220, 1995.
31. Eshak, E.S. and Arafa, A.E., Thiamine deficiency and cardiovascular science. *Nutr. Metab. Cardiovasc. Dis.*, 28, 965–972, 2018.
32. Farhangi, M.A., Nameni, G., Hajiluian, G., Mesgari-Abbasi, M., Cardiac tissue oxidative stress and inflammation after vitamin D administrations in high fat- diet induced obese rats. *BMC Cardiovasc. Disord.*, 17, 161, 2017.
33. Farrell, P.M., Deficiency states, pharmacological effects, and nutrient requirements, in: *Vitamin E: A Comprehensive Treatise, Basic and Clinical Nutrition*, L.J. Machlin (Ed.), pp. 20–630, Marcell Dekker, New York, 1980.
34. Fedelesova, M., Sulakhe, P.V., Yates, J.C., Dhalla, N.S., Biochemical basis heart function. IV. Energy metabolism and calcium transport in hearts of vitamin E deficient rats. *Can. J. Physiol. Pharmacol.*, 49, 909–918, 1971.
35. Feingold, K.R., *Triglyceride Lowering Drugs*, NCBI, Marylan, 2000, https://www. ncbi.nlm.nih.gov/books/NBK425699/.
36. Fitch, C.D., Experimental anemia in primates due to vitamin E deficiency. *Vitam. Horm.*, 26, 501–514, 1968.
36. Friso, S., Girelli, D., Martinelli, N., Olivieri, O., Lotto, V., Bozzini, C. et al., Low plasma vitamin B-6 concentrations and modulation of coronary artery disease risk. *Am. J. Clin. Nutr.*, 79, 992–998, 2004.
37. Gale, C.R., Martyn, C.N., Winter, P.D., Cooper, C., Vitamin C and risk of death from stroke and coronary heart disease in cohort of elderly people. *Brit. Med. J.*, 310, 1563–1566, 1995.
38. Gatz, A.J. and Houchin, O.B., Studies on the heart of vitamin E deficient rabbits. *Anat. Rec.*, 110, 249–265, 1951.
39. Gominak, S.C., Vitamin D deficiency changes the intestinal microbiome reducing B vitamin production in the gut. The resulting lack of pantothenic acid adversely affects the immune system, producing a "pro-inflammatory" state associated with atherosclerosis and autoimmunity. *Med. Hypotheses*, 94, 103–107, 2016.
40. Gori, T. and Münzel, T., Oxidative stress and endothelial dysfunction: Therapeutic implications. *Ann. Med.*, 43, 259–272, 2011.

41. Grandi, N.C., Brietling, L.P., Brenner, H., Vitamin D and cardiovascular disease: Systematic review and meta-analysis of prospective studies. *Prev. Med.*, 51, 228–233, 2010.
42. Grigoreva, V.A. and Medovar, E.N., Studies on the components of the adenylic system in skeletal and cardiac muscles in experimental muscular dystrophy (Russian text). *Ukr. Biokhim, Zh.*, 31, 351–368, 1959.
43. Gullickson, T.W., The relation of vitamin E to reproduction in dairy cattle. *Ann. N. Y. Acad. Sci.*, 52, 256–259, 1949.
44. Gullickson, T.W. and Calverley, C.E., Cardiac failure in cattle on vitamin E-free rations as revealed by electrocardiograms. *Science*, 104, 312–313, 1946.
45. Guthikonda, S. and Haynes, W.G., Homocysteine: Role and implications in atherosclerosis. *Curr. Atheroscler. Rep.*, 8, 100–106, 2006.
46. Hagar, H.H., Folic acid and vitamin B(12) supplementation attenuates isoprenaline-induced myocardial infarction in experimental hyperhomocysteinemic rats. *Pharmacol. Res.*, 46, 213–219, 2002.
47. Haynes, W.G., Hyperhomocysteinemia, vascular function and atherosclerosis: Effects of vitamins. *Cardiovasc. Drugs Ther.*, 16, 391–399, 2002.
48. Herzlich, B.C., Plasma homocysteine, folate, vitamin B6 and coronary artery diseases risk. *J. Am. Coll. Nutr.*, 15, 109–110, 1996.
49. Hodzic, E., Potential anti-inflammatory treatment of ischemic heart disease. *Med. Arch.*, 72, 94–98, 2018.
50. Ingles, D.P., Cruz Rodriguez, J.B., Garcia, H., Supplemental vitamins and minerals for cardiovascular disease prevention and treatment. *Curr. Cardiol. Rep.*, 22, 22, 2020.
51. Ivey, M., Nutritional supplement, minerals and vitamin products, in: *Handbook of Non-Prescription Drugs*, 6th Edn., J. Welch, M.T. Rasmussen, S.W. Goldstein, J. Kelly (Eds.), pp. 141–174, American Pharmaceutical Association, Washington, 1979.
52. Jarrah, M.I., Mhaidat, N.M., Alzoubi, K.H., Alrabadi, N., Alsatari, E., Khader, Y. et al., The association between the serum level of vitamin D and ischemic heart disease: A study from Jordan. *Vasc. Health Risk Manage.*, 14, 119–127, 2018.
53. Judd, S.E. and Tangpricha, V., Vitamin D deficiency and risk for cardiovascular disease. *Am. J. Med. Sci.*, 338, 40–44, 2009.
54. Kandzari, D.E., Dery, J.P., Armstrong, P.W., Douglas, D.A., Zettler, M.E., Hidinger, G.K. et al., MC-1 (pyridoxal 50-phosphate): Novel therapeutic applications to reduce ischaemic injury. *Expert. Opin. Investig. Drugs*, 14, 1435–1442, 2005.
55. Kandzari, D.E., Labinaz, M., Cantor, W.J., Madan, M., Gallup, D.S., Hasselblad, V. et al., Reduction of myocardial ischemic injury following coronary intervention (the MC-1 to eliminate necrosis and damage trial). *Am. J. Cardiol.*, 92, 660–664, 2003.

56. Kannan, K. and Jain, S.K., Effect of vitamin B6 on oxygen radicals, mitochondrial membrane potential, and lipid peroxidation in H2O2-treated U937 monocytes. *Free Radic. Biol. Med.*, 36, 423–428, 2004.
57. Keith, M.E., Walsh, N.A., Darling, P.B., Hanninen, S.A., Thirugnanam, S., Leong-Pi, H. et al., B-vitamin deficiency in hospitalized patients with heart failure. *J. Am. Diet. Assoc.*, 109, 1406–1410, 2009.
58. Khadangi, F. and Azzi, A., Vitamin E – the next 100 years. *IUBMB Life*, 71, 411–415, 2019.
59. Kheiri, B., Abdalla, A., Osman, M., Ahmed, S., Hassan, M., Bachuwa, G., Vitamin D deficiency and risk of cardiovascular diseases: A narrative review. *Clin. Hypertens.*, 24, 9, 2018.
60. Kim, M.K., Sasaki, S., Sasazuki, S., Okubo, S., Hayashi, M., Tsugane, S., Lack of long-term effect of vitamin C supplementation on blood pressure. *Hypertension*, 40, 797–803, 2002.
61. Knekt, P., Ritz, J., Pereira, M.A., O'Reilly, E., Augustsson, K., Fraser, G.E. et al., Antioxidant vitamins and coronary heart disease risk: A pooled analysis of 9 cohorts. *Am. J. Clin. Nutr.*, 80, 1508–1520, 2004.
62. Kok, F.J., Schrijver, J., Hofman, A., Witteman, J.C.M., Kruyssen, D., Remme, W.J. et al., Low vitamin B6 status in patients with acute myocardial infarction. *Am. J. Cardiol.*, 63, 513–513, 1989.
63. Ku, Y.C., Liu, M.E., Ku, C.S., Liu, T.Y., Lin, S.L., Relationship between vitamin D deficiency and cardiovascular disease. *World J. Cardiol.*, 5, 337–346, 2013.
64. Kushi, L.H., Folsom, A.R., Prineas, R.J., Mink, P.J., Wu, Y., Bostick, R.M., Dietary antioxidant vitamins and death from coronary heart disease in postmenopausal women. *N. Engl. J. Med.*, 334, 1156–1162, 1996.
65. Lal, K.J., Dakshinamurti, K., Thliveris, J., The effect of vitamin B6 on the systolic blood pressure of rats in various animal models of hypertension. *J. Hypertens.*, 14, 355–363, 1996.
66. Latic, N. and Erben, R.G., Vitamin D and cardiovascular disease, with emphasis on hypertension, atherosclerosis, and heart failure. *Int. J. Mol. Sci.*, 21, 6483, 2020.
67. Legarth, C., Grimm, D., Krüger, M., Infanger, M., Wehland, M., Potential beneficial effects of vitamin D in coronary artery disease. *Nutrients*, 12, 99, 2019.
68. Lin, L., Zhang, L., Li, C., Gai, Z., Li, Y., Vitamin D and vitamin D receptor: New insights in the treatment of hypertension. *Curr. Protein Pept. Sci.*, 20, 984–995, 2019.
69. Liu, C., Liu, C., Wang, Q., Zhang, Z., Supplementation of folic acid in pregnancy and the risk of preeclampsia and gestational hypertension: A meta-analysis. *Arch. Gynecol. Obstet.*, 298, 697–704, 2018.
70. Liu, R., Mi, B., Zhao, Y., Li, Q., Yan, H., Dang, S., Effect of B vitamins from diet on hypertension. *Arch. Med. Res.*, 48, 187–194, 2017.

71. Long, P., Liu, X., Li, J., He, S., Chen, H., Yuan, Y. et al., Circulating folate concentrations and risk of coronary artery disease: A prospective cohort study in Chinese adults and a Mendelian randomization analysis. *Am. J. Clin. Nutr.*, 111, 635–643, 2020.
72. Lu, G.D., Emerson, G.A., Evans, H.M., Phosphorus metabolism of the musculature of E-deficient suckling rats. *Am. J. Physiol.*, 133, 367–368, 1941.
73. Machado, A.D., Andrade, G.R.G., Levy, J., Ferreira, S.S., Marchioni, D.M., Association between vitamins and minerals with antioxidant effects and coronary artery calcification in adults and older adults: A systematic review. *Curr. Pharm. Des.*, 25, 2474–2479, 2019.
74. MacKenzie, J.B. and MacKenzie, C.G., Vitamin E activity of alphatocopherylhydroquinone and muscular dystrophy. *Proc. Soc. Exp. Biol. Med.*, 84, 388–392, 1953.
75. Madsen, L.L., McCay, C.M., Maynard, L.A., Possible relationship between cod liver oil and muscular degeneration of herbivora fed synthetic diets. *Proc. Soc. Exp. Biol. Med.*, 30, 1434–1438, 1933.
76. Maulik, S.K. and Kumar, S., Oxidative stress and cardiac hypertrophy: A review. *Toxicol. Mech. Methods*, 22, 359–366, 2012.
77. McGreevy, C. and Williams, D., New insights about the vitamin D and cardiovascular disease. *Ann. Intern. Med.*, 155, 820–826, 2011.
78. McNulty, P.H., Robertson, B.J., Tulli, M.A., Hess, J., Harach, L.A., Scott, S. et al., Effect of hyperoxia and vitamin C on coronary blood flow in patients with ischemic heart disease. *J. Appl. Physiol.*, 102, 2040–2045, 2007.
79. Mehta, R.H. et al., High-risk coronary artery bypass graft surgery: MC-1 eliminate necrosis and damage in coronary artery bypass graft surgery trial (MEND-CABG) II– study design and rationale. *Am. Heart J.*, 155, 600–608, 2008.
80. Moat, S.J., Clarke, Z.L., Madhavan, A.K., Lewis, M.J., Lang, D., Folic acid reverses endothelial dysfunction induced by inhibition of tetrahydrobiopterin biosynthesis. *Eur. J. Pharmacol.*, 530, 250–258, 2006.
81. Moser, M.A. and Chun, O.K., Vitamin C and heart health: A review based on findings from epidemiologic studies. *Int. J. Mol. Sci.*, 17, 1328, 2016.
82. Mozos, I. and Marginean, O., Links between vitamin D deficiency and cardiovascular diseases. *Biomed. Res. Int.*, 2015, 109275, 2015.
83. Mulder, A.G., Gatz, A.J., Tigerman, B., Phosphate and glycogen determination in the hearts of vitamin E deficient rabbits. *Am. J. Physiol.*, 196, 246–248, 1954.
84. Murray, J.C., Fraser, D.R., Levene, C.I., The effect of pyridoxine on lysyl oxidase activity in the chick. *Exp. Mol. Pathol.*, 28, 301–308, 1978.
85. Muscogiuri, G., Annweiler, C., Duval, G., Karras, S., Tirabassi, G., Salvio, G. et al., Vitamin D and cardiovascular disease: From atherosclerosis to myocardial infarction and stroke. *Int. J. Cardiol.*, 230, 577–584, 2017.

86. Myung, S.K., Ju, W., Cho, B., Oh, S.W., Park, S.M., Koo, B.K. et al., Efficacy of vitamin and antioxidant supplements in prevention of cardiovascular disease: Systematic review and meta-analysis of randomized controlled trials. *Brit. Med. J.*, 346, f10, 2013.
87. Nagel, E., Meyer zu Vilsendorf, A., Bartels, M., Pichlmayr, R., Antioxidative vitamins in prevention of ischemia/reperfusion injury. *Int. J. Vitam. Res.*, 67, 298–306, 1997.
88. Nam, C.M., Oh, K.W., Lee, K.H., Jee, S.H., Cho, S.Y., Shim, W.H. et al., Vitamin C intake and risk of ischemic heart disease in a population with a high prevalence of smoking. *Null*, 22, 372–378, 2003.
89. National Research Council (US) Committee on Diet and Health, *Diet and health: Implications for reducing chronic disease risk*, National Academies Press, Washington, 1989.
90. Nemerovski, C.W., Dorsch, M.P., Simpson, R.U., Bone, H.G., Aaronson, K.D., Bleske, B.E., Vitamin D and cardiovascular disease. *Pharmacotherapy*, 29, 691–708, 2009.
91. Neri, M., Fineschi, V., Di Paolo, M., Pomara, C., Riezzo, I., Turillazzi, E. et al., Cardiac oxidative stress and inflammatory cytokines response after myocardial infarction. *Curr. Vasc. Pharmacol.*, 13, 26–36, 2015.
92. NyyssOnen, K., Parviainen, M.T., Salonen, R., Tuomilehto, J., Salonen, J.T., Vitamin C deficiency and risk of myocardial infarction: Prospective population study of men from eastern Finland. *BMJ*, 314, 634–638, 1997.
93. Olson, R.E., Vitamin E and its relation to heart disease. *Circulation*, 48, 179–184, 1973.
94. Osganian, S.K., Stampfer, M.J., Rimm, E., Spiegelman, D., Hu, F.B., Manson, J.E. et al., Vitamin C and risk of coronary heart disease in women. *J. Am. Coll. Cardiol.*, 42, 246–252, 2003.
95. Oski, F.A. and Barness, L.A., Vitamin E deficiency: A previously unrecognized cause for hemolytic anemia in the premature infant. *J. Pediatr.*, 70, 211–220, 1969.
96. Ozkanlar, S. and Akcay, F., Antioxidant vitamins in atherosclerosis–animal experiments and clinical studies. *Adv. Clin. Exp. Med.*, 21, 115–123, 2012.
97. Palace, V.P., Khaper, N., Qin, Q., Singal, P.K., Antioxidant potential of vitamin A and carotenoids and their relevance to heart disease. *Free Radic. Biol. Med.*, 26, 746–761, 1999.
98. Vanga, S.R., Good, M., Howard, P.A., Vacek, J.L., Role of vitamin D in cardiovascular health. *Am. J. Cardiol.*, 106, 6, 798–805, 2010.
99. Nitsa, A., Toutouza, M., Machairas, N., Mariolis, A., Philippou, A., Koutsilieris, M., Vitamin D in cardiovascular disease. *In Vivo*, 32, 5, 977–981, 2018.
100. Norman, P.E. and Powell, J.T., Vitamin D and cardiovascular disease. *Circ. Res.*, 114, 2, 379–393, 2014.

101. Verhave, G. and Siegert, C.E., Role of vitamin D in cardiovascular disease. *Neth. J. Med.*, 68, 3, 113–8, 2010.
102. Lavie, C.J., DiNicolantonio, J.J., Milani, R.V., O'Keefe, J.H., Vitamin D and cardiovascular health. *Circulation*, 128, 22, 2404–2406, 2013.
103. Ahire, E.D., Sonawane, V.N., Surana, K.R., Talele, G.S., Drug discovery, drug-likeness screening, and bioavailability: Development of drug-likeness rule for natural products, in: *Applied Pharmaceutical Practice and Nutraceuticals*, pp. 191–208, Apple Academic Press, Canada, 2021.
104. Surana, K.R., Ahire, E.D., Sonawane, V.N., Talele, S.G., Talele, G.S., Molecular modeling: Novel techniques in food and nutrition development, in: *Natural Food Products and Waste Recovery*, pp. 17–31, Apple Academic Press, Canada, 2021.
105. Surana, K.R., Ahire, E.D., Sonawane, V.N., Talele, S.G., Biomolecular and molecular docking: A modern tool in drug discovery and virtual screening of natural products, in: *Applied Pharmaceutical Practice and Nutraceuticals*, pp. 209–223, Apple Academic Press, Canada, 2021.
106. Keservani, R.K., Kesharwani, R.K., Vyas, N., Jain, S., Raghuvanshi, R., Sharma, A.K., Nutraceutical and functional food as future food: A review. *Der Pharm. Lett.*, 2, 1, 106–116, 2010a.
107. Keservani, R.K., Kesharwani, R.K., Sharma, A.K., Vyas, N., Chadoker, A., Nutritional supplements: An overview. *Int. J. Curr. Pharm. Rev. Res.*, 1, 1, 59–75, 2010b.
108. Keservani, R.K. and Sharma, A.K., Flavonoids: Emerging trends and potential health benefits. *J. Chin. Pharm. Sci.*, 23, 12, 815, 2014.
109. Keservani, R.K., Sharma, A.K., Kesharwani, R.K., Nutraceutical and functional foods for cardiovascular health, in: *Food Process Engineering*, pp. 291–312, 2016a.
110. Keservani, R.K., Sharma, A.K., Kesharwani, R.K., Medicinal effect of nutraceutical fruits for the cognition and brain health. *Scientifica*, 2016, 10 pages, 2016b, Article ID 3109254.
111. Keservani, R.K., Sharma, A.K., Kesharwani, R.K., An overview and therapeutic applications of nutraceutical and functional foods, in: *Recent Advances in Drug Delivery Technology*, pp. 160–201, 2017.
112. Keservani, R.K., Sharma, A.K., Kesharwani, R.K. (Eds.,) *Nutraceuticals and dietary supplements: Applications in health improvement and disease management*, CRC Press, Canada, 2020.

113. Singh, P., Kesharwani, R.K., Keservani, R.K., Antioxidants and vitamins: Roles in cellular function and metabolism, in: *Sustained Energy for Enhanced Human Functions and Activity*, pp. 385–407, Academic Press, Canada, 2017.
114. Keservani, R.K., Kesharwani, R.K., Sharma, A.K., Jarouliya, U., Dietary supplements, nutraceutical and functional foods in immune response (immunomodulators), in: *Nutraceutical and Functional Foods in Human Life and Disease Prevention*, D. Bagchi, H.G. Preuss, A. Swaroop (Eds.), pp. 343–358, CRC Press, Taylor and Francis, Boca Raton, Fl., 2015, Chapter 20.

4

Impact of Vitamins on Immunity

Abhijeet G. Parkhe[1], Khemchand R. Surana[2*], Eknath D. Ahire[3], Sunil K. Mahajan[4], Dhananjay M. Patil[5] and Deepak D. Sonawane[5]

[1]In Vivo Pharmacology Department, Glenmark Pharmaceutical Ltd., Navi Mumbai, Maharashtra, India
[2]Department of Pharmaceutical Chemistry, Shreeshakti Shaikshanik Sanstha, Divine College of Pharmacy, Satana, Nashik, India
[3]Department of Pharmaceutics, MET's Institute of Pharmacy, Adgaon, Nashik, India
[4]Department of Pharmaceutical Chemistry, MGV's Pharmacy College, Panchavati, Nashik, India
[5]Department of Pharmaceutics, Shreeshakti Shaikshanik Sanstha, Divine College of Pharmacy, Satana, Nashik, India

Abstract

Human beings were blessed with two kinds of immunity, born immunity and acquired immunity. As a multisystem organism, we have distinct functions to carry out for the duration of our life. We are not the simplest ones residing on earth; however, different microorganisms coexist with us in near proximity. In a manner, we are making a symbiotic relationship with the opposite microorganism. Sometimes those can become dominant species and might invade the human body. As we are blessed with our immune system, we are able to prevent them. In a contemporary situation, nutrients and minerals have played a considerable function in immunity booster within the COVID-19. Wuhan changed the origin of this deadly virus, which brought on a pandemic in 2020. Basically, COVID-19 virus attacks the immune system and turns on distinct inflammatory modulators, which seriously affect the human body. A scientific practitioner and a team of researchers observed that multivitamins and some micronutrients can assist to enhance the immune system. Vitamins, including A, B, C, D, K and micro vitamins together with zinc, sodium, potassium, and calcium, play a main function in

---

Corresponding author: khemchandsurana411@gmail.com

Eknath D. Ahire, Raj K. Keservani, Khemchand R. Surana, Sippy Singh and Rajesh K. Kesharwani (eds.) *Vitamins as Nutraceuticals: Recent Advances and Applications*, (87–106) © 2023 Scrivener Publishing LLC

such deadly diseases. In this chapter, we have focused at the function of nutrients within the immunity and immune associated diseases.

Keywords: Vitamins, immunity, autoimmune diseases, arthritis, psoriasis

4.1 Introduction

In the present day, internationally, we are prone to be multitaskers, however at the same time we are ignoring our health [1]. In this context, we would like to cite a few immune associated disorder names, which are rheumatoid arthritis, systemic lupus erythematosus, inflammatory bowel sicknesses, type 1diabetes mellitus, Guillain Barre syndrome, and psoriasis. Among all of the nutrients diet, A and D stay the maximum dependent on nutrients in terms of treating immune-related sicknesses within the essential time [2]. Rheumatoid arthritis is an autoimmune disorder and mainly impacts joints and reasons irritation of joints and thereby swelling. Some nutrients were studied within the beyond as effective treatment for the arthritis. Vitamins A, C, E, and D were examined and discovered

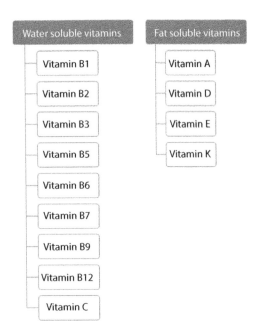

Figure 4.1 Classification of the fat-soluble and water-soluble vitamins.

to have good efficacy within the identical. Several researches have proven that this multivitamin therapy is helpful for the patients with arthritis [3]. Vitamin D and vitamin K are essential in bone strength, and vitamin K is concerned in cartilage structure formation. On the flip side, psoriasis nutrients are not the most effective manner to deal with psoriasis; there is no change manner to deal with it without traditional remedy. These sicknesses stated above are taken into consideration to be a very not unusual place within the elderly population [4]. Figure 4.1 indicates the classification of the fat-soluble and water-soluble vitamins.

4.2 Vitamin-Rich Foods for the Management of Immune System-Related Diseases

It is reported in the literature that the mentioned vitamins in Table 4.1 provide significant improvement in the immune system-related diseases. Some of them are easily available for common people, which significantly

Table 4.1 Specific vitamins have impact on the immune system-related diseases or auto-immune diseases and its food source.

Sr. no.	Vitamin	Food source	Disease	Reference
1	Vitamin A	Fish, meat, and dairy products	Psoriasis	[3]
2	Vitamin D	Fatty fish, dairy products, orange juice, cereals, beef liver, cheese and egg yolks	Auto-immune diseases example Psoriasis	[4–8]
3	Vitamin E	Sunflower seeds, Almonds, Mango, Avocado & Peanuts	Type 1 diabetes, Rheumatoid arthritis (RA), Psoriasis/psoriatic arthritis, Multiple sclerosis	[7–10]

(Continued)

Table 4.1 Specific vitamins have impact on the immune system-related diseases or auto-immune diseases and its food source. (*Continued*)

Sr. no.	Vitamin	Food source	Disease	Reference
4	Vitamin K	Green leafy vegetables, Soybean, Smaller amounts in meat, cheese & eggs	Rheumatoid arthritis & Systemic lupus erythematosus	[11–14]
5	Vitamin B1	Peas, fresh fruits, nuts & wholegrain breads	Rheumatoid arthritis & Psoriasis	[15, 16]
6	Vitamin B2	Milk and dairy products & dark-green vegetables	Multiple sclerosis & Systemic lupus erythematosus	[17, 18]
7	Vitamin B3	Whole grains, eggs, milk, nuts & avocados	Cancer & Multiple sclerosis	[19, 20]
8	Vitamin B5	Cereals, Mushrooms, Avocado, Nuts, seeds, dairy milk, yogurt, Potatoes, Eggs, Brown rice, Oats, & Broccoli	Lupus & Multiple sclerosis	[21, 22]
9	Vitamin B6	Fish, potatoes, vegetables, and fruit	Huntington disease, Lupus & Multiple sclerosis	[23, 24]

(*Continued*)

Table 4.1 Specific vitamins have impact on the immune system-related diseases or auto-immune diseases and its food source. (*Continued*)

Sr. no.	Vitamin	Food source	Disease	Reference
10	Vitamin B7	Cooked eggs, Salmon, Avocados, Beef liver, Pork, Sweet potato, & Nuts	Multiple sclerosis & Psoriasis	[25, 26]
11	Vitamin B9	Dark green leafy vegetables like spinach, Asparagus, broccoli, Beans, Whole grains, Sunflower seeds Peanuts, & Fresh fruits	Cytokine storm & Multiple sclerosis	[27, 28]
12	Vitamin B12	Fish, Meat, Milk, Eggs & Cheese	Autoimmune gastritis & Lupus	[29, 30]
13	Vitamin C	Citrus fruit, orange, Strawberries, sprouts, broccoli & potatoes.	Systemic lupus erythematosus & Multiple sclerosis	[31, 32]

impact the life of the patients with such immune system-related diseases. Immune system-related diseases are type 1 diabetes, inflammatory bowel disease, systemic lupus erythematosus (SLE), rheumatoid arthritis (RA), psoriasis/psoriatic arthritis, multiple sclerosis (MS), Graves' disease, and Addison's disease [5, 6]. Figure 4.2 indicates the role of vitamins in the immune system-related diseases.

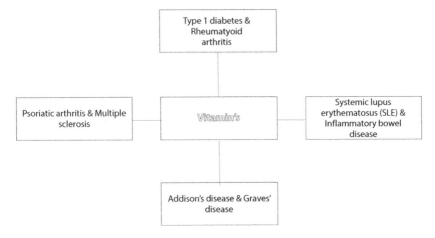

Figure 4.2 Role of vitamins in the immune system-related diseases.

4.3 Fat-Soluble Vitamins Reported in the Literature Commonly Used in the Treatment of the Immune System-Related Diseases

According to the literature, here are a few lists of the fat-soluble nutrients definitely studied for the remedy of the system-related illness and their effect at the immune system [7].

4.3.1 Vitamin A

Nerve fiber cells, the microbe-sensing alarms of the immune system, will channelize a "red alert" to stimulate immunity, or a "calm down" message that tones down immoderate immunity that can damage the host. The "calm down" message uses axerophthol, imparting an evidence for the link among vitamin A deficiency and reaction diseases. Microorganism and viruses that purpose continual infections, reminiscent of tuberculosis, viral hepatitis and HIV, might also additionally have developed methods that skew this stability of signals of their favor [8]. Nerve fiber cells, the microbe sensing indicator of the immune system, will channelize a "red alert" to stimulate immunity, or a "calm down" message that tones down immoderate immunity which can damage the host. The "calm down" message uses vitamin imparting an evidence for the link among vitamin A deficiency and reaction diseases. Microorganism and viruses that cause continual infections, resembling tuberculosis, viral hepatitis and HIV, might also additionally have developed techniques that skew this stability of alerts of their favor. The consequences of zymosan and TLR2 will deter white blood cells from assaultive worried tissue in a very mouse version of multiple sclerosis, the authors found. In the version, mice are immunized in opposition to myelin, that forms a defensive sheath round nerves. Injecting the mice with zymosan at an equivalent time as immunization decreased the damage to their nerves [9].

4.3.2 Vitamin D

Vitamin D at once and circuitously regulates the differentiation, activation of CD4+ T-lymphocytes and might save you the improvement of autoimmune processes. Dendritic cells (DC) are expert antigen-providing cells (APC), which have vital function within the initiation and renovation of T cell–based immune responses. *In vitro* 1, 25(OH)2D3 nutrition inhibits the differentiation of monocytes to DC, consequently reduces the variety of those expert APC to stimulate T cells. D3 will increase the extent of acid phosphatase and augments oxidative burst. Moreover, 1, 25(OH)2D3 intensifies the antimicrobial peptide interest in human monocytes, neutrophils and different cell lines. Endogenous antibiotics, inclusive of defensin and cathelicidin, have direct microbe-detrimental function. Cathelicidin, as an antimicrobial peptide, may even damage the intracellular mycobacterium [10]. Besides neutrophils and macrophages, herbal killer cells and epithelial cells of the respiration machine are able to secrete antimicrobial peptides and feature a pivotal function within the defence mechanism in opposition to airborne pathogens. The impact of nutrition D is in reference to the stimulation of those antimicrobial proteins and UVB radiation, which induces the manufacturing of the nutrition. D3 will increase the extent of acid phosphatase and augments oxidative burst. Moreover, 1, 25(OH)2D3 intensifies the antimicrobial peptide interest in human monocytes, neutrophils and different cell lines [11]. Endogenous antibiotics, inclusive of defensin and cathelicidin, have direct microbe-detrimental function. Cathelicidin, as an antimicrobial peptide, may even damage the intracellular mycobacterium. Besides neutrophils and macrophages, herbal killer cells and epithelial cells of the respiration machine are able to secrete antimicrobial peptides and feature a pivotal function within the defence mechanism in opposition to airborne pathogens. The impact of nutrition D is in reference to the stimulation of those antimicrobial proteins and UVB radiation, which induces the manufacturing of the nutrition [12]. The significance of comparing serum degrees of nutrition D in those sufferers wishes in addition potential research, however, can be envisaged as a probable destiny biomarker contributing to the evaluation of ailment interest and development in those diseases [13]. Vitamin D remedy has the capacity to lessen the transition to a well-described systemic autoimmune ailment in sufferers with undifferentiated connective tissue ailment, or as a minimum slows down the progress. We accept as true with that via way of means of coming across new elements of the immune-suppressive results of vitamin D within the local and adaptive immune machine, a potential, new utility of the nutrition might be advanced in future remedy regime of autoimmune diseases [14].

4.3.3 Vitamin E

The impact of vitamin E at the immune system is reportedly associated with its functionality within the stimulation of the protection mechanism thru antioxidant activity. The modern literature is suggestive of a relationship among nutrition E deficiency and rheumatic sicknesses [15]. Accordingly, there are numerous research investigating rheumatologic conditions, consisting of rheumatoid arthritis (RA), systemic lupus erythematosus (SLE), Sjögren syndrome, Behçet's disorder, celiac disorder, inflammatory bowel sicknesses (IBD), and systemic sclerosis (i.e., scleroderma), on this regard. In view of the stated research, nutrition E become counseled as an extrinsic issue able to affecting autoimmune sicknesses [16]. Almost all of the reviewed articles within the present literature confirmed an affiliation among the serum stages of vitamin E and autoimmune sicknesses. According to the effects of the reviewed research, autoimmune sicknesses, like scleroderma and SLE, might be correctly managed with the aid of using nutrition E management. Nevertheless, the modern to be had statistics approximately such autoimmune sicknesses do now no longer specify whether or not nutrition E deficiency is the reason of the disorder or its consequence [17]. Therefore, similarly research is required to deal with the mechanisms with the aid of using which vitamin E popularity impacts autoimmunity in every autoimmune disorder. In addition, it is far crucial to behavior massive epidemiological research on this regard. Nonetheless, the proof supplied right here indicated the useful results of vitamin E management on autoimmune sicknesses, specifically the amelioration of inflammatory reactions [18]. Furthermore, given the truth that vitamin E is liable for stopping in opposition to lipid peroxidation, which contributes to the etiology of autoimmune sicknesses, nutritional consumption of vitamin E might be used as a critical issue for the control of autoimmune sicknesses and their progress [19].

4.4 Water Soluble Vitamins Reported in the Literature Commonly Used in the Treatment of the Immune System-Related Diseases

4.4.1 Vitamin B1

Madden's treatment resulted from a maximum complete research of a few 259 instances of psoriasis. He divided those into small companies and dealt with every institution with the aid of using a extraordinary method, making use of the following: vitamin B1, vitamin B2, vitamin B entire complex, brewers' yeast, vitamin C, oestrogenic substances, sulphanilamide, bismuth salicylate in oil, anterior pituitary extract, adrenal cortex extract, low-fat weight loss plan with vitamin B1, low-fat weight loss plan and liver extract, low-fat diet with vitamin B, and anterior pituitary extract, and low-fat weight loss plan with vitamin B, anterior pituitary extract, and adrenal cortex extract. Authors arrived at a belief that the satisfactory effects have been received with a low-fats weight loss plan plus 1,000 global devices of vitamin B1 day by day with the aid of using mouth, blended with an exfoliating ointment. Madden, however, says he realizes that now no longer all instances will reply to this remedy [20, 21]. An aggregate of psoralen taken orally and UV irradiation (UVA) 2 h later reasons that a phototoxic response is beneficial. Long wave UV is received from solar lamps. Methotraxate. This cytotoxic, folic acid antagonist is used to retard the epidermal cell turnover charge with the aid of using blockading the synthesis of DNA. Methotraxate may be given orally, intramuscularly or intravenously, consistent with requirements. Retinoic Acid. In excessive instances fragrant retinoids are used with sizable benefit. Unfortunately, aspect consequences may be excessive, and consist of cheilitis, xerosis, facial dermatitis and hair loss. The drug is teratogenic and ought to know no longer accept in pregnancy. Peritoneal dialysis and hemodialysis were powerful within the remedy of psoriasis; nonetheless, taken into consideration heroic methods. Physicians on occasion prescribe diet arrangements as lesser adjuncts [22, 23]. One hundred and twelve sufferers have been dealt with from October 1937 to October 1939 with vitamin D, vitamin B1, vitamin B complex, brewers' yeast, vitamin C, liver extract, diluted hydrochloric acid, estrogenic substance, sulfanilamide, bismuth salicylate, anterior pituitary extract or adrenal cortex extract on my own or in aggregate with each other or in aggregate with a low fats weight loss plan. All the sufferers have been ambulatory, a few obtained numerous sorts of remedy, and simplest people with specific medical and microscopic psoriasis have been studied within the literature. The sufferers have began out at the sort of remedy getting used after they have been first examined. If an alternate becomes disregarded within, the psoriasis after a sure time had elapsed. At the identical time the affected person takes 1,000 devices of vitamin B, with the aid of using mouth day by day. In a few instances, the ointment is so eliminated with the aid of using motion in mattress at night time that it needs to be reapplied within the morning earlier than going to the radiation department. In different instances wherein there are specifically thickened lesions I upload 20 to 30 grains of salicylic acid to the tar ointment and endorse the affected person to clean off the scales with a stiff brush or with the aid of using pumice stone. The ointment is reapplied after this exfoliating remedy, after which the radiation remedy is achieved as above [24–27].

4.4.2 Vitamin B2

Riboflavin, additionally called vitamin B2, is a micronutrient with a key function in retaining human health. It has additionally been proven to enhance host resistance to bacterial infections in mice. The purpose of this observation is to evaluate the function of vitamin B2 remedy in inflammatory conditions. Three fashions of inflammatory states have been assessed. One of them encompasses neutrophil mediated however T cell/macrophage independent cutaneous inflammation. Another one is behind a scheduled kind allergic reaction response (DTH), a T cell/macrophage structured, however, neutrophil unbiased inflammatory response. The 1/3 is collagen-triggered arthritis, having additives from each of the above-defined reactions. Mice have been handled with vitamin B2, administered through peritoneal injections, for the duration of the direction of the experiments. The granulocyte structured response to olive oil became drastically decreased in nutrition B2-handled mice. In contrast, DTH reactivity and collagen II arthritis have been now no longer laid low with the remedy [28–32]. It is with apprehension that one reviews any new shape of remedy for psoriasis. However, the consequences with a brand new shape of riboflavin have been so encouraging in a confined range of instances that this initial file is issued. Relatively latest discoveries at the mode of motion of riboflavin have cautioned its use in a number of the scaly pores and skin sicknesses of a person. B2 deficiency in monkeys every now and then consequences in the advent of a scaly dermatitis in guy eruptions of this kind also are related to the B2 deficiency state, leading one to wonder whether or not any of the not unusual place maculo- or papulo-squamous eruptions are associated with abnormalities of riboflavin metabolism.

Rheumatoid arthritis (RA) is an autoimmune inflammatory disorder. Highly reactive oxygen unfastened radicals are believed to be worried within the pathogenesis of the sickness. RA sufferers have been subgrouped relying on the presence or absence of rheumatoid factor, sickness interest rating, and sickness duration. RA patients and wholesome controls have been evaluated for the oxidant-antioxidant popularity through tracking ROS production, biomarkers of lipid peroxidation, protein oxidation, and DNA harm. The degree of diverse enzymatic and nonenzymatic antioxidants became additionally monitored. Rheumatoid arthritis (RA) is an autoimmune inflammatory disorder. Highly reactive oxygen unfastened radicals are believed to be worried within the pathogenesis of the sickness. In this observation, RA sufferers have been subgrouped relying on the presence or absence of rheumatoid factor, sickness interest rating and sickness duration. RA patients and wholesome controls [33, 34] have been evaluated for the oxidant-antioxidant popularity through tracking ROS production, biomarkers of lipid peroxidation, protein oxidation, and DNA harm. The degree of diverse enzymatic and nonenzymatic antioxidants became additionally monitored. RA sufferers confirmed a marked growth in ROS formation, lipid peroxidation, protein oxidation, DNA harm and reduce within the interest of antioxidant defence system main to oxidative strain which can also additionally make a contribution to tissue harm and subsequently to the chronicity of the sickness [35–38].

4.4.3 Vitamin B3

Damage to the medullary sheath (demyelination) is one in all the principal manifestations of one pathology (MS). Interestingly, every MS and B complex deficiency evokes extreme myeline degeneration, main to loss in neural sign transmission. Deficiency in vitamin B sophisticated vary, even supposing not unusual place signs and symptoms comprises fatigue, extended aerophilic stress, infection and demyelination. In particular, cobalamin (cobalamin) has had extended interest for its performance within the methylation process, involvement in myelination and remyelination, and reversal of MS signs and symptoms [39–42].

Method: Here, we communicate the characteristic of nutrition B complex (B1, B2, B3, B4, B5, B6, B7, B9 and B12) in MS. The anti-inflammatory and remyelinating attributes of nutrition B complex people are promising, no matter confined medical studies. There is an urgent need for massive studies to determine the characteristic of nutrients B supplementation alone, or in mixture with one-of-a-kind recuperation agents, in prevention or reversal of MS, and useful resource in improved top notch of life of MS patients [43, 44].

4.4.4 Vitamin B6

The active form of vitamin B6, pyridoxal 5′-phosphate (PLP), serves as a co-element in extra than a hundred and fifty enzymatic reactions. Plasma PLP has constantly been showed to be low in inflammatory conditions; there can be a parallel cut price in liver PLP, however minor adjustments in erythrocyte and muscle PLP and in practical diet B6 biomarkers [45–48]. Plasma PLP furthermore predicts the hazard of persistent ailments like cardiovascular illness and a few cancers, and is inversely related to several inflammatory markers in scientific and population-primarily based totally absolutely studies. Vitamin B6 consumption and supplementation beautify a few immune features in vitamin B6-poor human beings and experimental animals. A viable mechanism worried is mobilization of vitamins B6 to the sites of infection in which it could function a co-issue in pathways generating metabolites with immunomodulating effects. Relevant vitamin B6-established inflammatory pathways embody vitamin B6 catabolism, the kynurenine pathway, sphingosine 1-phosphate metabolism, the trans-sulfuration pathway, and serine and glycine metabolism [49–52].

4.4.5 Vitamin B9

Amyotrophic lateral sclerosis (ALS) is an incurable persistent revolutionary neurodegenerative sickness with the revolutionary degeneration of motor neurons within the motor cortex and decrease motor neurons within the spinal wire and the mind stem. The etiology and pathogenesis of ALS are being actively studied; however, there is nevertheless no single concept. The observation of ALS chance elements can assist to apprehend the mechanism of this sickness improvement and, possibly, sluggish down the charge of its development in sufferers and additionally lessen the chance of its improvement in human beings with a predisposition closer to familial ALS [53–55]. The hobby of researchers and clinicians within the defensive position of vitamins within the improvement of ALS has been growing in current years. However, the position of a number of them is not always well understood or disputed. The goal of this observation is to investigate research at the position of vitamins as environmental elements affecting the chance of growing ALS and the charge of motor neuron degeneration development. Research, together with randomized scientific trials, scientific cases, and meta-analyses, regarding ALS sufferers and research on animal fashions of ALS [56, 57].

This bankruptcy established that the subsequent nutrients are the maximum tremendous protectors of ALS improvement: vitamin B12, vitamin E > vitamin C > vitamin B1, vitamin B9 > vitamin D > vitamin B2, vitamin B6 > vitamin A, and vitamin B7. In addition, observed outcomes suggest that the position of meals with an excessive content material of cholesterol, polyunsaturated fatty acids, urates, and purines performs a large component in ALS improvement. The inclusion of nutrients and a ketogenic weight-reduction plan in sickness-enhancing ALS remedy can lessen the development charge of motor neuron degeneration and sluggish the charge of sickness development; however the method to nutrient choice should be personalized. The roles of vitamins C, D, and B7 as ALS protectors want similarly observed [58–61].

4.4.6 Vitamin B12

Serum and cerebrospinal fluid vitamin B12 stages had been anticipated in 46 patients with more than one sclerosis and 23 patients with miscellaneous problems had been used as a manipulate group. No sizable distinction among more than one sclerosis and manipulated organizations may be determined both within the absolute values of serum or cerebrospinal fluid vitamin B12 and within the serum/cerebrospinal fluid ratio. There turned into a sizable correlation among serum and cerebrospinal fluid vitamin B12 stages, however, now no longer among vitamin B12 and protein concentrations in cerebrospinal fluid. Vitamin B12 binding in serum and cerebrospinal fluid is discussed. It was referred to some sufferers with more than one sclerosis on this and former reviews have abnormally low serum vitamin B12 stages despite the fact that this is not statistically considerable [62–67].

4.4.7 Vitamin C

Epidemiological research has cautioned an affiliation among vitamin C (and different antioxidant vitamins) and most cancer risks. However, the mechanisms accounting for prevention have now no longer been considerably investigated. In skin, vitamin C (ascorbic acid) exerts distinct organic roles, which include photoprotective consequences and participation in collagen synthesis. This paper reviews new findings, approximately extra features of the vitamin. Vitamin C counteracts oxidative pressure thru transcriptional and post-translational mechanisms; this modulation might also additionally intervene with the interest of redox-sensitive transcription factors, dedication to differentiation or cell cycle arrest, and apoptosis in reaction to DNA damage. All of those nutrition C-mediated responses are probably vital in distinct cell types, bearing in mind the protection of body homeostasis [68–70]. Defective DNA damage processing has been said in systemic lupus erythematosus (SLE). Vitamin C may moreover modulate formation/removal of the oxidative DNA lesion 8-oxo-2'-deoxyguanosine (8-oxodG). Baseline ranges of 8-oxodG measured in SLE serum, urine and PBMC DNA now no longer fluctuate appreciably from healthful subjects. In assessment to wholesome subjects, no extensive lower in PBMC 8-oxodG or growth in urinary 8-oxodG turned into in vitamin C supplemented SLE patients. A extensive, even though attenuated, growth in serum 8-oxodG turned into detected in SLE patients, as compared to healthful subjects [71–73].

4.5 Conclusion

Vitamins are an important component of the human diet. Humans need to take in a well-balanced diet or raw food needed to make such important vitamins consumed by the body. In this chapter, we made an effort to summarize all the important vitamins under one roof. Vitamins have a crucial impact on the human body and play a major role in daily life. We do not realize their importance until we face their deficiency. In this chapter, we tried to cover water-soluble vitamins and fat-soluble vitamins and their role in daily life functions. Also, we focused on the diseases involved in this matter. Some immune-related diseases were focused on and how vitamins can play a major role in the treatment of them. For example, psoriasis disease can be treated with medicines but if patients take vitamin D and E supplements with them, the patient can recover fast from the psoriasis disease. Vitamins have huge potential in the future as a nutraceutical in various diseases and long-term scope in immune-related conditions.

Acknowledgment

The authors thank MET's Institute of Pharmacy, BKC, which is affiliated with Savitribai Phule Pune University, Nashik. EDA wishes to express gratitude to the NFST/RGNF/UGC, Government of India, for providing financial assistance in the form of a fellowship (award no 202021-NFST-MAH-01235).

References

1. Kriegel, M.A., Manson, J.E., Costenbader, K.H., Does vitamin D affect risk of developing autoimmune disease?: A systematic review. *Semin. Arthritis Rheumatol.*, 40, 6, 512–531, 2011, June, WB Saunders.
2. Mora, J.R., Iwata, M., Von Andrian, U.H., Vitamin effects on the immune system: Vitamins A and D take centre stage. *Nat. Rev. Immunol.*, 8, 9, 685–698, 2008.
3. Girgis, C.M., Baldock, P.A., Downes, M., Vitamin D, muscle and bone: Integrating effects in development, aging and injury. *Mol. Cell. Endocrinol.*, 410, 3–10, 2015.
4. Cantorna, M.T., Vitamin D and autoimmunity: Is vitamin D status an environmental factor affecting autoimmune disease prevalence?(44485). *Proc. Soc. Exp. Biol. Med.*, 223, 3, 230–233, 2000.
5. Illescas-Montes, R., Melguizo-Rodríguez, L., Ruiz, C., Costela-Ruiz, V.J., Vitamin D and autoimmune diseases. *Life Sci.*, 233, 116744, 2019.
6. Adorini, L. and Penna, G., Control of autoimmune diseases by the vitamin D endocrine system. *Nat. Clin. Pract. Rheumatol.*, 4, 8, 404–412, 2008.
7. Rezaieyazdi, Z., Sahebari, M., Saadati, N., Khodashahi, M., Vitamin E and autoimmune diseases: A narrative review. *Rev. Clin. Med.*, 5, 2, 42–48, 2018.
8. Ayres Jr., S. and Mihan, R., Is vitamin E involved in the autoimmune mechanism? *Cutis*, 21, 3, 321–325, 1978.
9. Whittam, J., Jensen, C., Hudson, T., Alfalfa, vitamin E, and autoimmune disorders. *Am. J. Clin. Nutr.*, 62, 5, 1025–1026, 1995.
10. Ramadan, R., Tawdy, A., Hay, R.A., Rashed, L., Tawfik, D., The antioxidant role of paraoxonase 1 and vitamin E in three autoimmune diseases. *Skin Pharmacol. Physiol.*, 26, 1, 2–7, 2013.
11. Itzhaki Ben Zadok, O. and Eisen, A., Use of non-vitamin K oral anticoagulants in people with atrial fibrillation and diabetes mellitus. *Diabet. Med.*, 35, 5, 548–556, 2018.
12. Shishavan, N.G., Gargari, B.P., Kolahi, S., Hajialilo, M., Jafarabadi, M.A., Javadzadeh, Y., Effects of vitamin K on matrix metalloproteinase-3 and rheumatoid factor in women with rheumatoid arthritis: A randomized, double-blind, placebo-controlled trial. *J. Am. Coll. Nutr.*, 35, 5, 392–398, 2016.
13. Harrison, S.R., Li, D., Jeffery, L.E., Raza, K., Hewison, M., Vitamin D, autoimmune disease and rheumatoid arthritis. *Calcif. Tissue Int.*, 106, 1, 58–75, 2020.
14. Recarte-Pelz, P., Tàssies, D., Espinosa, G., Hurtado, B., Sala, N., Cervera, R., Reverter, J.C., de Frutos, P.G., Vitamin K-dependent proteins GAS6 and protein S and TAM receptors in patients of systemic lupus erythematosus: Correlation with common genetic variants and disease activity. *Arthritis Res. Ther.*, 15, 2, 1–9, 2013.

15. Riyapa, D., Rinchai, D., Muangsombut, V., Wuttinontananchai, C., Toufiq, M., Chaussabel, D., Ato, M., Blackwell, J.M., Korbsrisate, S., Transketolase and vitamin B1 influence on ROS-dependent neutrophil extracellular traps (NETs) formation. *PLoS One*, 14, 8, e0221016, 2019.
16. Blitshteyn, S., Vitamin B1 deficiency in patients with postural tachycardia syndrome (POTS). *Neurol. Res.*, 39, 8, 685–688, 2017.
17. Mikkelsen, K. and Apostolopoulos, V., Vitamin B1, B2, B3, B5, and B6 and the immune system, in: *Nutrition and Immunity*, pp. 115–125, Springer, Cham, 2019.
18. Kalarn, S.P. and Watson, R.R., Effects of B vitamins in patients with multiple sclerosis, in: *Nutrition and Lifestyle in Neurological Autoimmune Diseases*, pp. 261–265, Academic Press, US, 2017.
19. Cornell, L. and Arita, K., Water soluble vitamins: B1, B2, B3, and B6, in: *Geriatric Gastroenterology*, pp. 1–28, 2020.
20. Ortí, J.E.D.L.R., Cuerda-Ballester, M., Drehmer, E., Carrera-Juliá, S., Motos-Muñoz, M., Cunha-Pérez, C., Benlloch, M., López-Rodríguez, M.M., Vitamin B1 intake in multiple sclerosis patients and its impact on depression presence: A pilot study. *Nutrients*, 12, 9, 2655, 2020.
21. Zaringhalam, J., Akbari, A., Zali, A., Manaheji, H., Nazemian, V., Shadnoush, M., Ezzatpanah, S., Long-term treatment by vitamin B1 and reduction of serum proinflammatory cytokines, hyperalgesia, and paw edema in adjuvant-induced arthritis. *Basic Clin. Neurosci.*, 7, 4, 331, 2016.
22. Chiba, A., Murayama, G., Miyake, S., Mucosal-associated invariant T cells in autoimmune diseases. *Front. Immunol.*, 9, 1333, 2018.
23. Stene-Larsen, G., Mosvold, J., Ly, B., Selective vitamin B12 malabsorption in adult coeliac disease: Report on three cases with associated autoimmune diseases. *Scand. J. Gastroenterol.*, 23, 9, 1105–1108, 1988.
24. Theofylaktopoulou, D., Ulvik, A., Midttun, Ø., Ueland, P.M., Vollset, S.E., Nygård, O., Hustad, S., Tell, G.S., Eussen, S.J., Vitamins B2 and B6 as determinants of kynurenines and related markers of interferon-γ-mediated immune activation in the community-based hordaland health study. *Br. J. Nutr.*, 112, 7, 1065–1072, 2014.
25. Wang, Z., Long, H., Chang, C., Zhao, M., Lu, Q., Crosstalk between metabolism and epigenetic modifications in autoimmune diseases: A comprehensive overview. *Cell. Mol. Life Sci.*, 75, 18, 3353–3369, 2018.
26. Hajianfar, H., Mirmossayeb, O., Mollaghasemi, N., Nejad, V.S., Arab, A., Association between dietary inflammatory index and risk of demyelinating autoimmune diseases. *Int. J. Vitam. Nutr. Res.*, 92, 2022.
27. Zouali, M., DNA methylation signatures of autoimmune diseases in human B lymphocytes. *Clin. Immunol.*, 222, 108622, 2021.
28. Hill, L.J. and Williams, A.C., Meat intake and the dose of vitamin B3–nicotinamide: Cause of the causes of disease transitions, health divides, and health futures? *Int. J. Tryptophan Res.*, 10, 1178646917704662, 2017.

29. Nijhuis, L., van de Wetering, R., Houtzager, I., Lalmohamed, A., Vastert, S., van Loosdregt, J., SAT0031 vitamin B3 (nam) suppresses t cell activation in and production of pro-inflammatory cytokines *in vitro* in a dose dependent manner indicating therapeutic potential for the treatment of JIA. *Scientific Abstract*, 1080, 2019.
30. Nazarali, S. and Kuzel, P., Vitamin B derivative (nicotinamide) appears to reduce skin cancer risk. *Skin therapy letter*, 22, 1–4, 2017.
31. Prousky, J.E., Efficacy of vitamin B3 and its related coenzymes for the treatment of bell's palsy, huntington's disease, migraine and chronic tension-type headaches, multiple sclerosis, parkinson's disease, and tinnitus. *J. Orthomol. Med.*, 27, 2, 69–86, 2012.
32. Khanna-Gupta, A. and Berliner, N., Vitamin B3 boosts neutrophil counts. *Nat. Med.*, 15, 2, 139–141, 2009.
33. Penberthy, W.T., Pharmacological targeting of IDO-mediated tolerance for treating autoimmune disease. *Curr. Drug Metab.*, 8, 3, 245–266, 2007.
34. Freitas, L.M., Antunes, F.T.T., Obach, E.S., Correa, A.P., Wiiland, E., de Mello Feliciano, L., Reinicke, A., Amado, G.J.V., Grivicich, I., Fialho, M.F.P., Rebelo, I.N., Anti-inflammatory effects of a topical emulsion containing Helianthus annuus oil, glycerin, and vitamin B3 in mice. *J. Pharm. Investig.*, 51, 2, 223–232, 2021.
35. Brown, M.J., Ameer, M.A., Beier, K., *Vitamin B6 deficiency*, StatPearls Publishing, Treasure Island (FL), 2017.
36. Hemminger, A. and Wills, B.K., *Vitamin B6 toxicity*, StatPearls Publishing, Treasure Island (FL), 2020.
37. Rail, L.C. and Meydani, S.N., Vitamin B6 and immune competence. *Nutr. Rev.*, 51, 8, 217–225, 1993.
38. Cheng, C.H., Chang, S.J., Lee, B.J., Lin, K.L., Huang, Y.C., Vitamin B6 supplementation increases immune responses in critically ill patients. *Eur. J. Clin. Nutr.*, 60, 10, 1207–1213, 2006.
39. Chandra, R.K. and Sudhakaran, L., Regulation of immune responses by vitamin B6. *Ann. N. Y. Acad. Sci.*, 585, 1, 404–423, 1990.
40. Selhub, J., Byun, A., Liu, Z., Mason, J.B., Bronson, R.T., Crott, J.W., Dietary vitamin B6 intake modulates colonic inflammation in the IL10−/− model of inflammatory bowel disease. *J. Nutr. Biochem.*, 24, 12, 2138–2143, 2013.
41. Gheita, A.A., Gheita, T.A., Kenawy, S.A., The potential role of B5: A stitch in time and switch in cytokine. *Phytother. Res.*, 34, 2, 306–314, 2020.
42. Mikkelsen, K. and Apostolopoulos, V., Vitamin B1, B2, B3, B5, and B6 and the immune system, in: *Nutrition and Immunity*, pp. 115–125, Springer, Cham, 2019.
43. Mikkelsen, K., Stojanovska, L., Prakash, M., Apostolopoulos, V., The effects of vitamin B on the immune/cytokine network and their involvement in depression. *Maturitas*, 96, 58–71, 2017.

44. Debourdeau, P.M., Djezzar, S., Estival, J.L.F., Zammit, C.M., Richard, R.C., Castot, A.C., Life-threatening eosinophilic pleuropericardial effusion related to vitamins B5 and H. *Ann. Pharmacother.*, 35, 4, 424–426, 2001.
45. Yoshii, K., Hosomi, K., Sawane, K., Kunisawa, J., Metabolism of dietary and microbial vitamin B family in the regulation of host immunity. *Front. Nutr.*, 6, 48, 2019.
46. Kalarn, S.P. and Watson, R.R., Effects of B vitamins in patients with multiple sclerosis, in: *Nutrition and Lifestyle in Neurological Autoimmune Diseases*, pp. 261–265, Academic Press, US, 2017.
47. Kavian, N., Mehlal, S., Marut, W., Servettaz, A., Giessner, C., Bourges, C., Nicco, C., Chéreau, C., Lemaréchal, H., Dutilh, M.F., Cerles, O., Imbalance of the Vanin-1 pathway in systemic sclerosis. *J. Immunol.*, 197, 8, 3326–3335, 2016.
48. Evans, E., Piccio, L., Cross, A.H., Use of vitamins and dietary supplements by patients with multiple sclerosis: A review. *JAMA Neurol.*, 75, 8, 1013–1021, 2018.
49. He, W., Hu, S., Du, X., Wen, Q., Zhong, X.P., Zhou, X., Zhou, C., Xiong, W., Gao, Y., Zhang, S., Wang, R., Vitamin B5 reduces bacterial growth via regulating innate immunity and adaptive immunity in mice infected with Mycobacterium tuberculosis. *Front. Immunol.*, 9, 365, 2018.
50. Nemazannikova, N., Mikkelsen, K., Stojanovska, L., Blatch, G.L., Apostolopoulos, V., Is there a link between vitamin B and multiple sclerosis? *Med. Chem.*, 14, 2, 170–180, 2018.
51. Pape, K., Steffen, F., Zipp, F., Bittner, S., Supplementary medication in multiple sclerosis: Real-world experience and potential interference with neurofilament light chain measurement. *Mult. Scler. J.-Exp. Transl. Clin.*, 6, 3, 2055217320936318, 2020.
52. Agrawal, S., Agrawal, A., Said, H.M., Biotin deficiency enhances the inflammatory response of human dendritic cells. *Am. J. Physiol.-Cell Physiol.*, 311, 3, C386–C391, 2016.
53. Salomon, B., Lenschow, D.J., Rhee, L., Ashourian, N., Singh, B., Sharpe, A., Bluestone, J.A., B7/CD28 costimulation is essential for the homeostasis of the CD4+ CD25+ immunoregulatory T cells that control autoimmune diabetes. *Immunity*, 12, 4, 431–440, 2000.
54. Scott, W.C., Literature review of both classic and novel roles of biotin (Vitamin B7) in cellular processes. *UTSC's J. Nat. Sci.*, 1, 1, 45–51, 2020.
55. Windhagen, A., Newcombe, J., Dangond, F., Strand, C., Woodroofe, M.N., Cuzner, M.L., Hafler, D.A., Expression of costimulatory molecules B7-1 (CD80), B7-2 (CD86), and interleukin 12 cytokine in multiple sclerosis lesions. *J. Exp. Med.*, 182, 6, 1985–1996, 1995.
56. Miller, S.D., Vanderlugt, C.L., Lenschow, D.J., Pope, J.G., Karandikar, N.J., Dal Canto, M.C., Bluestone, J.A., Blockade of CD28/B7-1 interaction prevents epitope spreading and clinical relapses of murine EAE. *Immunity*, 3, 6, 739–745, 1995.

57. Shakya, A.K. and Nandakumar, K.S., Antigen-specific tolerization and targeted delivery as therapeutic strategies for autoimmune diseases. *Trends Biotechnol.*, 36, 7, 686–699, 2018.
58. Kunisawa, J., Hashimoto, E., Ishikawa, I., Kiyono, H., A pivotal role of vitamin B9 in the maintenance of regulatory T cells *in vitro* and *in vivo*. *PLoS One*, 7, 2, e32094, 2012.
59. Mansouri, R., Moogooei, M., Moogooei, M., Razavi, N., Mansourabadi, A.H., The role of vitamin D3 and vitamin B9 (Folic acid) in immune system. *Int. J. Epidemiol. Res.*, 3, 1, 69–85, 2016.
60. Kurniawan, H., Soriano-Baguet, L., Brenner, D., Regulatory T cell metabolism at the intersection between autoimmune diseases and cancer. *Eur. J. Immunol.*, 50, 11, 1626–1642, 2020.
61. Kalarn, S.P. and Watson, R.R., Effects of B vitamins in patients with multiple sclerosis, in: *Nutrition and Lifestyle in Neurological Autoimmune Diseases*, pp. 261–265, Academic Press, US, 2017.
62. Miceli, E., Lenti, M.V., Padula, D., Luinetti, O., Vattiato, C., Monti, C.M., Di Stefano, M., Corazza, G.R., Common features of patients with autoimmune atrophic gastritis. *Clin. Gastroenterol. Hepatol.*, 10, 7, 812–814, 2012.
63. Emamifar, A. and Hansen, I.M.J., The influence of thyroid diseases, diabetes mellitus, primary hyperparathyroidism, vitamin B12 deficiency and other comorbid autoimmune diseases on treatment outcome in patients with rheumatoid arthritis: An exploratory cohort study. *Medicine*, 97, 21, 777–780, 2018.
64. Morel, S., Georges, A., Bordenave, L., Corcuff, J.B., Thyroid and gastric autoimmune diseases. *Ann. Endocrinol.*, 70, 1, 55–58, 2009, March, Elsevier Masson.
65. Ness-Abramof, R., Nabriski, D.A., Shapiro, M.S., Shenkman, L., Shilo, L., Weiss, E., Reshef, T., Braverman, L.E., Prevalence and evaluation of B12 deficiency in patients with autoimmune thyroid disease. *Am. J. Med. Sci.*, 332, 3, 119–122, 2006.
66. Gonul, M., Cakmak, S., Soylu, S., Kilic, A., Gul, U., Serum vitamin B12, folate, ferritin and iron levels in Turkish patients with vitiligo. *Indian J. Dermatol. Venereol. Leprol.*, 76, 4, 448, 2010.
67. Dickey, W., Low serum vitamin B12 is common in coeliac disease and is not due to autoimmune gastritis. *Eur. J. Gastroenterol. Hepatol.*, 14, 4, 425–427, 2002.
68. Ahire, E.D., Sonawane, V.N., Surana, K.R., Talele, G.S., Drug discovery, drug-likeness screening, and bioavailability: Development of drug-likeness rule for natural products, in: *Applied Pharmaceutical Practice and Nutraceuticals*, pp. 191–208, Apple Academic Press, USA, 2021.
69. Surana, K.R., Ahire, E.D., Sonawane, V.N., Talele, S.G., Talele, G.S., Molecular modeling: Novel techniques in food and nutrition development, in: *Natural Food Products and Waste Recovery*, pp. 17–31, Apple Academic Press, USA, 2021.

70. Surana, K.R., Ahire, E.D., Sonawane, V.N., Talele, S.G., Biomolecular and molecular docking: A modern tool in drug discovery and virtual screening of natural products, in: *Applied Pharmaceutical Practice and Nutraceuticals*, pp. 209–223, Apple Academic Press, USA, 2021.
71. Kodama, M. and Kodama, T., Vitamin C and the genesis of autoimmune disease and allergy. *In Vivo (Athens, Greece)*, 9, 3, 231–238, 1995.
72. Babri, S., Mehrvash, F., Mohaddes, G., Hatami, H., Mirzaie, F., Effect of intrahippocampal administration of vitamin C and progesterone on learning in a model of multiple sclerosis in rats. *Adv. Pharm. Bull.*, 5, 1, 83, 2015.
73. Tam, L.S., Li, E.K., Leung, V.Y., Griffith, J.F., Benzie, I.F., Lim, P.L., Whitney, B., Lee, V.W., Lee, K.K., Thomas, G.N., Tomlinson, B., Effects of vitamins C and E on oxidative stress markers and endothelial function in patients with systemic lupus erythematosus: a double blind, placebo controlled pilot study. *J. Rheumatol.*, 32, 2, 275–282, 2005.

5
Nutraceuticals Potential of Fat-Soluble Vitamins

Jagannath Gaikwad[1], Shweta Jogdand[1], Afsar Pathan[2], Ashwini Mahajan[1]*, Anmol Darak[3], Eknath D. Ahire[4] and Khemchand R. Surana[5]

[1]Department of Drug Regulatory Affair, R.C. Patel Institute of Pharmaceutical Education and Research Shirpur, MH, India
[2]Department of Pharmacology, R.C. Patel Institute of Pharmaceutical Education and Research Shirpur, MH, India
[3]R.C. Patel Institute of Pharmaceutical Education and Research Shirpur, MH, India
[4]Department of Pharmaceutics, METs, Institute of Pharmacy, BKC, Adgaon, Affiliated to SPPU, Nashik, MH, India
[5]Department of Pharmaceutical Chemistry, SSS's Divine College of Pharmacy, Satana, Nashik, MH, India

Abstract

Nutraceuticals are the most common part of daily life. In the last few years, the use of nutraceuticals has increased drastically due to their cost effectiveness and minimal or no side effects. In the recent pandemic situation, the world is moving toward nutraceuticals, such as multivitamin tablets, Nutraceuticals is the combination of nutrition and pharmaceuticals that is categorized in three major parts as nutrients, dietary supplement and herbals. They can be used as food, as well as medicines; Vitamins are also comes under the class of Nutraceuticals as nutrients and classified into two categories as fat-soluble and water-soluble vitamins. Fat-soluble vitamins are further classified as vitamins A, D, E, and K. These vitamins are used in treatments of many diseases like cardiovascular (CVS), hemophilia, immunomodulatory, and immunity booster. We may use vitamins as nutraceuticals, which do not show the side effects as frequently as other medicines, and it is been founded that the vitamin has greater medicinal potential than synthetic drugs. It is our need to know deep about vitamins and their nutraceuticals potential, in this chapter, we are focused on fat-soluble vitamins and their potential as nutraceuticals.

Corresponding author: abmahajan9@gmail.com

Eknath D. Ahire, Raj K. Keservani, Khemchand R. Surana, Sippy Singh and Rajesh K. Kesharwani (eds.) *Vitamins as Nutraceuticals: Recent Advances and Applications*, (107–128) © 2023 Scrivener Publishing LLC

Keywords: Nutraceuticals, vitamins, dietary supplements, nutrients, nutrition, anti-oxidants, dietary fibers

5.1 Introduction

Every single person absolutely needs to have an immune system that is robust and well developed in order to survive. There is a significant and positive correlation between adequate intakes of vitamins and trace elements and the physiology of the immune system. The maintenance of a well-functioning immune system is dependent on maintaining a balanced diet that includes the consistent consumption of vitamins, minerals, and trace elements. Since vitamins can affect and strengthen the immune system, it is important that we get enough of these nutrients at each of our three daily meals [1]. Albert Szent statement Gyorgyi's encapsulates the effect of vitamins on the body's key organs, particularly the immune system. Vitamins (vital amines) are chemical molecules that must be consumed in trace amounts since they are not generated at significant levels by the body [2]. Nutraceuticals are substances that became more popular in the early years, since they have been recognised as very beneficial to the human race. Nutraceuticals are classified into three major parts: nutrients; herbals; and dietary supplements. Vitamins, which show nutraceuticals properties, are gaining more and more attention in the medicinal market. They are reliable and effective components and have been used in many disease treatments as well. Vitamins are also categorized into two parts: water-soluble vitamins and fat-soluble vitamins. In this chapter, the potential properties of fat-soluble vitamins as nutraceuticals have been enlightened.

Definition
Nutraceuticals are defined as any substance that is food and provides medical or health benefits, including the prevention and treatment of disease.

Nutritional Supplements
Nutraceuticals help to treat and prevent almost any disease. It is derived from the merging of the terms nutrition and pharmaceutical [3]. Medical foods, nutritional supplements, and dietary supplements are all terms used to describe them. The father of medicine, Hippocrates, recognized the link between diet and health 2500 years ago. According to him, eating the appropriate foods may protect one's health against illnesses [4]. These are foods that have health advantages, such as minimizing the risk of chronic diseases and providing basic nutrition [5]. As a result, the term "nutraceuticals" was coined 20 years ago to describe a mix of nutrition and

pharmaceutics, both of which are vital to human health. In the previous 20 years, 87 scholarly articles have been published on so-called functional foods and Nutraceuticals [6]. Unlike pharmaceuticals, nutraceuticals are chemicals that are not often covered by patents. Although both pharmaceutical and nutraceuticals chemicals can be used to cure or prevent diseases, the government only approves pharmaceutical substances [7]. A dietary supplement is a substance that includes or carries one or more of the nutrients listed below: a concentration, metabolite, component, extract, or a mix of these substances for usage by humans to supplement their diet by escalating total daily consumption. Nutraceuticals are dietary supplements that provide health advantages, as well as nutrition. Prominent nutraceuticals comprise ginseng, Echinacea, green tea, glucosamine, omega-3, lutein, folic acid, and cod liver oil. The vast majority of nutraceuticals have an impressive array of therapeutic effects.

5.1.1 Categories of Nutraceuticals

These are divided into three major categories (Figure 5.1).

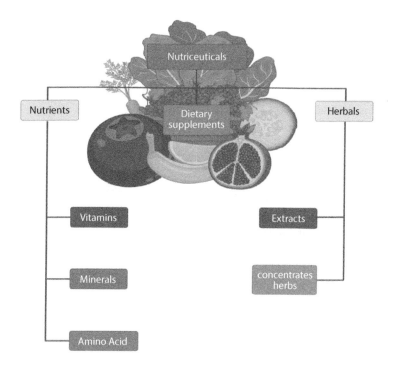

Figure 5.1 Classification of nutraceuticals.

a) **Nutrients:** vitamins, minerals, amino acids, and fatty acids are examples of substances having proven nutritional properties. Antioxidants, water, and fat-soluble vitamins are the most well-known nutrients. Antioxidant supplementation or dietary intake has been related to several potential advantages. High nutritional intake of vitamin E may prevent Parkinson's disease. Vitamin E, C, and beta carotene in combination have been have been demonstrated to reduce low-density lipoprotein oxidation and atherosclerosis [7].

b) **Herbals:** Extracts and concentrates herbs or botanical substances.

c) **Dietary supplements:** Reagents obtained from different sources (for example, pyruvate, chondroitin sulfate, and steroid hormone precursors) that are utilized in sports nutrition, weight-loss supplements, and meal replacements [7].

5.1.2 Vitamins

"Vitamins are organic compounds that are required in small amounts with our regular diet to carry out certain biological functions and for the maintenance of our metabolism" [8]. Vitamins are little amounts of nutrients that the body requires to function and stay healthy. It can be found in plant and animal foods, also in dietary supplements. Some vitamins are synthesized in the human body from diet. There are two types of solubility for vitamins: fat and water. When there is an excess of fat-soluble vitamins in the body, those vitamins are stored in the body's fatty tissue, while any excess of water-soluble vitamins is eliminated through the urine. Some vitamins that are fat-soluble are vitamin A, vitamin D, and vitamin E [8]. Vitamins, which aid in the development and efficient functioning of your body, Vitamins A, D, E, and K, together with the B vitamins (thiamine, riboflavin, niacin, pantothenic acid, biotin, and folate) all contribute to the proper nutrition of the body [9].

Vitamins Divide into two types:

1) Fat-soluble vitamins
2) Water-soluble vitamins

A, D, E, and K are fat-soluble vitamins that dissolve in fat and are then stored in the body. C and B complex are examples of water-soluble vitamins that dissolve in water before being absorbed by the body and hence cannot be stored. To avoid shortages or inadequacies in the body, they must be consumed regularly [9, 10].

5.1.2.1 Fat-Soluble Vitamins

Vitamins that are soluble in fat are necessary for a wide variety of bodily functions, including vision, bone health, immune function, and blood coagulation, among others. Vitamin A, D, E, and K are the four types (Table 5.1) of fat-soluble vitamins [11].

Sources of Vitamin A
Egg yolks, milk, liver, cheese, and butter are all rich sources of vitamin A. Vitamin A is derived from plants in the form of carotenoids, which are then converted to retinol during the digestive process. Vitamin A is abundant in dark green leafy vegetables (spinach, amaranth, and others), carrots, squash, yellow maize, mangoes, and papayas. Mangoes and papayas also contain a good amount of vitamin A [12].

Sources of Vitamin D
D2 and D3 are the most common types of vitamin D. Certain foods, such as salmon, tuna, and mackerel, contain vitamin D2 (ergocalciferol). Beef liver, cheese, and egg yolks have smaller amounts. Vitamin D is added to natural milk in many countries, This is a method used to reduce the incidence of rickets and osteomalacia. Vitamin D3 (cholecalciferol) is produced in the skin as a result of sun exposure, earning it the nickname "sunshine vitamin" [13].

Sources of Vitamin E
A-tocopherol is the most common type of vitamin E. Other tocopherols and tocotrienols, such as the alpha, gamma, beta, and delta forms, are also in circulation. Vitamin E can be found in vegetable oils, seeds, nuts, and whole grains [14].

Sources of Vitamin K
K1 and K2 are the two major types of vitamin K. Green leafy vegetables, cabbage, and cauliflower all contain vitamin K1 (phylloquinone). Fish, meat, and some fruits contain smaller amounts, vitamin K2 is produced by the gut bacteria (menaquinone) [15].

Functions
Vitamin A is a big part of all-trans retinoic acid, which is a nuclear hormone that forms heterodimers with retinoic acid receptors (RAR) in the nucleus. This is important for the growth and differentiation of epithelial cells in the eyes, salivary glands, and genitourinary tract. RAR-retinoid X receptor

Table 5.1 Fat-soluble vitamins and their health benefit.

Fat-soluble vitamins

Vitamin	Structure	Sources	Health benefits
A (retinol)	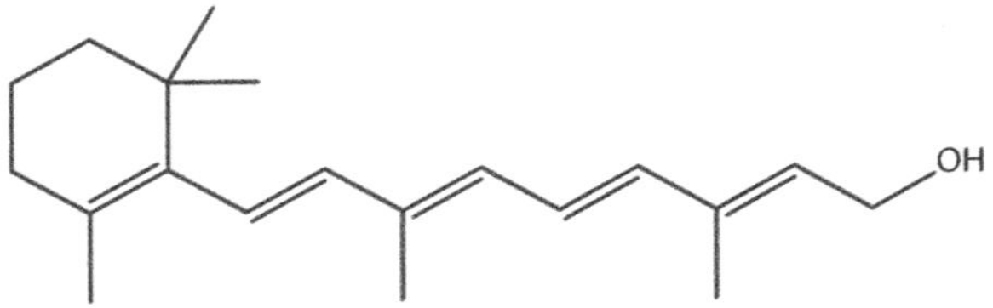	Liver, fish, eggs, fortified milk, dark green, yellow-orange vegetables	Essential nutrients for development and growth. Antioxidants help keep your eyes, skin, and mucous membranes healthy. They also help prevent some cancers and skin conditions and treat some of them.

(*Continued*)

Table 5.1 Fat-soluble vitamins and their health benefit. (*Continued*)

Fat-soluble vitamins

Vitamin	Structure	Sources	Health benefits
D (calcitriol)		Sunlight, fatty fish, fortified	Helps the body absorb and utilize calcium and is necessary for bone and tooth growth.
E (alpha-tocopherol)		Asparagus, almonds, peanuts, salad dressing	The antioxidant aids in the formation of blood cells, muscles, lung, and nerve tissue, as well as strengthen the immune system.

(*Continued*)

Table 5.1 Fat-soluble vitamins and their health benefit. (*Continued*)

Fat-soluble vitamins

Vitamin	Structure	Sources	Health benefits
K (phylloquinone)	*[Chemical structure of phylloquinone with CH₃ group]*	Green leafy vegetables, broccoli, peas, green beans, bacteria in colon	It is crucial for blood clotting.

heterodimers function as transcription factors by binding to specific regions in gene promoters. Throughout the body, these genes encode essential structural proteins, extracellular matrix proteins, and enzymes. Retinal, a vitamin A component, gets its name from its capacity to create rhodopsin in the retina, which aids vision in low-light situations. In response to immunological stimuli, vitamin A also promotes T-lymphocyte differentiation and B-lymphocyte activation [16]. Retinol and similar substances that demonstrate retinol's biological activity are referred to as vitamin A. Retinol, retinoic acid, and retinal are the most widespread forms of vitamin A, while retinyl palmitate is the most common liver storage form [17].

The major purpose of vitamin D is to boost plasma levels of calcium and phosphate, which, in turn, helps in the mineralization of osteoid in the bone. This is accomplished by the vitamin's ability to bind to calcium and phosphate. The ability to cause an increase in calcium levels is essential for the proper functioning of neuromuscular junctions, neuronal transmission, and hormone secretion and action. Both vitamin D3 as from skin and vitamin D2 from the nutrition are considered to be prohormones. The enzyme 25-hydroxylase in the liver is responsible for converting these prohormones into 25-hydroxycholecalciferol. The kidney converts 25-hydroxycholecalciferol to 1, 25-dihydroxycholecalciferol, which is the physiologically active form. 1-a-Hydroxylase, an enzyme tightly regulated by parathyroid hormone, converts water into a physiologically active form in the kidney.

The active form of vitamin D works to improve calcium and phosphate uptake in the duodenum and also calcium intestinal absorption from the distal convoluted tubule. This is accomplished by increasing the activity of calcium transporters, which are responsible for transporting calcium across epithelial cells. Vitamin D triggers osteoclasts, which are bone-resorbing cells in our bodies. Bone production and resorption are in balance in the human body. Some bone resorption is required to successfully mineralize bone [18]. Vitamin D is a prohormones that has been linked to a variety of diseases, both directly and indirectly [19].

Vitamin E is best known for its antioxidant properties and can only be derived from the diet. During fat oxidation, vitamin E prevents the formation of reactive oxygen species. It protects polyunsaturated fatty acids in cell membranes against oxidative degradation, allowing them to remain fluid and stable. Supplementation has not resulted in a decrease in cardiovascular events, even though it reduces lipid peroxidation, particularly LDL oxidation [20]. Vitamin E is necessary for the correct shape of erythrocytes and is hypothesized to take part in the role of reducing the aging process since it is required for the removal of reactive oxygen species (ROS), which are responsible for cell death [21]. Furthermore, because this

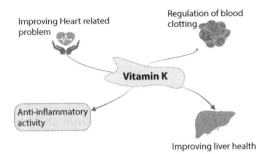

Figure 5.2 Function of vitamin K.

vitamin suppresses platelet aggregation, it may protect against atherosclerosis and cardiovascular disease [22, 23]. It has also been suggested that vitamin E has a protective role against arthritis, cataracts, neurological disease, and immunological disorders [21, 24].

Vitamin K is required for the activation of clotting factors in the liver (Figure 5.2) which is involved in coagulation. The clotting proteins must bind calcium to activate. Certain glutamic acid residues are gamma-carboxylated by vitamin K, allowing the proteins to bind calcium and carry out the coagulation cascade. Vitamin K is a cofactor for gamma-glutamyl carboxylase, which catalyzes the formation of gamma-carboxy-glutamyl residues after translation. Prothrombin, factors VII, IX, X, protein C, and S are all activated during this process. These carboxylation processes are powered by the oxidation of vitamin K hydroquinone. Vitamin K epoxide reductase and vitamin K quinone reductase are required for the regeneration of vitamin K hydroquinone [13], as shown in Figure 5.2.

5.1.2.2 Fat-Soluble Vitamins in Covid-19

In the year 2020, coronavirus is expected to be the primary agent responsible for lung infections and deaths. In the meantime, there is much controversy surrounding the identification of the factors that influence an improvement in therapeutic performance and a strengthening of the immune system [25].

Vitamin A: is still very important since it can help guard against life-threatening consequences and infections like malaria, HIV, and lung diseases [26]. This keeps vitamin A at the top of the list of priorities. Impact of vitamin A to COVID-19 infection has been more evident in its action against the infectious bronchitis virus (IBV), vitamin A is envisioned to be a potential choice in addressing the COVID-19 pandemic by suppressing lung infections.

Vitamin D: Vitamin D has multiple activities, including involvement with nonspecific defensive systems, activation of Toll-like receptors, and/or an increase in cathelicidins and -defensins levels. This affects acquired immunity by lowering the amount of immunoglobulin made by plasma cells and the amount of proinflammatory cytokines made [27]. It is possible that the protective effect that vitamin D has against the SARS-CoV-2 infection is related to the effect that it has had in the past on other respiratory infections. This theory received additional backing from a metaanalysis that provided clear evidence that vitamin D consumption is effective in the treatment of acute respiratory tract infections [28].

Vitamin E: Because of immunosenescence, elderly people with severe diabetes, cardiovascular diseases, cancer, and other diseases such as these are more likely to become infected with COVID-19 [29]. Administration of vitamin E to older individuals is likely to improve immunological function, which enhances the likelihood of infection resistance and decreases infection-related mortality. Multiple investigations into the potential advantages of vitamin E for COVID-19 patients suggested that a combination of vitamin E and vitamin C might be an effective antioxidant medication for the cardiac complications of COVID-19 [30].

5.1.2.3 Properties of Fat-Soluble Vitamins (Potential)

Vitamin A

Vitamin A is a vital nutrient that our systems cannot create and must be obtained through our diet. The first vitamin to be given an official name was vitamin A [31]. It is fat-soluble, which means it is kept in the body and accumulates to lethal levels when consumed in large amounts. It is a group of retinoid compounds that comprise retinol, retinal, retinoic acid, and numerous provitamins A carotenoids, as well as beta-carotene, which has all-trans retinol's biologic activity [32]. According to Green and Mellan by in 1928, although vitamin A was then acknowledged as a growth-promoting vitamin, data from the animal study revealed it was an anti-infective vitamin. Four years later, Ellison published the results of a controlled trial involving 600 hospitalized English children with measles, which revealed that cod liver oil lowered mortality by 58%. However, vitamin A's potential anti-infective properties were overshadowed by its significance in preventing xerophthalmic blindness, which occurred around the same time as antibiotics were discovered. Vitamin A can be present in a wide range of foods. Vitamin A is essential for many functions, including vision, embryonic development and reproduction, bone metabolism, hematopoiesis, skin and cellular health, immunity, gene transcription, and antioxidant activity. Vitamin A also plays a role in hematopoiesis [33]. Vitamin A is an anti-inflammatory vitamin that inhibits apoptosis and helps to preserve the mucosal lining of the gastrointestinal and respiratory tracts. Vitamin A is essential for normal metabolism and immune function. It has pleiotropic benefits that range from a variety of physiological functions in preserving our system's vital biological needs to a well-known truth in improving eyesight. Because of its critical role in supporting the immune system's response, vitamin A is also known as an anti-inflammatory vitamin [34]. Vitamin A is primarily used to treat dermatological disease and lesions (due to keratin synthesis and mucous secretion suppression), xerophthalmia, cold, warts, corns, and calluses (skin infections), acne, psoriasis, and persistent follicular hyperkeratosis of the arms, night blindness, breast cancer, and vision [35]. Through surface IgA, T helper cell regulation, and the production of cytokines, it regulates humoral and cell-mediated immunity. A has been extensively studied as part of the possible supporting therapy for preventing the incidence of acute lower respiratory tract infections (ALRTIs), as well as decreasing the severity and speeding up recovery. Other synthetic retinoids, such as retinamide or fenretinide, have been found to be quite successful in breast, prostate, and ovarian carcinoma, with minimal toxicity in humans [36]. One of the most researched nutrients for the immune function is vitamin A. It is a reliable antioxidant for cancer prevention, particularly in the treatment of skin cancer and lung cancer. It also aids in the avoidance of other diseases. Males should consume 900 g per day, while ladies should consume 700 g/day. Although vitamin A is essential for our bodies, it can have several acute and chronic side effects. Vitamin A insufficiency results in abdominal pain, vomiting, migraine headaches, lethargy, dermatitis, patchy hair loss, edema, anaemia, respiratory tract infection, and chronic liver disease [31].

Vitamin D
Vitamin D is a fat-soluble vitamin, belongs to the secosteroids family. Vitamin D's key activities in humans include calcium, iron, magnesium, phosphate, and zinc absorption. Because vitamin D acquired from sunshine is physiologically inert, its activation requires enzymatic conversion in the liver and kidney. Vitamin D is divided into two types: vitamin D2 (ergocalciferol) and vitamin D3 (cholecalciferol) (cholecalciferol) [37]. Recent studies indicate that low serum concentrations of vitamin D are associated with prevalent AD, dementia, and cognitive impairment. Deficiency in vitamin D has also been linked to vascular dysfunction, ischemic stroke risk, brain shrinkage, and putative anti-inflammatory activity. Vitamin D is a steroid hormone and immune system modifier that decreases the levels of cytokines and boosts macrophage activity. It also makes the natural

killer cells, monocytes, neutrophils, and respiratory epithelial cells make more antimicrobial peptides (AMPs) [33]. Vitamin D has multiple effects, including the suppression of infection and the enhancement of the body's natural defenses against pathogens. There is some evidence from a few trials that vitamin D supplementation may play a role in reducing infections in the upper respiratory tract [38]. In addition to this, it reduces the expression of cytokines and transforms growth factor beta (TGF-b), both of which have the effect of favorably attenuating virus-induced pathological cellular processes [39]. However, in spite of these limitations, the research demonstrates that vitamin D (increased IL-1bin cell culture) is an indispensable component in the process of warding off viral infections. Moreover, the findings have not been validated in clinical settings. According to the findings of the study, maintaining serum 25-hydroxy vitamin D levels in the range of >50 to 80 ng/ml may be beneficial in reducing morbidity caused by COVID-19. Research is limited to laboratory scale, is not established clinically, and shows that vitamin D (increased IL-1bin cell culture) plays an essential role in fighting viral infections. The study suggested that a range of >50 and <80 ng/ml serum 25-hydroxy vitamin D might prove helpful in mitigating morbidity from COVID-19. According to the current research, vitamin D influences the immune system's innate responses to respiratory viral infections, such as RSV, para influenza 1 and 2, and influenza A and B. vitamin D ingestion notably reduced the incidence of respiratory infections in persons who already had a shortage, as well as lowering infection risk in those with sufficient levels of vitamin D, according to an RCT involving 11,321 people from 14 countries [39].

Vitamin E

The naturally occurring vitamin E forms are eight lipophilic molecules, which include α-, β-, γ-, and δ-tocopherol (αT, βT, γT,δT)1 and α-, β-, γ-, and δ-tocotrienol (αTE, βTE, γTE, δTE) Tocopherols are saturated, and tocotrienols have three double bonds. All vitamin E forms have a chromanol ring and a 16-carbon sphytyl-like side chain. Tocopherols and tocotrienols are powerful antioxidants that scavenge lipoperoxyl radicals [40]. (a-Tocopherol) vitamin E is an antioxidant that can modulate the immunological response of the host, and its deficiency is known to impair humoral and cell-mediated immunity [11]. Vitamin forms and carboxy chromanols have antioxidant properties. All forms of vitamin E are powerful antioxidants, as they scavenge lipid peroxy radicals by donating hydrogen from the chromanol ring's phenolic group. Because their phenolic moieties are identical, all vitamin E forms are considered to have potential antioxidant activities. Vitamin E is an antioxidant that protects proteins and membrane fatty acids, regulates humoral and cell-mediated immunity, and modulates host immunological processes [41]. It also affects innate immunity, the creation, proliferation, and differentiation of antibodies and lymphocytes [40]. Vitamin E supplementation (200 IU/day) had little effect on lower respiratory tract infections in senior people but had a protective effect on upper respiratory tract infections, particularly common colds. Considerable evidence suggests that high oxidative stress may play a role in the onset of Parkinson's disease. Antioxidants such as vitamin E are likely to prevent the onset of Parkinson's disease. This has been investigated in numerous epidemiologic studies. In the Rotterdam Study, De Rijk *et al.*, discovered that a high vitamin E intake may defend against the progress of Parkinson disease [42]. Although exploratory studies have shown some promising benefits with nutritional supplements, it is vital to remember that there is currently insufficient scientific evidence to prescribe them for Parkinson's disease. Patients should be informed that over-the-counter medications have negative effects, interact with other prescriptions, and are costly [43].

Vitamin K
Vitamin K is sometimes called the "coagulation vitamin." Vitamin K has long been known as a pharmacological agent, particularly vitamin K2 (menaquinones), which has been used in clinical studies all over the world to treat brittle bones, and research suggests that it also acts as a transcriptional regulator and hormone. Recent research has discovered that vitamin K2 possesses anti-calcification, anti-diabetic, and anti-cancerous characteristics. In the traditional diet, vitamin K2 is hard to come by [44]. Vitamin K2 is only found in fermented foods like Natto and Sauerkraut, hence supplements are required to meet K2 requirements.

Types of Vitamin K
Vitamin K is available in two bioactive forms: Vitamin K1 (phytonadione/phylloquinone) and vitamin K2 (phytonadione/phylloquinone) (menaquinones). Even though 2-methyl-1 and 4-naphthoquinone (vitamin K3) have the same ring structure, they differ in key ways. Leafy green foods and fruits are high in vitamin K1. Phylloquinone concentrations in animal tissues are modest compared to vitamin K2, which is predominantly obtained from animals, fermented foods, and gut flora. Vitamin K2 can also be generated in the liver by converting K3 (Menadione), however, due to its toxicity, the FDA has banned the use of K3 as a nutritional supplement [44].

Biological Cycle of Vitamin K
Vitamin K is absorbed in the small intestine and then transported throughout the body by the blood, including to the liver. The small intestine absorbs

vitamin K and then transported throughout the body by the blood, including to the liver. To lessen nutritional dependency, the human body recycles and repurposes the limited levels of vitamin K stored in the body only through the vitamin K-epoxide cycle. Because of their high lipophilicity, long-chain menaquinones have superior intestinal absorption to MK-4 and phylloquinone [44]. Vitamin K2 also has a longer half-life than vitamin K1, which only stays in the blood for 8 hours.

Sources of Vitamin K2

Fermented dairy products, cheese, natto, cheonggukjang, and other fermented foods are high in vitamin K2. Microorganisms in the stomach, primarily Bacteroides, produce a little amount of vitamin K2 inside the body. Extraction, chemical, and microbiological methods are used to make vitamin K2. Long-chain MKs is produced by lactic acid bacteria such as Lactobacillus, Streptococcus, Leuconostoc, and Lactococcus. *Lactococcus lactis* strains produce huge amounts of long-chain MKs [45]. Because it is mostly produced in the distal colon, and its main absorption site is the terminal ileum, where bile salts carry out its solubilization, only a little amount is functionally available. Vitamin K's lipophilicity determines how well it is absorbed. Recent research has underlined the importance of vitamin K2 consumption, as intestinal menaquinones may not be enough [45, 46].

Biological Activity of Vitamin K Series

Vitamin K is a versatile vitamin that plays an important role in a variety of processes, including blood coagulation, blood vessel calcification prevention, signal transduction, and more. Many VKDPs are post-transnationally changed because vitamin K is a cofactor for the enzyme GGCX, which Carboxylated glutamate into carboxyglutamate. Vitamin K insufficiency is linked to the rapid progression of several age-related disorders, including osteoporosis, diabetes, cancer, cardiovascular, neurological, and pulmonary conditions [47].

Blood Coagulation

VKDP—Factor II, VII, IX, X, protein S, protein X, and protein Z—are seven of the 12–13 blood-clotting factors activated during the process of blood coagulation. VK1 regulates the synthesis of vitamin K-dependent coagulation proteins in the liver. Abnormal coagulation is not caused by a high vitamin consumption [48]. A blood clot that travels around the body and lodges in an organ is known as an embolism. Some oral anticoagulants (vitamin K anticoagulants), such as warfarin, disrupt the vitamin K cycle by suppressing vitamin K 2,3-epoxide reductase activity, resulting in reduced gamma-carboxylation of VKDPs implicated in coagulation and thereby preventing hemostasis. Vitamin K can be administered to patients to prevent excessive blood thinning or to offset the effects of warfarin before surgery [47, 49].

Bone Health
A bone is constantly remodelled, and good bones replace the human skeleton every 8 to 10 years. Vitamin K2, along with vitamin D3, is emerging as a key player in bone homeostasis and calcium management. By adjusting the actions of osteoclasts and osteoblasts, vitamin K supplementation could repair the degeneration of bones caused by obesity. Osteocalcin (OC) is a calcium ion-binding vitamin K2-dependent protein generated by osteoblasts in the bones [50]. It has two key domains: one calcium-dependent "Gla helix" that binds to hydroxyapatite, the principal component of bone matrix, and another "–COOH-terminal beta-sheet" that attracts monocytes, which are thought to be the precursors of osteoclasts. The silent osteoporotic illness progression is characterized by weak and brittle bones, which can be fractured simply by a little fall or coughing [50]. It affects males and females of all ethnicities, but white and Asian women, particularly older women post-menopause, are more susceptible [46].

Diabetes Mellitus
The condition is linked to several micro and macrovascular problems, as well as other significant consequences such as bone demineralization, decreased quality of life, and increased mortality. It has been found that vitamin K2 can improve insulin sensitivity, control the glycemic index, and lower the risk of developing type 2 diabetes through a variety of mechanisms. The most important of these mechanisms are the incretin effect, the post-translational modification of VKDP, and the obstruction in inflammation [51, 52]. Vitamin K2 has been shown to increase insulin sensitivity, control the glycemic index, and lower the risk of developing type 2 diabetes mellitus. It does this in a number of ways, but the most important ones are the action of incretin, the post-translational modification of VKDP, and the reduction of inflammation [53].

Vitamin K2 supplementation was found to upregulate OC gene expression and reduce the severity of diabetes mellitus and obesity in later trials [54]. Vitamin K2 improves glucose sensitivity by inhibiting the release of the cytokines interleukin (IL)-1, IL-6, and tumor necrosis factor-alpha (TNF-), which enhance insulin resistance [51]. Vitamin K has been found to inhibit inflammation, which affects insulin sensitivity, secretion, and glucose levels.

Vitamin K2 as a Hormone
By interacting with the steroid and xenobiotic receptor (SXR), an intranuclear receptor, vitamin K2 functions as a transcriptional regulator or modulator, upregulating the expression of numerous genes for bone markers, cell phenotype, and proteins involved in cell signaling and extracellular matrix proteins [46]. Furthermore, these vitamin K2 analogs (MK-7 and MK-4) can upregulate target gene expression by activating transcription factors from the Fox A and Fox O families, similar to insulin and growth hormones [46]. Vitamin K2 was also discovered to boost testosterone production in the testes by upregulating testosterone-producing gene expression. MK-4 promotes the manufacture of the CPA11A enzyme in testes, which catalyzes the rate-limiting translation of cholesterol to testosterone [55].

Spermatogenesis Regulation
Vitamin K's antioxidant properties protect the testes from oxidative damage. Both vitamin K isoforms have an antioxidant effect on the testes, and vitamin K deficiency in the diet causes spermatogenesis to be impaired [56].

5.2 Prospective Market Potential of Vitamin K2

Beyond blood coagulation, the vitamin K series is now regarded as a vital nutraceuticals. Vitamin K2 has carved out a niche for itself among food supplements, with its applications extending to the management of modern lifestyle disorders, such as osteoporosis [57], arteriosclerosis [58], and diabetes [59]. As a result, vitamin K2's market potential is rising and predicted to grow rapidly, as medications used to treat these diseases have the greatest market sector. Furthermore, vitamin K2's regulatory status demonstrates that it is safe and has no recognized harm, The FDA, Japan, and European regulatory organizations have officially approved MK-7, the most versatile vitamin K2 [60–63].

5.3 Conclusion

Vitamins are a vital part of human life, which is required for all daily activities in the human body. By adding vitamin-rich foods to our daily diet, we can create a good and healthy lifestyle. Fruits, meat, and grains are the best sources of vitamins. We have a large number of nutraceuticals that contain a variety of nutrients and vitamins. Most fat-soluble vitamins have good properties that can be used to treat a wide range of illnesses and nutritional deficiencies.

Acknowledgment

The authors thank R.C. Patel Institute of Pharmaceutical Education and Research Shirpur and MET's Institute of Pharmacy, BKC, which is affiliated with Savitribai Phule Pune University, Nashik. EDA wishes to express gratitude to the NFST/RGNF/UGC, Government of India, for providing financial assistance in the form of a fellowship (Award No - 202021-NFST-MAH-01235).

References

1. Mora, J.R., Iwata, M., Von Andrian, U.H., Vitamin effects on the immune system: Vitamins A and D take centre stage. *Nat. Rev. Immunol.*, 8, 9, 685–698, 2008.
2. Buettner, G.R. and Schafer, F.Q., Albert Szent-Gyorgyi: Vitamin C identification. *Biochem. J.*, 28, 5, October 2006, c5, 2006.
3. Chanda, S., Tiwari, R.K., Kumar, A., Singh, K., Nutraceuticals inspiring the current therapy for lifestyle diseases. *Adv. Pharmacol. Sci.*, 2019, 1–5, 2019.
4. Singh, J. and Sinha, S., Classification, regulatory acts and applications of nutraceuticals for health. *Int. J. Pharm. Biol. Sci.*, 2, 1, 177–187, 2012.
5. Drug, H., Subject, T., Food, H., Module -2.
6. Cassels, J.W.S., Advanced analysis, in: *Local Fields*, pp. 280–312, 2012.
7. Sandra, I., Oghenekeno, G., Odiba, J., Advances in nutraceuticals. *Int. J. Med. Plants Nat. Prod.*, 5, 2, 8–22, 2019.
8. Facts, Q., Fat-soluble vitamins: A , D , E , and K., 9. Fact sheet.
9. Rafeeq, H. *et al.*, Biochemistry of fat soluble vitamins, sources, biochemical functions and toxicity. *Haya: The Saudi Journal of Life Sciences*, 6221, 188–196, 2020.
10. Vitamins, W., Vitamins 10.1. *Module of Biochemistry Notes*, 6, 142–154.
11. Albahrani, A.A. and Greaves, R.F., Fat-soluble vitamins: Clinical indications and current challenges for chromatographic measurement. *Clin. Biochem. Rev.*, 37, 1, 27–47, 2016, [Online]. Available: http://www.ncbi.nlm.nih.gov/pubmed/27057076%0Ahttp://www.pubmedcentral.nih.gov/articlerender.fcgi?artid=PMC4810759.
12. Gilbert, C., Jceh_26_84_065. *Community eye health journal*, 2013.
13. Reddy, P. and Jialal, I., *Biochemistry, fat soluble vitamins*, Treasure Island (FL), StatPearls Publishing LLC, 2022.

14. Shahidi, F. and De Camargo, A.C., Tocopherols and tocotrienols in common and emerging dietary sources: Occurrence, applications, and health benefits. *Int. J. Mol. Sci.*, 17, 10, 1–29, 2016.
15. Booth, S.L., Vitamin K: Food composition and dietary intakes. *Food Nutr. Res.*, 56, 1–5, 2012.
16. Herschel Conaway, H., Henning, P., Lerner, U.H., Vitamin A metabolism, action, and role in skeletal homeostasis. *Endocr. Rev.*, 34, 6, 766–797, 2013.
17. J. & B. L., 2020, J. 10. Ross AC, Caballero B, Cousins RJ, "scholar." T. K. M. nutrition in health and disease.
18. Ross, A.C., Taylor, C.L., Yaktine, A.L., Del Valle, H.B. (Eds.), National Academy of Sciences, Washington (DC), 2011.
19. Norman, A.W., From vitamin D to hormone D: Fundamentals of vitamin D endocrine system essential for good health. *Am. J. Clin. Nutr.*, 88, February, 491S–499S, 2008.
20. Singh, U., Devaraj, S., Jialal, I., Vitamin E, oxidative stress, and inflammation. *Annu. Rev. Nutr.*, 25, 151–174, 2005.
21. Packer, L. and After, V., Role of vitamin E in biological ,2. *Am. J. Clin. Nutr.*, 53, 1050S–5S, 7, 1991.
22. Clarke, M.W., Burnett, J.R., Croft, K.D., Vitamin E in human health and disease. *Crit. Rev. Clin. Lab. Sci.*, 45, 5, 417–450, 2008.
23. Kline, K., Lawson, K.A., Yu, W., Sanders, B.G., Vitamin E and breast cancer prevention: Current status and future potential. *J. Mammary Gland Biol. Neoplasia*, 8, 1, 91–102, 2003.
24. Dror, D.K. and Allen, L.H., Vitamin e deficiency in developing countries. *Food Nutr. Bull.*, 32, 2, 124–143, 2011.
25. Sharami, S., Shahgheibi, S., Nokhostin, F., The role of fat-soluble vitamins A and D in the pathogenesis of coronavirus: With a focus on pregnant mothers. *J. Complement. Med. Res.*, 11, 3, 131, 2020.
26. Villamor, E. *et al.*, Vitamin A supplements ameliorate the adverse effect of HIV-1, malaria, and diarrheal infections on child growth. *Pediatrics*, 109, 1, 1-12, 2002.
27. Panfili, F.M., Roversi, M., D'Argenio, P., Rossi, P., Cappa, M., Fintini, D., Possible role of vitamin D in COVID-19 infection in pediatric population. *J. Endocrinol. Invest.*, 44, 1, 27–35, 2021.
28. Ilie, P.C., Stefanescu, S., Smith, L., The role of vitamin D in the prevention of coronavirus disease 2019 infection and mortality. *Aging Clin. Exp. Res.*, 32, 7, 1195–1198, 2020.
29. Mueller, A.L., McNamara, M.S., Sinclair, D.A., Why does COVID-19 disproportionately affect older people? *Aging (Albany. NY)*, 12, 10, 9959–9981, 2020, [Online]. Available: https://www.aging-us.com/article/103344/pdf.
30. Samad, N. *et al.*, Fat-soluble vitamins and the current global pandemic of covid-19: Evidence-based efficacy from literature review. *J. Inflamm. Res.*, 14, April, 2091–2110, 2021.

31. Korah, M.C., Junaid Rahman, P.V., Rajeswari, R., Behanan, A., Paul, E.P., Sivakumar, T., Adverse effects and side effects on vitamin therapy: A review. *Asian J. Pharm. Clin. Res.*, 10, 5, 19–26, 2017.
32. Gregory, J.F., Fennemas_food_chemistry, 4th_edition_.pdf.pdf., CRC press, Taylor and Francis, Boca Raton, London, NY, p. 460, 2007.
33. Glasziou, P.P. and Mackerras, D.E.M., Vitamin A supplementation in infectious diseases: A meta-analysis. *Br. Med. J.*, 306, 6874, 366–370, 1993.
34. Singh, S., Kola, P., Kaur, D., Singla, G., Mishra, V., Therapeutic potential of nutraceuticals and dietary supplements in the prevention of viral diseases: A review. *Front. Nutr.*, 8, September, 1–16, 2021.
35. Ravisankar, P., Reddy, A.A., Nagalakshmi, B., Koushik, O.S., Kumar, B.V., Anvith, P.S., The comprehensive review on fat soluble vitamins. *IOSR J. Pharm.*, 5, 11, 12–28, 2015.
36. Jain, A., Tiwari, A., Verma, A., Jain, S.K., Vitamins for cancer prevention and treatment: An insight. *Curr. Mol. Med.*, 17, 5, 79–88, 2017.
37. Fedotova, J.O., Vitamin D 3 treatment differentially affects anxiety-like behavior in the old ovariectomized female rats and old ovariectomized female rats treated with low dose of 17β-estradiol. *BMC Med. Genet.*, 20, Suppl 1, 45–56, 2019.
38. Amy S Rasor, K.M.P., A nutritionally meaningful increase in vitamin D in retail mushrooms is attainable by exposure to sunlight prior to consumption. *J. Nutr. Food Sci.*, 03, 06, 1–8, 2013.
39. Martineau, A.R. et al., Vitamin D supplementation to prevent acute respiratory infections: Individual participant data meta-analysis. *Health Technol. Assess. (Winchester, England)*, 23, 2, 1–44, Jan. 2019.
40. Jiang, Q., Natural forms of vitamin E: Metabolism, antioxidant, and anti-inflammatory activities and their role in disease prevention and therapy. *Free Radic. Biol. Med.*, 72, 76–90, 2014.
41. Moyersoen, I. et al., Intake of fat-soluble vitamins in the belgian population: Adequacy and contribution of foods, fortified foods and supplements. *Nutrients*, 9, 8, 1–22, 2017.
42. Vatassery, G.T., Bauer, T., Dysken, M., High doses of vitamin E in the treatment of disorders of the central nervous system in the aged. *Am. J. Clin. Nutr.*, 70, 5, 793–801, 1999.
43. Garima, V. and Manoj, K.M., A review on nutraceuticals:classification and its role in various diseases. *Int. J. Pharm. Ther.*, 7, 4, 152–160, 2016.
44. Mladěnka, P. et al., Vitamin K - sources, physiological role, kinetics, deficiency, detection, therapeutic use, and toxicity. *Nutr. Rev.*, 80, 4, 677–698, 2022.
45. Zhang, Z., Liu, L., Liu, C., Sun, Y., Zhang, D., New aspects of microbial vitamin K2 production by expanding the product spectrum. *Microb. Cell Fact.*, 20, 1, 1–12, 2021.
46. Aggarwal, S. et al., Vitamin K2: An emerging essential nutraceutical and its market potential. *J. Appl. Biol. Biotechnol.*, 10, 2, 173–184, 2022.

47. Geleijnse, J.M. et al., Dietary intake of menaquinone is associated with a reduced risk of coronary heart disease: The Rotterdam Study. *J. Nutr.*, 134, 11, 3100–3105, 2004.
48. de Vries, J.J.V., Chang, A.B., Bonifant, C.M., Shevill, E., Marchant, J.M., Vitamin A and beta (β)-carotene supplementation for cystic fibrosis. *Cochrane Database Syst. Rev.*, 2018, 8, 1–6, 2018.
49. Katayama, T. et al., Blood coagulation changes with or without direct oral anticoagulant therapy following transcatheter aortic valve implantation. *Am. J. Cardiol.*, 147, 88–93, 2021.
50. Al-Suhaimi, E.A. and Al-Jafary, M.A., Endocrine roles of vitamin K-dependent- osteocalcin in the relation between bone metabolism and metabolic disorders. *Rev. Endocr. Metab. Disord.*, 21, 1, 117–125, 2020.
51. Ho, H.J., Komai, M., Shirakawa, H., Beneficial effects of vitamin k status on glycemic regulation and diabetes mellitus: A mini-review. *Nutrients*, 12, 8, 1–16, 2020.
52. Li, Y., Chen, J.P., Duan, L., Li, S., Effect of vitamin K2 on type 2 diabetes mellitus: A review. *Diabetes Res. Clin. Pract.*, 136, November, 39–51, 2018.
53. Choi, H.J. et al., Vitamin K2 supplementation improves insulin sensitivity via osteocalcin metabolism: A placebo-controlled trial. *Diabetes Care*, 34, 9, 2011, 2011.
54. Bourron, O., Phan, F., Vitamin, K., A nutrient which plays a little-known role in glucose metabolism. *Curr. Opin. Clin. Nutr. Metab. Care*, 22, 2, 174–181, 2019.
55. Ito, A. et al., Menaquinone-4 enhances testosterone production in rats and testis-derived tumor cells. *Lipids Health Dis.*, 10, 1, 158, 2011.
56. Ma, X. et al., Sublethal dose of warfarin induction promotes the accumulation of warfarin resistance in susceptible Norway rats. *J. Pestic. Sci. (2004)*, 94, 3, 805–815, 2021.
57. Surana, K.R., Ahire, E.D., Sonawane, V.N., Talele, S.G., Biomolecular and molecular docking: A modern tool in drug discovery and virtual screening of natural products, in: *Applied Pharmaceutical Practice and Nutraceuticals*, pp. 209–223, Apple Academic Press, New York, 2021.
58. Plaza, S.M. and Lamson, D.W., Vitamin K2 in bone metabolism and osteoporosis. *Altern. Med. Rev.*, 10, 1, 24–35, 2005.
59. Surana, K.R., Ahire, E.D., Sonawane, V.N., Talele, S.G., Talele, G.S., Molecular modeling: Novel techniques in food and nutrition development, in: *Natural Food Products and Waste Recovery*, pp. 17–31, Apple Academic Press, New York, 2021.
60. Bellinge, J.W. et al., Vitamin k intake and atherosclerotic cardiovascular disease in the danish diet cancer and health study. *J. Am. Heart Assoc.*, 10, 16, 2021.
61. Dahlberg, S., Diabetes management and metabolism. *Adv. Nutr.*, 2, 439–446, March, 2019.

62. Sato, T., Inaba, N., Yamashita, T., MK-7 and its effects on bone quality and strength. *Nutrients*, 12, 4, 1–9, 2020.
63. Ahire, E.D., Sonawane, V.N., Surana, K.R., Talele, G.S., Drug discovery, drug-likeness screening, and bioavailability: Development of drug-likeness rule for natural products, in: *Applied Pharmaceutical Practice and Nutraceuticals*, pp. 191–208, Apple Academic Press, New York, 2021.

6

Marine-Derived Sources of Nutritional Vitamins

Neelam L. Dashputre[1], Rahul R. Sable[1], Mayur Sawant[2], Shubham J. Khairnar[1], Eknath D. Ahire[2], Surabhi B. Patil[1] and Jayesh D. Kadam[1]*

[1]Department of Pharmacology, MET's Institute of Pharmacy, Bhujbal Knowledge City, Adgaon, Nashik, MH, India
[2]Department of Pharmaceutics, MET's Institute of Pharmacy, Bhujbal Knowledge City, Adgaon, Nashik, MH, India

Abstract

The oceans have long been the world's most significant food source. They have developed into an important and varied source of bioactive chemicals. Marine creatures are becoming increasingly important as a natural source of new substances that could improve the food industry and human health. This review summarizes recent research on functional seafood compounds (chitin and chitosan, algae pigments, fish lipids, omega-3 fatty acids, bioactive proteins/peptides, phenolic compounds, polysaccharides, EAAs, and minerals), with a focus on their potential use as nutraceuticals and health benefits. This study provides an overview of a number of recently studied beneficial compounds with marine origin that show great potential as nutraceuticals or for use in the food industry. These include gelatin, dopamine, peptides, polysaccharides, polyphenols, FAs, fish oil, EAAs, chitin, chitosan, polysaccharides, polyphenols, pigments from algae, and vitamins and minerals. Although not all of them are strictly speaking bioactive molecules, their advantageous nutritional traits have a good effect on human health.

Keywords: Bioactive compounds, functional foods, marine resources, nutraceuticals, pharmaceuticals

---

Corresponding author: jayeshkadam21s@gmail.com

Eknath D. Ahire, Raj K. Keservani, Khemchand R. Surana, Sippy Singh and Rajesh K. Kesharwani (eds.) *Vitamins as Nutraceuticals: Recent Advances and Applications,* (129–166) © 2023 Scrivener Publishing LLC

6.1 Introduction

Nutraceuticals are raw foods, functional foods, or dietary supplements that contain bioactive molecules that can provide health advantages (prevention and treatment of disease) in addition to their nutritional value [1]. The phrases nutrition and medicinal component are combined in this name (pharmaceutical). In recent years, functional and bioactive compounds from natural sources, such as terrestrial and marine plants, animals, or even microorganisms, have become sustainable solution that offers new molecules with strong biological activity. With the increase in the field of health-based research, these new molecules are gaining more importance. In industrialized countries, modern food habits and lifestyles have resulted in an increase in diseases, such as type 2 diabetes, obesity, metabolic syndrome, cancer, and neurological disorders [2]. Bioactive components from natural sources with an ability to contribute to the overall health have become an interesting alternative to potentially harmful synthetic ingredients.

The ocean ecosystem's tremendous biodiversity and dynamics make it a suitable reservoir for discovering novel compounds and developing marine nutraceuticals. Although 20,000 marine bioactive components have been identified, only a small percentage of them have been properly researched and used in some way [3]. Marine habitats have been dubbed the "New Millennium Natural Medicine Chest," and they are rapidly becoming a significant market worldwide. The international market for marine-derived compounds was worth more than $10 billion in 2018, and it is predicted to increase to $22 billion at a compound annual growth rate of 11.3% from 2019 to 2025. Protein and peptides, PUFAs, enzymes, polyphenolic compounds, polysaccharides, pigments, and vitamins are some of the components from marine sources that have proven beneficial health effects and could be used in food and medical applications.

Generally, synthetic chemical drugs are still used in medical practice to treat diverse acute or chronic diseases, mainly various disorders involving the immune system's chronic inflammatory states, allergic reactions, diabetes, cardiovascular diseases, severe human tumors, and cancers or as immunosuppressant during transplantation. Despite their effectiveness, many of these synthetic chemical medications and conventional antibiotics have considerable human health risks as a result of their abuse, uncontrolled application, and overuse, as well as their proper usage. The usage, and especially the misuse, of some synthetic antimicrobial medications may be a major contributor to the spread of antibiotic-resistant bacteria (ARM). Natural nutraceuticals' strength is in their ability to improve quality of life, prevent or even treat some diseases without causing negative side effects. Because marine nutraceuticals are more appealing due to their safety, developing non-toxic yet effective natural compounds as alternatives to chemical chemicals may be beneficial. Fish, sponges, algae, crustaceans, mollusks, actinomycetes, fungus, and microbes have all been employed as natural component sources in the past [4].

This overview presents an overview of a variety of marine-based beneficial chemicals that have recently been the subject of research and have significant promise as nutraceuticals or applications in the food business. Chitin, chitosan, polysaccharides, polyphenols, pigments from algae, FAs, fish oil, EAAs, gelatin, dopamine, peptides, vitamins and minerals are some of these. Although not all of them are bioactive molecules in the strict sense, their favorable nutritional characteristics have a positive impact on human health. Because many of them have strong biological qualities yet are susceptible to deterioration, nanotechnology has been proposed as a means of protecting these compounds and improving their bioavailability after application.

6.2 Marine-Based Beneficial Molecules

6.2.1 Chitin and Chitosan

Chitin is a polymer that occurs naturally in crystalline forms, because the polysaccharide chains are oriented anti-parallel, -chitin is the most stable form of this polymer. Chitosan ((1-4)-2-amino-2-deoxy-D-glucan) is the most common and naturally occurring cationic polysaccharide found in crustaceans, mollusks, insects, and fungal exoskeletons. Chitin deacetylation removes acetyl groups (CH_3–CO) from the molecule, allowing the biopolymer to dissolve in most dilute acids. During the deacetylation process, the amine (NH) groups are freed, giving chitosan cationic properties [5]. The most common sources of chitosan are seafood by-products processing, such as crab shells and shrimp/prawn exoskeletons.

Chitin and chitosan are polymers found in nature with the same chemical structure. Both consist of a mixture of mainly N-acetyl-D-glucosamine and a small amount of D-glucosamine. Chitin is insoluble in water, but chitosan is acid-soluble due to the presence of free protonable amino groups in D-glucosamine units [6]. COS (chitooligomers) are chitin or chitosan degradation byproducts acquired from chemical or enzymatic chitosan hydrolysis. Anamine/acetamide, as well as primary and secondary hydroxyl groups in positions C-2, C-3, and C-6, is all present in chitosan. Differences in structure and physicochemical qualities are mostly influenced by amino acid content. The seafood processing business generates a lot of trash and by-products (shells, scales, tails, heads, and guts) that can be used as useful components. Shell material, for example, is a good source of chitin and chitosan. In this section, the health-promoting properties of chitin and chitosan, as well as their derivatives, are discussed [7].

6.2.1.1 Anti-Oxidant Properties

Oxidative stress could cause unanticipated enzyme activation and oxidative damage to cellular macromolecules, leading to a range of health disorders, including many cardiovascular diseases, inflammation, diabetes, neurodegenerative diseases and cancer. Antioxidants, such as chitosan and its derivatives, reduce oxidative damage by interrupting the chain reaction of radical oxidation [8].

In healthy people, the antioxidant impact of a dietary supplement (high molecular weight (MW) chitosan, trade name: Chitosamin®, 100 kDa, 90% degree of deacetylation [DD]) was investigated. The treatment reduced lipid hydroperoxides and uremic toxins in the GI tract, which helped to prevent oxidative stress from developing in the human systemic circulation. Chitosamin is an antioxidant supplement that can be used to treat a variety of ailments, including kidney failure [9].

Chitosan's antioxidant activity is determined by its MW, DD, and origin [10] investigated three MW (5-10, 1-5, and 1 kDa) chitosan variants derived from partly deacetylated chitosan preparations (90%, 75%, and 50%) The 1- to 5-kDa chitosan preparation containing 90% deacetylated chito-oligosaccharides was found to capture the most O2, OH, and DPPH Anraku *et al.* [21] employed high (HMWC; 1000 kDa) and low MW (LMWC; 30 kDa) chitosan to examine its influence on oxidative stress in normal and metabolic syndrome model rats and found similar results. In rats fed LMWC, there was a significant increase in antioxidant activity. HMWC-rich diets, on the other hand, lowered the amounts of pro-oxidants in the gastrointestinal tract, such as low-density lipoprotein cholesterol (LDL), avoiding oxidative stress in the systemic circulation. The antioxidant and protective effects of surface-deacetylated chitin nanofibers were investigated. In rats, (SDACNF) has an effect on the liver. SDACNF (80 mg/kg/day) administration for

8 weeks decreased liver damage and oxidative stress in rats compared to untreated animals [11].

6.2.1.2 Anti-Microbial Properties

The antibacterial effect of chitosan and chitin is thought to be based on the biopolymer's polycationic nature (i.e., the presence of NH3+ groups), which interact with negatively charged surface components of many microbes, resulting in cellular material leakage and cell death [12]. Gram-negative bacteria's lipopolysaccharides and Gram-positive bacteria's teichoic acid both have a function in chitosan interaction [13]. The bigger the number of positive charged amino groups in the structure of a biopolymer, the greater its antimicrobial activity. Chitosan contains a greater number of positive charged amino groups than chitin, and therefore, has higher antimicrobial activity [14] affected by many different factors, i.e., MW, pH, degree of polymerization, and DD. Moreover, the origin source of chitosan and chitin affects their antimicrobial properties [15]. Raw chitin from crab shells had little antibacterial action, but following purification, it showed antibacterial activity against *Escherichia coli*. Chitin from shiitake stipes outperformed chitin from crab shell in antibacterial action against infections. The antibacterial activity of chitin may be affected by the process of discoloration. After being cleaned, chitosan from shiitake stipes and crab shells demonstrated good antibacterial activity against eight pathogens [16].

Chitosan from shiitake stipes, on the other hand, was more effective than chitosan from crab shells. Chitosan's usage may be limited due to its weak solubility in organic solvents. Chitosan's amino and hydroxyl groups can be modified to tailor its physicochemical qualities for certain purposes. Schiff bases are formed when amine groups combine with aldehydes and ketones. With reactions with a pyrazole heterocycle molecule, [17] developed three novel Shiff base chitosan derivatives. The chitosan derivatives showed *E. coli*-specific antibacterial activity and *Klebsiella* as Gram-negative bacteria, *Staphylococcus aureus*, and *Streptococcus mutans* as Gram-positive bacteria as well as *Aspergillus fumigatus*, and *Candida albicans* as fungi. Furthermore, the MMT test revealed no cytotoxic action in normal retinal cells. N-methylchitosan (NMC), trimethylchitosan (TMC), diethylmethyl chitosan (DEMC), and carboxymethyl chitosan (CMC) are N-selective chitosan derivatives (CMC). Chitosan's antibacterial properties were improved by replacing the alkyl groups. TMC, on the other hand, had the best antibacterial reaction against

E. coli and S. aureus, which could be related to positive charges on the chitosan skeleton [18, 19]. The antibacterial activity of N-guanidinium chitosan acetate against E. coli, P. aeruginosa, S. aureus, B. subtilis, and C. albicans was the best of the four derivatives, with low minimum inhibitory concentration (MIC) values for all pathogens [20, 21].

6.2.1.3 Anti-Hypertensive Activity

Hypertension causes the development of heart disease. In the human blood, angiotensin-I converting enzyme (ACE) contributes relating to blood pressure control by converting inactive angiotensin I into its active form, angiotensin II, and this causes small blood vessels to narrow and blood pressure to rise. Reduction of ACE function may be advantageous in preventing hypertension [22]. Chitosan derivatives—COS, exhibited antihypertensive effects in particular. Their ability to block ACE is determined by the compound's DD and MW [140]. Huang et al. [121] modified COS with -COCH$_2$CH$_2$COO- groups. Renin converts angiotensinogen in the blood to angiotensin-I, which will then be converted to angiotensin-II by ACE. Renin inhibition is a potential antihypertensive strategy [23]. COS with varied MW (10–5, 5–1, and 1 kDa) and DD were produced (90% and 50%). Both DD and MW have an effect on renin inhibitory activity, according to the data.

6.2.1.4 Anti-Allergy and Anti-Inflammatory Activity

Allergies are caused by an interaction between an antigen and the antigen-specific IgE. Asthma, on either hand, is an allergic illness accompanied by high respiratory tract sensitivity. COS with three distinct MW ranges (1–3, 3–5, and 5–10 kDa) decreased allergy reactions by decreasing degranulation and cytokine release in mast cells, according to [24, 25]. *In vivo* and *in vitro*, researchers looked at the anti-inflammatory effects of LWM COS made from HMW chitosan as a result of enzymatic digestion against allergic responses and allergic asthma. The anti-inflammatory effects of LMW-COS were linked to the modulation of Th2 and proinflammatory cytokines, suggesting that it could be a promising option for developing an effective allergic asthma treatment medication [26].

6.2.1.5 Anti-Obesity and Anti-Diabetic Activity

The increase in the number of people with obesity is becoming a global burden on public health. In epidemiological studies, it has been shown that a lower incidence of obesity-related diseases has been observed in populations where seafood is consumed. Certain compounds found in seafood are thought to aid in the fight against obesity [27]. Obesity-related disorders are treated with chitosan and its derivatives. The use of chitosan in dietary supplementation effectively lowers plasma levels of total cholesterol (TC) and LDL-C, as well as liver and plasma levels of triacylglycerol (TG). Lowering the level of lipids in the plasma results from the ability of chitosan to bind dietary lipids and bile acids, and inhibit the activity of pancreatic lipase, thus reducing the absorption of intestinal fat in the gastrointestinal tract [28].

Chitosan with a high DD and MW has a higher fat binding capability than chitosan with a low DD and MW. Chitosan has been proved to be a safe nutritional supplement that benefits human health in tablet form. The ability of hypolipidemic chitosan to bind to lipids, lipids, and bile salts is thought to be the mechanism of action Chitosan's hypolipidemic effects are caused by hydrophobic interactions and hydrogen bonding between chitosan and lipids, as well as electrostatic interaction among charged amino groups of chitosan and charged negatively carboxyl groups of FA and bile salts [29]. In the diets of rats, surface-deacetylated chitin nanofibers (SDCH-NF) were used. By stimulating the intestinal microbiota, oral treatment of low molecular weight chitosan elevated plasma levels of ATP and 5-HT. Their findings suggested that alterations in the gut microbiota population may be responsible for SDCH-anti-obesity NF's action. Weight gain decrease in overweight patients has been confirmed in several researches. However, it was also reported that chitosan/chitin had just a small weight-loss effect and was unlikely to be clinically relevant [30].

A recent study looked at the impact of low-molecular-weight chitosan in the diet of mice with type 1 diabetes. In mice, daily injection of 0.8% chitosan in their drinking water reduced serum glucose, urine glucose, and serum triglycerides, resulting in a reduction in hyperglycemia, hypertriglyceridemia, polydipsia, and polyuria [31].

6.2.1.6 Anti-Cancer and Anti-Tumor Activity

Chitosan also has an anti-cancer effect by limiting cancer cell proliferation. The anti-tumor activity stems from the immune system's potential stimulation [32]. DNA fragmentation inhibits angiogenesis and apoptosis, as well as inhibiting angiogenesis and apoptosis [144]. MMP-2 melanoma cells were suppressed by chitosan (500 kDa, 70% DD). Despite the fact that MMP-2 expression was unaffected, the amount of MMP-2 in the cell supernatant was reduced. This behavior can be attributed to the post-transcriptional effect of chitosan on MMP-2Using atomic force microscopy, researchers discovered a direct molecular contact between MMP-2 and chitosan, as well as non-competitive suppression of MMP-2 by chitosan (using a colorimetric test) [33]. Chitin was extracted from N. norvegicus by-products, and chitosan was produced by 50% deacetylation of chitin. The biopolymer inhibited the proliferation of HCT116 colon cancer cells. After 24 hours of treatment with 0.5–6 mg/mL chitosan, HCT116 cell growth was considerably reduced by 13.5% to 67.5% [34]. Extracted chitosan nanoparticles waste from shrimp shells using two successive steps: demineralization and deproteinization. Chitosan NP inhibited the proliferation of MCF-7 breast cancer cells and had low cytotoxicity in normal L929 fibroblast cells when compared to chemically produced chitosan [35]. Freshwater crayfish waste (*Procambarus clarkii*) was employed as a precursor to get chitin, which was then deacetylated to produce chitosan. Chitosan NP and Schiff bases were created from the chitosan. When evaluated against three strains (HepG-2, HCT-116, and MCF-7), chitosan Schiff bases had the best anti-tumor effectiveness, followed by chitosan NP. Chitosan showed the lowest anti-tumor activity of all the tested compounds [36] prepared nanofibers of chitosan derivatives. The MMT test revealed that the material 4T1 breast cancer cells have good activity and have no harmful effects on normal cells, indicating that nanofibers may have a promising application in the prevention of breast cancer recurrence [37].

6.3 Beneficial Molecules from Marine Macroalgae

6.3.1 Pigments

Marine algae are one of the most primitive producers of complete aquatic biomass, giving them a supply of biologically active substances among biological species. Several valuable compounds derived from marine algae have been discovered to offer health benefits for humans. Bioactive natural algal pigments (NPM) are found in chlorophyceae, rhodophyceae, and phaeophyceae. The three types of NPM produced by marine algae are carotenoids, chlorophylls, and phycobiliproteins [38]. Their chemical structures determine their stability, which can be altered by a variety of elements including oxygen, light, heat, air, and pH. The NPM are also distinguished by their photosynthetic functions [39]. NMP has been applied in the food, nutraceuticals, and cosmetics industries due to their antioxidant, antimicrobial, antidiabetic, antimalarial, anticancer, antiviral, anti-inflammatory, and anti-obesity activities [40].

Carotenoids are a type of fat-soluble NPM found in algal biomass, and they are part of the tetraterpenoids category, which consists of a linear polyene chain (C40). Carotenoids are classed as unsaturated hydrocarbon carotenoids, usually known as carotenes, such as lycopene, -carotene, and -carotene pigments, and oxygenated carotenoids, such as astaxanthin, lutein, canthaxanthin, -cryptoxanthin, and zeaxanthin, based on their chemical structure. Generally, fucoxanthin and astaxanthin are the most frequent and natural carotenoid pigments produced in seaweeds or marine algae [41]. Alternatively, the stability of carotenoid pigments is mostly influenced by environmental factors such as oxidation, dehydrogenation, and hydrogenation processes, which can cause structural changes [42]. These NPMs are regarded antioxidants because they protect cells, retinal epithelium, and skin from oxidative damage, lowering the risk of CVD, atherosclerosis, neurological, and other non-communicable diseases (NCD) [43]. A fucoxanthin-rich fraction derived from brown algae *Sargassum siliquosum* and *S. polycystum*, ACE, was reported to have -amylase inhibitory activity and -glucosidase, which may help to minimize the risk of cardiovascular disease. Macular degeneration is protected by lutein and zeaxanthin derived from macroalgae. Furthermore, carotenoid pigments, By acting as antitumor, anti-inflammatory, anticancer, anti-obesity, and neuroprotective agents, fucoxanthin, in particular, can be utilized to treat rheumatoid arthritis, osteoporosis, and diabetes disorders [44]. Figure 6.1 indicating the biological properties of beneficial molecules derived from marine source.

The proteinase activity, which is liquid proteins and highly luminous substances generated by blue-green and red algae, is another major algal pigment. Phycoerythrins, allophycocyanins, and phycocyanins are the three types of NPM that have been identified [45]. Among other pharmaceutical and health-improving applications, these photosynthetic pigments are used in histochemistry, immunoassays, flow cytometry, and cell imaging. When isolated from *Porphyra* sp., they could be used to detect reactive oxygen substances (ROS) due to their antioxidant characteristics. Natural colorings made from macroalgal phycobiliproteins can be found in chewing gums, dairy products, cosmetics, and other items [46]. Chlorophyll, a tetrapyrrole and greenish lipid soluble pigment is another basic NPM made up of algae species. Generally, there are four major categories of chlorophylls found in marine algae: chlorophyll a, b, c, and d. Chlorophyll pigments and their derivatives have cancer protective and anti-mutagenic effects and may be taken into consideration for replacing the synthetic pigments that are used in the food business [47].

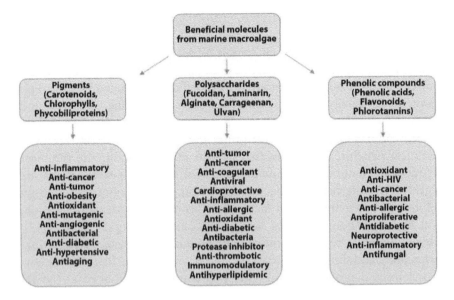

Figure 6.1 Biological properties of beneficial molecules derived from marine macroalgae.

6.3.2 Polysaccharides

Polysaccharides are sugar polymers, a biological macromolecule with varying degrees of sulfation found in many species of marine algae, but also crabs and krill [141]. Polysaccharides extracted from sea creatures are considered safer and less costly than mammalian polysaccharides, thus more suitable for application in drug development, cosmetics, and functional food products [48]. Alginates, carrageenan, fucoidan, agar, furcelleran, ascophyllan, laminarin, polyuronides carrageenan, agar-agar, fucans, fucanoids, chitin and chitosan are marine-origin bioactive polysaccharides with anti-tumor, anti-coagulant, anti-virus, cardioprotective, anti-inflammatory, anti-allergic, anti-oxidant, anti-diabetic, antibacterial, and protease inhibitor activities. Marine polysaccharides have antioxidant capacity through their scavenging of ROS [49].

The composition of polysaccharides in marine algae, the primary non-animal supply of sulfated polysaccharides, varies according to the season, species, and geographic location [50]. Fucoidan, laminarin, and alginate are the principal sulfated carbohydrates found in brown algae, whereas carrageenan and ulvan are present in red and green algae, accordingly [51].

Fucoidan is a sulfated carbohydrate found in brown macroalgae cell walls that have been researched for its biological functions [52].

Fucoidan's structural complexity ranges from the basic structure that contains sulfate groups attached to fucose units to macromolecules containing a range of different monosaccharide units such as mannose, galactose, glucose, and xylose. Various factors, including type, harvesting time, and environmental conditions, influence its intricacy [53]. Fucoidan extracts have been approved by the FDA for use in meals and dietary supplements at doses up to 250 mg per day [54]. Anticancer effects of fucoidans on different cancer cell lines have been reported including inducing apoptosis in 5637 human bladder cancer cells, in human breast (MCF-7) and colon cancer cell (HCT15) lines, and the colon cancer adenocarcinoma (Caco-2) cell line. Fucoidans from brown algae also have an inhibitory role in colony formation in human melanoma and colon cancer cells [55].

Laminarin is a polymer from brown algae with a low molecular weight (MW) of 5 kDa. It can be present in Laminaria and Saccharina species, as well as Ascophyllum and Fucus. Laminarin is a reserve beta-glucan made up of (1,3)-D-glucan and some -(1,6)-intrachain linkages. Laminarin's anti-cancer actions have recently been identified, including increased apoptotic cellular death, reduction of angiogenic potential, and colony formation suppression [56]. Other than anticancer effects, laminarin from *Cystoseira barbata* (5% cream) significantly enhanced the *in vivo* healing process, improved wound contraction, accelerated re-epithelization, and allowed restitution of mice skin tissue. Photo-cross-linkable laminarin-based hydrogels for cell encapsulation and/or drug delivery have also been created. Alginate is a natural polysaccharide made up of (1-4) linked -D-mannuronic acid (M) and -L-guluronic acid (G) monomers that form M-, G-, and MG-block structures. It can be found in the cell walls of brown macroalgae. Alginates are being used in various applications, such as alginate fiber wound dressings, as excipients in drug delivery, as dental impression materials, and preventing gastric reflux. Alginates are also used for food protection, as gelling, thickening, and coating, emulsifying, and stabilizing agents in food product [56].

Carrageenan is sulfated polysaccharide with high molecular weight that consists of alternating linear chains of α-1,3-galactose and β-1,4,3,6-anhydrogalactose with ester sulfates (15–40%), and it is structural component of red macroalgae cell membranes. It has anti-thrombotic, anti-cancer, anti-viral, and immunomodulatory properties, among others. Carrageenan is used in medication administration, bone and cartilage tissue regeneration, and wound healing due to its gelling process and physiochemical features [57]. Ulvan, a water-soluble polysaccharide, is found in green macroalgae of the order Ulvales (*Ulva* and *Enteromorpha* sp.). Sulfate, rhamnose, xylose, iduronic, and glucuronic acids are the main constituents. Ulvan has been demonstrated to have antioxidant, antiviral, anticancer, immunomodulating, and antihyperlipidemic properties, as well as the ability to modify cellular signaling processes in plant and animal systems, resulting in improved productivity and health. Ulvan has also been shown to lower total serum cholesterol, LDL cholesterol, and triglycerides while increasing high density lipoprotein (HDL) cholesterol levels. Ulvan was tested *in vitro* tests on a human breast cancer cell line (MCF-7) and an *in vivo* animal model of breast carcinogenesis, and it was discovered to have a possible chemopreventive effect [58].

6.3.3 Phenolic Compounds

Phenolics can be defined as substances with an aromatic ring having one or more hydroxyl groups, including their functional derivatives. Plants contain a large variety of phenolic derivatives including simple phenols, benzoic acid derivatives, phenylpropanoids, flavonoids, tannins, stilbenes, lignans, and lignins [59]. The phenolics from terrestrial sources have been well studied, but information on aquatic species is limited Environmental factors like salinity, UV radiation, availability of nutrients, and temperature influence the natural generation of phenolic content in marine organisms. Phenolics in marine macroalgae range from basic molecules like phenolic acids to extremely complex ones like phlorotannins (PHT). Bromophenols and PHT are two phenolic chemicals that have only been found in marine sources. Brown algae have large levels of PHT, which is formed by polymerizing phloroglucinol units. They are found in cell walls, cytoplasm, and cellular components [60]. PHT's excellent oxidation resistance has sparked interest in food preservation and antiaging products, as well as high-value commercial items in medicinal, cosmetic, nutritional, and agricultural products. Phenolics from macroalgae are used as natural anti-allergic substances for allergy remission, as bioactive components in pharmaceuticals and foods for the treatment and/or protection of neurodegenerative disease and cardiovascular disease, and as compounds with potential antidiabetic effects by inhibiting both -amylase and -glucosidase [61].

Besides pigments, polysaccharides, and phenolics, marine macroalgae also contain other beneficial molecules such as fatty acids, proteins and vitamins. Various researchers did *in vivo* studies on the beneficial effects of algae ingestion in rats. For example, [62] reported that supplementation of *Gelidium amansii* in the diet will help the increased insulin resistance

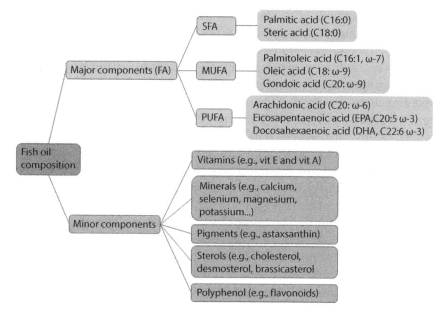

Figure 6.2 Composition of fish oil.

and hypercholesterolemia induced by feeding high fructose diet in rats [63]. Discovered that giving rats 1 g of wakame (Undaria Pinnatifida) per 100 g diet resulted in lower serum total cholesterol levels and less body fat buildup. However, in both studies identification of the components from the algae responsible for the results was not determined [64]. Figure 6.2 showing the different composition of fish oil.

6.4 Fish Oil

Many health advantages have been linked to the ingestion of marine seafood, primarily due to the uptake of fish oil. Fish oil is mostly composed of -3 FA, which comprises long-chain (LC) -3 PUFA, primarily eicosapentaenoic acid (EPA) and docosahexaenoic acid (DHA), both of which are favorable to human health [65].

Fish oil has been used in the food, biomedical, and pharmaceutical sectors. Several studies have reported that fish oil will become used to treat various disorders and prevent the progression of several chronic diseases. Human ingestion of fish oil is possible either by directly eating fish (and algae) or by consuming different formulations, such as tablets or capsules. Earlier studies reported that fish oil enriched with EPA and

DHA can be applied in the form of capsules to prevent CVD, by reducing the risk of high TG, hypertension, dyslipidemia, heart disorders, while decreasing blood levels of low-density cholesterol. The regular use of fish oil capsules can help prevent cancers, especially for patients with progressive cancers. Fish oil enriched with ω-3 FA has been recommended to optimize the functions of the human brain, kidney, liver and heart, and hence, to decrease the progression of cardiovascular, hypertension, cancer, neurodegenerative, auto-immune and renal diseases. Also, fish oil enriched with LC ω-3 PUFA can reduce the amounts of C-reactive protein (CRP) and pro-inflammatory cytokines, and thus, reduce the risk of inflammatory diseases, such as rheumatoid arthritis. De Souza *et al.* [70] have reported that the FA of fish oil capsules is suitable for medication of other disorders, such as type-2 diabetes mellitus (T2DM) and obesity, and also to decrease the atherogenic factors, principally the atherogenic index of plasma (AIP) in patients with T2DM who suffer from obesity. Earlier studies have reported that fish oil will became to lower the risk of Alzheimer's disease [66].

6.5 EAA in Protein Supplement Systems

Proteins have several important functions in living system such as protecting the immune system, the storage and transit of other molecules, and also as catalysts. Biologically active enzymes and peptides found in marine organisms supply EAA. EAA such as arginine, leucine, isoleucine, gamma-aminobutyric acid (GABA), glycine, glutamic acid, methionine, and phenylalanine are abundant in crustaceans, fish, and mollusks [67].

EAA nutrients of "cysteine, leucine, histidine, methionine, proline, hydroxyproline, tyrosine, threonine, trans-4-hydroxy-proline, and valine" showed antioxidant activity due to scavenging activity and lipid peroxidation suppression, and aid in human homeostasis, owing to their role in regulation of various cellular mechanisms and as precursors of other molecules (e.g., nitrogenous bases and hormones) and also as protein building blocks. *Rapana venosa* and *Mytilus galloprovincialis* (L.) EAAs had good anti-inflammatory action [68].

GABA, a neurotransmitter inhibitor generated by marine organisms such as marine bacteria, can reduce hypertension by lowering blood pressure. GABA can also help cure autonomic illnesses and depression by stimulating the immune system and regulating diabetes through its anti-hyperglycemic impact [69].

The biological active EAA taurine, on the other hand, is a "β-aminosulphonic acid" that can be obtained from crustaceans and mollusks. Taurine has been demonstrated to have a variety of physiological and biological effects in humans, including cell membrane stabilization, retina and central nervous system development, and immunomodulatory actions [70].

6.6 Minerals in Seafood for Human Diet

In the human diet, seafood can be an important source of vital minerals. Although the flesh of fish and other seafood can be a good source of Ca, phosphorus, magnesium, zinc, iron, selenium and iodine, even greater heights of minerals can be obtained from the seafood industry's by-products. Ca is the main mineral obtained from seafood by-products, mainly fish bones and shells [71].

Calcium carbonate is the most common form of calcium in shells, whereas hydroxyapatite or tricalcium phosphate is the most common form of calcium in bones. Ca is commonly extracted from shells using the calcination process, which involves heating the shell, which became largely argonite, to produce particular structural changes. If the temperature is increased to >600°C to 800°C, the argonite structure is reorganized into the trigonal-rhombohedral configuration of calcite and calcium oxide (CaO). The calcinations of fish bones using temperature in the range of 600°C to 1200°C results in calcium phosphates the mineral hydroxyapatite the mineral hydroxyapatite and tricalcium phosphate. The higher the temperature of calcination the higher the rate of transformation of hydroxyapatite to tricalcium phosphate. Those compounds have a number of health benefits and can be used in tissue engineering scaffolds, implants, dietary supplements or food additives. Both hydroxyapatite and tricalcium phosphate have been used in bioceramics to produce scaffolds for tissue engineering and bone regeneration as well as substrates for coatings of metallic implants. Hydroxyapatite can also be a helpful source of nutrient supplements for humans, with better efficiency and tolerability than regularly utilized calcium carbonate and also no acute or chronic toxicity [72–74].

Although fish bones consist mostly of Ca and P, which constitute >95% of fish bone minerals, various other microelements are also obtained during the preparation process, resulting in a product with potential food supplement applications. Bubel *et al.,* [43] developed a simple method for Ca preparations from cod and salmon backbone containing 24.9–27.8% Ca and 12.5–13.4% P but also relatively high levels of Mg (4.6–6.6 g/kg) and microelements: 3.9–6.2 mg/kg Cu, 11–24 mg/kg Fe, 28–53 mg/kg Mn and 50–57 mg/kg Zn. Even higher levels of Ca (38.2%) and P (23.3%) have been found in tuna bone powder. Aside from those two elements the bone powder also contained elevated levels of Fe (62 mg/kg) and Mg (4700 mg/kg). Boiling hake bones enhanced the Ca and P content of the bone powder while dramatically decreasing the Na and K content, according to [75]. This powder had a high cell bioavailability and led in a considerable increase in rat bone mineralization, similar to that seen with commercial supplements. The size and solubility of Ca in fishbone affect its bioavailability. Furthermore, lowering the size of the particles of bone powders to the nanoscale can increase bioavailability even more and experiments with rats revealed no harmful effects at the nano calcium carbonate level [76].

Other than fish bones and seafood shells, no other seafood by-product is employed as a potential mineral source. Fish by-products, such as fish viscera, on the other hand, may supply a considerable amount of minerals if correctly removed, as the ash level of fish viscera ranges from 7% to 11% of dry weight, with high Ca, K, and Mg content. However, little is known about the actual mineral makeup of fish viscera, leaving room for further investigation [77].

6.7 Marine-Based Vitamin Sources

Seafood can supply all of the vitamins that people require, including vitamins A, D, E, and B12, as well as vitamin C in the case of some algae. This section will focus on recent findings because the utilization of seafood as a source of nutrients has been well researched. Omega-3 fatty acids and fat-soluble vitamins are abundant in the lipid part of seafood. A summary of recent findings on fat-soluble vitamin sources derived from shellfish [78]. Table 6.1 comprising the recent results on seafood-based fat-soluble vitamin sources.

Despite the fact that vitamin D serves a variety of functions in humans, insufficiency has been recorded in a variety of groups around the world. Seafood, primarily oily fish species or non-fatty fish liver, is the primary source of vitamin D in the human diet, as it is the only food product that contains this vitamin in relatively high amounts, except from mushrooms

Table 6.1 Recent results on seafood-based fat-soluble vitamin sources.

Vitamin	Source	Key findings	Reference
E	Tuna liver oil that has been farmed. Crude oil extracted from the gills and guts of farmed tuna. Sardine heads, guts, and fins are used to make crude oil. Oil extracted from a whole sardine. Crude oil extracted from the heads and guts of farmed seabass and seabream.	All crude oils have significantly less -tocopherol than cod liver oil. Tuna by-product oil had the same amount of -tocopherol as tuna liver oil. The -tocopherol content of crude oil from sardine by-products was substantially greater than crude oil from whole sardines. There was no link discovered between increased -tocopherol levels and crude oil stability.	[79]
	Cod liver oil	The amount of -tocopherol in crude oil was reduced by 31–45% during refining.	[80]
	Oil from rainbow trout heads, bones and tails. Oil from rainbow trout intestines.	The temperature of oil extraction had no effect on the amount of -tocopherol in different oils. The amount of -tocopherol in oils ranged from 90 to 160 g/g of oil.	
	Fresh *Caulerpa* sp. leaves	Vitamin E content of 2.2 mg/kg.	[81]

(Continued)

Table 6.1 Recent results on seafood-based fat-soluble vitamin sources. (*Continued*)

Vitamin	Source	Key findings	Reference
	Rainbow trout flesh	Solid-liquid extraction with n-hexane outperformed the other five extraction methods for -tocopherol.	[82]
K	Meat of Atlantic salmon fed a diet with high vitamin D_3 and K_1	Improvement in several bone formation and resorption markers after consuming salmon fed with high vitamin D and K. The results were obtained despite using vitamin K_1 for supplementation.	[83]
D	Anchovy filleting wastes	Oil extracted using d-limonene as biosolvent contained 81 µg of vitamin D_3/kg of oil.	[84]
	Wakame and combu leaves	Vitamin D <0.05 µg/100 g in both fresh and dried leaves.	[85]
A	Pangasius catfish filleting wastes	Fish oil obtained as part of a zero-waste procedure, contained 334 µg of retinol/kg of oil.	[86]
	Fresh *Caulerpa sp.* leaves	High vitamin A reaching 4810 mg/kg.	[87]
	Dried *Ulva lactuca*	Vitamin A below detection limit.	[88]

and egg yolk. When choosing a type of seafood as a source of vitamin D, keep in mind that many processed seafood products, such as fish fingers (or sticks), do not have high quantities. Vitamin D2 levels are high in some edible seaweed, while they are low in others, such as combu and wakame [125] microgram/gram, which have levels below the detection limit (0.05 g/g). Vitamin D fortification of foods has been found to benefit both children and adults. However, according to [89], not all vitamin D-fortified products have received positive consumer feedback. The following issues must be addressed to successfully use food augmentation as a tool to combat vitamin D deficiency: consumers must have a positive attitude toward the food product, consumers must see a personal benefit from the fortified food, cultural appropriateness, and awareness of the prevalence of vitamin D deficiency in society [90, 91].

Obtaining this vitamin in fish oil via seafood by-products may be a cost-effective solution. Recent research has used bio solvents like d-limonene instead of typical organic solvents to enhance the quality of obtained fish oil. D-limonene is non-toxic and can be recovered completely by hydrodistillation at temperatures below 100 degrees Celsius. It is used to obtain high quality fish oil from anchovy filleting waste with a vitamin D_3 content of 81 μg/kg [92].

Seafood, especially seaweeds, can be a valuable source of vitamin A. For example, *Caulrepa sp.* have high levels of vitamin A (4.8 g/kg). On either hand, not all seaweeds are a rich source of vitamin A, as shown by [93], who reported that vitamin A in dried *Ulva lactuca* was below the detection limit. Vitamin A can also be obtained from fish and its by-products. Nam *et al.*, [145] used an enzymatic hydrolysis of Pangasius catfish filleting by-products which included head, trimmings, viscera, scales, liver, roe and skin, during a zero-waste procedure to obtain protein hydrolysate, hydroxyapatite and, after additional purification, fish oil with a vitamin A content of 334 μg/kg of oil. The vitamin A content, however, was relatively low, when compared to the retinol content in an unspecified fish wastes oil reported by (0.70 g/kg) [94].

Vitamin E is commonly associated with four tocotrienols and four tocopherols (α, β, γ and δ). This may, however, be inaccurate, since only α-tocopherol fulfills the definition of a "vitamin", while the other tocopherols and tocotrienols do not prevent ataxia, a vitamin E deficiency symptom. Fortunately, α-tocopherol is the main tocopherol found in seafood products [96].

α-Tocopherol is often obtained from seafood during crude oil extraction. Having strong antioxidant properties, α-tocopherol is often responsible for better oil stability during storage. Although low-temperature superior fish oil stability in general, [97] found that different oil refining temperatures yield varying levels of fish oil stability (70 vs. 90 °C) did not affect the α-tocopherol content of the oil extracted from rainbow trout by-products (head, bone, tail and intestine), with the content ranging from ~90 to 160 μg/g of oil. Crude oils with high levels of α-tocopherol can be obtained from various fish by-products. For example, [98] used tuna gill and gut to obtain crude oils with a high yield of 26.1%, which was an α-tocopherol content of 76 μg/g. On the other hand, extraction of crude oil from sardine head, gut and fin resulted in a yield of only 9.2% which was 36 μg/g of α-tocopherol. Therefore, the choice of fish species and type of by-product are important factors to recover high levels of α-tocopherol. Processing of crude oil also negatively affected the α-tocopherol content, as reported by [99] After refining crude oil from fish by-products, they discovered a 31% to 45% fall in -tocopherol content. Soxhlet extraction, Folch extraction, solid-liquid extraction with n-hexane and methanol-BHT, saponification with KOH and n-hexane extraction, and saponification with KOH with magnetic agitation were all compared [100]. After further adjustment, they determined that solid-liquid extraction with n-hexane was the most suited approach.

Depending on the source, the normal recommended daily intake (RDI) for vitamin K varies. The standard recommendations are 55 to 75 grams every day (1 gram per kilogram of body weight per day), although some sites recommend 600 grams per day. Vitamin K concentration calculated as the sum of K1 and K2 in fish is usually in the range of 1.8–11.3 g/kg [101].

Eel (644 g/kg) and dried seaweeds (1750–12,900 g/kg) are two seafood sources that have significantly more vitamin K. All of these microalgae and macroalgae have been suggested as potential sources of vitamin K1. Fish, on the other hand, usually contains vitamin K in the form of menaquinone (K2), whereas algae contain phylloquinone (K1). Because these two forms of vitamin K have different functions and health-promoting properties, algae should not be used to replace fish or other animal-based food products as a source of vitamin K, but rather should be used to supplement it [102–104].

Graff *et al.* [100] have investigated the use of Atlantic salmon fed with a high vitamin D_3 and K_1 diet on several bone formation markers of human subjects with additional Ca supplementation. They found that the consumption of such treated salmon improved more significantly the bone formation markers then in patients consuming salmon fed only high vitamin D_3. Surprisingly, these results were observed even though the form of vitamin K was of phylloquinone, meanwhile the positive effect on bone quality is usually associated with menaquinone [105].

Seafood can also be a valuable source of water-soluble vitamins. One of the most important water-soluble vitamins found in seafood is vitamin B_{12}, which can be found mainly in sources of animal origin or algae, with the latter being a potential source of vitamin B_{12} for food fortification and supplementation. The main source of vitamin B12 in the diets of adult Koreans and Canadians has been discovered to be seafood. Vitamin B12 levels are often higher in the dark flesh of fish muscle than in the light meat. Furthermore, fish by-products such as viscera, which can contain much higher levels of vitamin B12 than muscle, are a viable source for vitamin B12 extraction [106]. Vitamins can be found in abundance in seafood, which are often hard to supply from other food sources. Those include vitamin D or B_{12}. As in case of minerals, the seafood by-products seem to be a potential source of vitamins [107].

6.8 Dopamine in Seafood as Drug and Supplement

Dopamine (3,4-dihydroxyphenethylamine) is a neurotransmitter that has the potential to be employed as a medication. It plays a crucial role in cognitive functions. Some of the areas affected are ambition, thinking, resting state, penalty, memory, attention, and memory. Drugs derived from DA or its metabolites are also being used to treat clinical illnesses (bipolar disorder, Parkinson's disease, and several types of addiction, among others). DA can also be used to improve heart rate and urine production, and also for pediatric therapies, according to Pacific. The sourcing of DA is potentially important to the drug industry [108].

Black inks are found in cephalopods such as squid, cuttlefish, and octopus, and are made up of melanin, enzymes (tyrosinase), amino acids, and DA [95]. Although some inkless octopus species exist, cephalopods could be assessed for DA supply. According to, squid ink contains anticancer, antioxidant, anti-retroviral, and antibacterial properties [109]. Squid ink contains a significant amount of DA, according to Palumbo et al. [142]. Also, according to [110], the concentrations of L-DA and DA in squid ink were 1.15 and 0.19 mM, respectively. Ink from cuttlefish (Sepia officinalis) is also a good source of DA in different forms. According to HPLC analysis results based on crude ink obtained from the whole cuttlefish, the concentrations of dopa and DA were found to be 2.2 ± 0.8 and 0.06 ± 0.02 nmol/mg of protein, respectively. DA is obtained from L-tyrosine protein-rich foods. As a result, the DA content in the protein fraction should be determined. Naila *et al.*, [146] estimate that DA can be found in fish, meat, and their products, in addition to some cephalopod inks. As a result, these protein-rich foods could be considered as possibilities for someone who wants or needs to enhance their DA levels, because the brain requires tyrosine, which can be found in protein-rich foods like fish, to produce DA [111].

A DA hydrochloride and 5% dextrose injectable might be utilized to correct hemodynamics quickly in shock patients. Use of 800, 1600, or 3200 mcg/mL doses of DA by infusion depended on the patient's body weight from 10 to 100 kg. One of the primary causes of death is traumatic brain injury (TBI). TBI has been related with fluctuations in DA levels [112].

Establishing the DA level in the blood requires a well-balanced diet. If DA is required immediately, it can be injected. Probiotics, some minerals, vitamins, and fish oil supplements may also be used to assist enhance DA, but non-prescription techniques have not been encouraged. Soups made with squid, cuttlefish, or octopus ink, for example, may be appropriate. Pills containing DA derived from squid, cuttlefish, and octopus inks may be useful [113–115].

6.9 Bioactive Peptides From Marine Sources

Bioactive peptides are found in marine organisms such as sponges, tunicates, bryozoans, mollusks, bacteria, microalgae, macroalgae, cyanobacteria, fish, and crustaceans, and have antimicrobial, cardioprotective (anticoagulant, antihypertensive, antiatherosclerotic), antioxidant, radioprotective, antiparasitic, anti-inflammatory, and anti-cancerous properties [116].

The protein component of fish and other marine organisms and their by-products have ingredients with potentially important roles as functional and medicinal foods that may prevent and/or treat many chronic diseases. Marine macroalgae are a possible source of high-quality proteins with greater nutritional characteristics than terrestrial plants since they include all EAA in large concentrations. A variety of proteins, peptides, and amino acids found in marine species can help to reduce inflammation, boosting the immune system's ability to fight off infections and injuries. Anticancer therapy is being researched using marine proteins. New cytotoxic proteins, such as chondroitin from the common marine sponge *Chondrosia reniformis*, have been found [117–119].

Bioactive peptides are inert in their parent protein, but can be produced when big pre-propeptides are decomposed into particular protein fragments and changed to improve a variety of physiological activities [120].

The best sources of structurally diverse bioactive peptides with functions such as ACE inhibitory and anti-hypertensive, antioxidative, anticoagulant, and antimicrobial effects are marine organisms. Bioactive peptides from the sea can be made by solvent extraction, enzymatic hydrolysis, or microbial fermentation of proteins, resulting in fragments that usually contain 3–20 amino acid residues. Their amino acid sequence determines the biological activity. The bioactivity of peptide combinations in protein hydrolysates is influenced by their molecular size and physical elements, with small MW fractions (1 to 5 kDa) containing more effective antioxidative peptides in general. To get pure peptides, peptide portions can be isolated using column chromatography. For example, those with a tripeptide sequence at the C-terminal end of peptides with antihypertensive activity contain hydrophobic amino acid. They were demonstrated to be ACE-inhibitory peptides. ACE causes blood vessels to constrict increasing blood pressure. Coughs, high blood potassium levels, low blood pressure, skin rashes, headaches, fatigue, fetal and taste problems are all side effects of commercial ACE inhibitors (benazepril, captopril, enalapril, perindopril, trandolapril, quinapril, lisinopril, and moexipril). Natural components with ACE inhibitory properties have been a hot topic in hypertension research. The sequence of ACE-inhibitory peptides from marine creatures with high ACE inhibitor capacity has been investigated, and their activity has been characterized [122, 143].

6.10 Gelatin From Marine Sources

Gelatin is not a naturally occurring protein. It is, however, one among the most popular versatile biopolymers, an animal-based protein obtained by thermal denaturation with partial acid/alkaline hydrolysis or enzymatic hydrolysis of collagen. Protein content, moisture, and ash, together with certain carbs, make up the majority of marine gelatin. Its qualities are distinct from those derived from animal sources, and it has found use in the pharmaceutical and food industries, as well as for therapeutic purposes. In 2018 the global gelatin market was estimated at 4.5 billion USD, with an increased demand for gelatin from sources other than bovine and porcine. The raw materials commonly used for gelatin production are the bones, skins, and connective tissue of terrestrial animals Cattle and pigs, for example. The demand for new collagen sources stems from religious reasons as well as health concerns related to the bovine spongiform encephalopathy outbreak, which has caused some customers to want or desire alternative collagen sources [123]. Many of their problems are addressed by marine gelatins. The viscous liquid state of marine gelatins at room temperature is both a benefit and a disadvantage. Good absorption capacity, the survival of enzymatic digestion products in the git, enhanced digestibility, and good film-forming properties are some of the functional properties that are mostly an advantage of marine gelatins in some applications, especially in biomedical and food applications. Functional properties of gelatin such as gelling, foaming, stabilizing, or emulsifying ability determine its suitability for many applications in food production, directly or as an ingredient in food coatings, and an active component in packaging material [124]. Some features of sea gelatin, including gel strength, melting temperature, and MW, are lower than those of terrestrial gelatin, making commercialization of fish gelatin difficult. Also, cold- and hot fish have different gel strengths and melting temperatures, with warm-water fish gelatin being more akin to bovine or pig gelatins. This is owing to changes in protein properties and amino acid composition between cold- and warm-water species, as well as cold-water fish having a lower hydroxyproline level. Gelatin of marine origin has a gel strength of 98 to 600 g. The probable applications of a gelatin are determined by the combination of its qualities. Lower melting point gelatins derived from the sea have several advantages in food applications. They could be used as a food emulsifier, stabilizer, and foaming agent, as well as for microencapsulation of colorants and enhancement of sensory qualities of low-fat foods (flavor). Various approaches have been investigated to enhance the fundamental qualities of marine gelatins. Gelatin can be modified using transglutaminase to improve gelatin elasticity and cohesiveness of the gels as well as providing non-thermoreversible gels with lower gel strength. Furthermore, fish gelatin can be used as a powerful antibacterial agent when hydrolyzed with papain. Non-electrolytes (glycerol, sorbitol, sucrose) can improve the strength of gelatin gels, whereas co-enhancers (magnesium, sulphate, sucrose, and transglutaminase) can improve the strength and melting point of fish gelatin. Gel strength has improved significantly and reduction in viscosity can be obtained using ultraviolet irradiation. Jridi et al., 2013 found that cuttlefish gelatin prevents-carotene bleaching, implying its usefulness in food preservation from drying and light exposure, as well as its potential use in the manufacture of food packaging materials. Gelatin in food packaging would help to reduce drip loss as well as oxygen-induced alterations such lipid oxidation and color changes. Production of edible coatings that may carry antioxidants and/or antimicrobials might prolong the shelf-life including flavor and odor loss during storage and change the mechanical and the films barrier properties. Gelatin does not really satisfy the dietary requirements for proteins as it is nutritionally unbalanced but when combined with other proteins, the expectation is that it functions like any other protein. It can be utilized to enhance the functional qualities of a product of food and beverage products and to enhance the nutritional value of food products [126, 127].

Besides food applications, the properties of marine gelatin can be improved for other uses as well. The addition of phenolic compounds, such as caffeic acid, to gelatin derived from fish scales improved its mechanical biodegradability and cytocompatibility, making it a more effective tissue engineering material. Pacific cod skin gelatin was hydrolyzed with pepsin to produce two bioactive compounds that inhibited ACE in a considerable way. This enzyme is crucial in the management of T2DM and hypertension. Although the functional qualities of gelatin vary by species and extraction techniques, it is widely recognized as a non-carcinogenic, cost-effective protein when related to many other proteins. but significantly more expensive than bovine and porcine gelatin, and biocompatible for many pharmaceuticals. Collagen and gelatin-based biomedical products such as gels, scaffolds, microspheres, and films have been shown to be beneficial in tissue engineering, implants, and wound dressing [128, 129].

The use of oral administration, microcryogel injection, and biodegradable scaffolds to promote wound healing at different levels including superficial, deep layer, and systematic levels have been studied. Gelatin is also used as a wound dressing material and in the production of sterile sponges for medical and dental surgery. It is also the main ingredient in both soft and hard gel capsules with an increased viscosity that prolongs the release of trapped materials such as drugs, vitamins, and minerals from nanoparticles. More recently, gelatin nanoparticles obtained by nanoprecipitation, were tested for improved mechanical properties such as particle size, shape, and surface chemistry for drug delivery systems [130].

6.11 Health Benefit of Nano-Based Materials for Bioactive Compounds from Marine-Based Sources

Nanotechnology is a relatively recent technology that allows for the development of long-term crops and treatments. Nanofibers, for example, let fish meat retain lipids and peptides. Vitamin intake and stability are also important, and chitosan-based nanoparticles and thymol-loaded electrospun chitosan-based nanomaterials may successfully deliver nicotinamide acid, pyridoxal, pyridoxine, and pyridoxamine in fish fillets. Important marine-based substances for human health include EPA, DHA, and EAA, as well as tryptophan and B group vitamins. Probiotic microorganisms are beneficial to both food systems and human immune systems. Consumption of nanoprobiotic-coated fish meat (*L. reuteri* and *L. rhamnosus*) could be a suitable option. The fatty acids in fish meat become more stable because to these nanoprobiotics. Algae are high in essential fatty acids like -3 and -6, which are advantageous to the immune system on both sides. In addition, Au nanoparticles produced from brown algal seaweed have been shown to have anti-diabetic and anti-inflammatory characteristics in medical applications [131, 132].

Nanotechnology applications of marine-based products could be combined with other probiotic-friendly dietary ingredients. Nanoemulsion technology, for example, increased the physicochemical qualities of fish oil-enriched yoghurt. Nano-based materials can be made using microalgae-based medications and their therapeutic applications. Nanoparticles with maximum diameters of 29 and 60 nm, for example, were generated from marine fungi like *Aspergillus flavus* and seagrass like *Cymodocea* sp. and showed good anticancer and cytotoxic activities. The marine algal product fucoxanthin was found to be safe for humans, and its nanoparticulate delivery could improve supplement efficacy. Nanostructures generally provide a larger contact area on the surface of the materials and can provide a good controlled release profile [133, 134].

Krill are tiny crabs found in abundance in the polar oceans of the North (Arctic) and South (Antarctic). The Antarctic Euphausia Superba, the greatest of the krill species, is used to extract krill oil (KO). Krill is a sustainable source of ω-3 PUFA, including EPA and DHA. KO includes a significant amount of -3 PUFA attached to phospholipids (PL), the most abundant of which is phosphatidylcholine, whereas fish oil is largely made up of -3 PUFA linked to triacylglycerides (TAG) (PC). PC has more than 80% of the EPA and DHA found in KO. It is, nonetheless, a relatively costly product. Nanotechnology applications such as nanoparticles (130 nm) can be used to contain KO (Euphausia superba) as a nutritional supplement. Also improved was the oxidative stability of KO (1 wt %) produced from nanoliposomes (217 nm). Nanoliposomes could effectively control the release of KO in a simulated gastrointestinal system. These results showed that the nanoform of KO can be utilized to improve the release profile [135–139].

6.12 Conclusions

Marine organisms are becoming attractive sources of compounds that show value beyond the nutritional one. New discoveries of diverse biologically active compounds and the growth of their possible applications in food, functional food and supplement development are receiving more attention. Chitosan, chitin, fish oil, EPA and DHA, EAA, peptides, gelatin, polysaccharides, polyphenols, pigments, vitamins, minerals, and other materials have been characterized by their antimicrobial, antioxidant, anti-inflammatory, anti-cancer, anti-tumor, antiviral, antimalarial, anti-obesity, and immunomodulatory properties. Many of these compounds have been utilized as functional food ingredients, or their biological properties have been used to treat/prevent some type of health disorder. They have also been used in the food business to improve the nutritional value of foods (stabilizer, emulsifier, coating or thickening agent, texture modifier) or to enriched the foods with functional components (ω-3) and allow their application in health-promoting foods for direct consumption. The worldwide nutraceutical sector is rising in constant search of compounds to be implemented in the dietary, beverage and supplement industries. At the same time, the importance of the role of consumers is growing and benefits of the functional foods and supplements on overall health. Both the search for health promoting compounds from natural sources and the development of new functional products has intensified.

Bioavailability, development of environmentally acceptable technologies for elevated extractions, preservation from deterioration, and recognition of individual components that can be refined for usage in a specific form are all factors that influence the future of marine-derived components. The sustainability of marine sources should be considered when they are exploited on the industrial level. Farming and cultivation of the organisms for a particular component and determining the conditions needed for its high yield recovery is a complex undertaking that requires development of new cost-effective technologies. The nanotechnology techniques may be used for the production of nanosystems with marine-based bioactive molecules to protect these functional compounds against degradation. Also, clinical studies are needed, especially for newly discovered compounds to confirm their therapeutic effect, establish their role in health promoting and quantities for daily consummation. These would help the food industry develop functional foods appealing to the consumers.

Acknowledgment

The authors thank MET's Institute of Pharmacy, BKC, which is affiliated with Savitribai Phule Pune University, Nashik. EDA wishes to express gratitude to the NFST/RGNF/UGC, Government of India, for providing financial assistance in the form of a fellowship (award 202021-NFST-MAH-01235).

References

1. Aakre, I., Næss, S., Kjellevold, M., Markhus, M.W., Alvheim, A.R., Dalane, J.Ø., Kielland, E., Dahl, L., New data on nutrient composition in large selection of commercially available seafood products and its impact on micronutrient intake. *Food Nutr. Res.*, 63, 2019.
2. Abachi, S., Bazinet, L., Beaulieu, L., Antihypertensive and angiotensin-i-converting enzyme (ACE)-inhibitory peptides from fish as potential cardioprotective compounds. *Mar. Drugs*, 17, 613, 2019.
3. Abd-Ellatef, G.E.F., Ahmed, O.M., Abdel-Reheim, E.S., Abdel-Hamid, A.H.Z., Ulva lactuca polysaccharides prevent wistar rat breast carcinogenesis through the augmentation of apoptosis, enhancement of antioxidant defense system, and suppression of inflammation. *Breast Cancer Targets Ther.*, 9, 67–83, 2017.
4. Admassu, H., Gasmalla, M.A.A., Yang, R., Zhao, W., Identification of bioactive peptides with α-amylase inhibitory potential from enzymatic protein hydrolysates of red seaweed (Porphyra spp). *J. Agric. Food Chem.*, 66, 4872–4882, 2018.
5. Adrian, G., Mihai, M., Vodnar, D.C., The use of chitosan, alginate, and pectin in the biomedical and food sector—Biocompatibility, bioadhesiveness, and biodegradability. *Polym. (Basel)*, 11, 1837, 2019.
6. Afonso, C., Bandarra, N.M., Nunes, L., Cardoso, C., Tocopherols in seafood and aquaculture products. *Crit. Rev. Food Sci. Nutr.*, 56, 128–140, 2016.
7. Aguirre-Joya, J.A., Chacón-Garza, L.E., Valdivia-Najár, G., Arredondo-Valdés, R., Castro-López, C., Ventura-Sobrevilla, J.M., Aguilar-Gonzáles, C.N., Boone-Villa, D., Nanosystems of plant-based pigments and its relationship with oxidative stress. *Food Chem. Toxicol.*, 143, 111433, 2020.
8. Ahmad, S.I., Ahmad, R., Khan, M.S., Kant, R., Shahid, S., Gautam, L., Hasan, G.M., Hassan, M.I., Chitin and its derivatives: Structural properties and biomedical applications. *Int. J. Biol. Macromol.*, 164, 526–539, 2020.
9. Aidos, I., Van Der Padt, A., Boom, R.M., Luten, J.B., Quality of crude fish oil extracted from herring byproducts of varying states of freshness. *J. Food Sci.*, 68, 458–465, 2003.

10. Aissaoui, N., Abidi, F., Hardouin, J., Abdelkafi, Z., Marrakchi, N., Jouenne, T., Marzouki, M.N., ACE inhibitory and antioxidant activities of novel peptides from scorpaena notata by-product protein hydrolysate. *Int. J. Pept. Res. Ther.*, 23, 13–23, 2017.
11. Aksun Tumerkan, E.T., Cansu, U., Boran, G., Regenstein, J.M., Ozogul, F., Physiochemical and functional properties of gelatin obtained from tuna, frog and chicken skins. *Food Chem.*, 287, 273–279, 2019.
12. Al Khalifah, R., Alsheikh, R., Alnasser, Y., Alsheikh, R., Alhelali, N., Naji, A., Al Backer, N., The impact of vitamin D food fortification and health outcomes in children: A systematic review and meta-regression. *Syst. Rev.*, 9, 144, 2020.
13. Alaswad, K., Lavie, C.J., Milani, R.V., O'Keefe, J.H., Fish oil in cardiovascular prevention. *Ochsner J.*, 4, 83–91, 2002.
14. Alexa-Stratulat, T., Luca, A., Badescu, M., Bohotin, C.R., Alexa, I.D., Nutritional modulators in chemotherapy-induced neuropathic pain, in: *Nutritional Modulators of Pain in the Aging Population*, pp. 9–33, Elsevier Inc., Amsterdam, The Netherlands, 2017.
15. Aluko, R.E., Antihypertensive peptides from food proteins. *Annu. Rev. Food Sci. Technol.*, 6, 235–262, 2015.
16. Ambati, R.R., Gogisetty, D., Aswathanarayana, R.G., Ravi, S., Bikkina, P.N., Bo, L., Yuepeng, S., Industrial potential of carotenoid pigments from microalgae: Current trends and future prospects. *Crit. Rev. Food Sci. Nutr.*, 59, 1880–1902, 2019.
17. Anand, B.G., Thomas, C.K.N., Prakash, S., Kumar, C.S., Biosynthesis of silver nano-particles by marine sediment fungi for a dose dependent cytotoxicity against HEp2 cell lines. *Biocatal. Agric. Biotechnol.*, 4, 150–157, 2015.
18. Ande, M.P., Syamala, K., SrinivasaRao, P., MuraliMohan, K., Lingam, S.S., Marine nutraceuticals. *Mar. Omi. Princ. Appl.*, pp. 329–345, 2016.
19. Andryukov, B.G., Besednova, N.N., Kuznetsova, T.A., Zaporozhets, T.S., Ermakova, S.P., Zvyagintseva, T.N., Chingizova, E.A., Gazha, A.K., Smolina, T.P., Sulfated polysaccharides from marine algae as a basis of modern biotechnologies for creating wound dressings: Current achievements and future prospects. *Biomedicines*, 8, 301, 2020.
20. Anraku, M., Fujii, T., Furutani, N., Kadowaki, D., Maruyama, T., Otagiri, M., Gebicki, J.M., Tomida, H., Antioxidant effects of a dietary supplement: Reduction of indices of oxidative stress in normal subjects by water-soluble chitosan. *Food Chem. Toxicol.*, 47, 104–109, 2009.
21. Anraku, M., Fujii, T., Kondo, Y., Kojima, E., Hata, T., Tabuchi, N., Tsuchiya, D., Goromaru, T., Tsutsumi, H., Kadowaki, D. *et al.*, Antioxidant properties of high molecular weight dietary chitosan *in vitro* and *in vivo*. *Carbohydr. Polym.*, 83, 501–505, 2011.
22. Anraku, M., Gebicki, J.M., Iohara, D., Tomida, H., Uekama, K., Maruyama, T., Hirayama, F., Otagiri, M., Antioxidant activities of chitosans and its derivatives in *in vitro* and *in vivo* studies. *Carbohydr. Polym.*, 199, 141–149, 2018.

23. Antoniac, I.V., Filipescu, M., Barbaro, K., Bonciu, A., Birjega, R., Cotrut, C.M., Galvano, E., Fosca, M., Fadeeva, I.V., Vadalà, G. et al., Iron ion-doped tricalcium phosphate coatings improve the properties of biodegradable magnesium alloys for biomedical implant application. *Adv. Mater. Interfaces*, 7, 2000531, 2020.
24. Aparna, P., Muthathal, S., Nongkynrih, B., Gupta, S., Vitamin D deficiency in India. *J. Fam. Med. Prim. Care*, 7, 324, 2018.
25. Aranaz, I., Mengibar, M., Harris, R., Panos, I., Miralles, B., Acosta, N., Galed, G., Heras, A., Functional characterization of chitin and chitosan. *Curr. Chem. Biol.*, 3, 203–230, 2009.
26. Araújo, M., Alves, R.C., Pimentel, F.B., Costa, A.S.G., Fernandes, T.J.R., Valente, L.M.P., Rema, P., Oliveira, M.B.P.P., New approach for vitamin E extraction in rainbow trout flesh: Application in fish fed commercial and red seaweed-supplemented diets. *Eur. J. Lipid Sci. Technol.*, 117, 1398–1405, 2015.
27. Azuma, K., Ifuku, S., Osaki, T., Okamoto, Y., Minami, S., Preparation and biomedical applications of chitin and chitosan nanofibers. *J. Biomed. Nanotechnol.*, 10, 2891–2920, 2014.
28. Azzi, A., Tocopherols, tocotrienols and tocomonoenols: Many similar molecules but only one vitamin E. *Redox Biol.*, 26, 101259, 2019.
29. Bakshi, P.S., Selvakumar, D., Kadirvelu, K., Kumar, N.S., Comparative study on antimicrobial activity and biocompatibility of n-selective chitosan derivatives. *React. Funct. Polym.*, 124, 149–155, 2018.
30. Bales, J.W., Kline, A.E., Wagner, A.K., Dixon, C.E., Targeting dopamine in acute traumatic brain injury. *Open Drug Discovery J.*, 2, 119–128, 2010.
31. Balti, R., Bougatef, A., Sila, A., Guillochon, D., Dhulster, P., Nedjar-Arroume, N., Nine novel angiotensin I-converting enzyme (ACE) inhibitory peptides from cuttlefish (sepia officinalis) muscle protein hydrolysates and antihypertensive effect of the potent active peptide in spontaneously hypertensive rats. *Food Chem.*, 170, 519–525, 2015.
32. Bashir, K.M.I., Sohn, J.H., Kim, J.S., Choi, J.S., Identification and characterization of novel antioxidant peptides from mackerel (Scomber japonicus) muscle protein hydrolysates. *Food Chem.*, 323, 126809, 2020.
33. Bello, A.B., Kim, D., Kim, D., Park, H., Lee, S.H., Engineering and functionalization of gelatin biomaterials: From cell culture to medical applications. *Tissue Eng. Part B Rev.*, 26, 164–180, 2020.
34. Bemani, E., Ghanati, F., Rezaei, A., Jamshidi, M., Effect of phenylalanine on taxol production and antioxidant activity of extracts of suspension-cultured hazel (Corylus avellana L.) cells. *J. Nat. Med.*, 67, 446–451, 2013.
35. Besednova, N.N., Zaporozhets, T.S., Kuznetsova, T.A., Makarenkova, I.D., Kryzhanovsky, S.P., Fedyanina, L.N., Ermakova, S.P., Extracts and marine algae polysaccharides in therapy and prevention of inflammatory diseases of the intestine. *Mar. Drugs*, 18, 289, 2020.
36. Bhat, R. and Karim, A.A., Ultraviolet radiation improves gel strength of fish gelatin. *Food Chem.*, 113, 1160–1164, 2009.

37. Bilal, M. and Iqbal, H.M.N., Biologically active macromolecules: Extraction strategies, therapeutic potential and biomedical perspective. *Int. J. Biol. Macromol.*, *151*, 1–18, 2020.
38. Biris-Dorhoi, E.S., Michiu, D., Pop, C.R., Rotar, A.M., Tofana, M., Pop, O.L., Socaci, S.A., Farcas, A.C., Macroalgae—A sustainable source of chemical compounds with biological activities. *Nutrients*, *12*, 3085, 2020.
39. Bito, T., Tanioka, Y., Watanabe, F., Characterization of vitamin B12 compounds from marine foods. *Fish. Sci.*, *84*, 747–755, 2018.
40. Bondiolotti, G., Bareggi, S.R., Frega, N.G., Strabioli, S., Cornelli, U., Activity of two different polyglucosamines, L112® and FF45®, on body weight in male rats. *Eur. J. Pharmacol.*, *567*, 155–158, 2007.
41. Bougatef, A., Nedjar-Arroume, N., Manni, L., Ravallec, R., Barkia, A., Guillochon, D., Nasri, M., Purification and identification of novel antioxidant peptides from enzymatic hydrolysates of sardinelle (Sardinella aurita) by-products proteins. *Food Chem.*, *118*, 559–565, 2010.
42. Bruno, S.F., Ekorong, F.J.A.A., Karkal, S.S., Cathrine, M.S.B., Kudre, T.G., Green and innovative techniques for recovery of valuable compounds from seafood by-products and discards: A review. *Trends Food Sci. Technol.*, *85*, 10–22, 2019.
43. Bubel, F., Dobrzański, Z., Bykowski, P.J., Chojnacka, K., Opaliński, S., Trziszka, T., Production of calcium preparations by technology of saltwater fish by product processing. *Open Chem.*, *13*, 1333–1340, 2015.
44. Burri, L., Hoem, N., Banni, S., Berge, K., Marine omega-3 phospholipids: Metabolism and biological activities. *Int. J. Mol. Sci.*, *13*, 15401–15419, 2012.
45. Byun, H.-G., Lee, J.K., Park, H.G., Jeon, J.-K., Kim, S.-K., Antioxidant peptides isolated from the marine rotifer, brachionus rotundiformis. *Process Biochem.*, *44*, 842–846, 2009.
46. Cashman, K.D., Dowling, K.G., Škrabáková, Z., Gonzalez-Gross, M., Valtueña, J., De Henauw, S., Moreno, L., Damsgaard, C.T., Michaelsen, K.F., Mølgaard, C. et al., Vitamin D deficiency in Europe: Pandemic? *Am. J. Clin. Nutr.*, *103*, 1033–1044, 2016.
47. Castelo-Branco, C., Cancelo Hidalgo, M.J., Palacios, S., Ciria-Recasens, M., Fernández-Pareja, A., Carbonell-Abella, C., Manasanch, J., Haya-Palazuelos, J., Efficacy and safety of ossein-hydroxyapatite complex versus calcium carbonate to prevent bone loss. *Climacteric*, *23*, 252–258, 2020.
48. Ceylan, Z., Yaman, M., Sağdıç, O., Karabulut, E., Yilmaz, M.T., Effect of electrospun thymol-loaded nanofiber coating on vitamin B profile of gilthead sea bream fillets (Sparus aurata). *LWT*, *98*, 162–169, 2018.
49. Ceylan, Z., Meral, R., Cavidoglu, I., Yagmur Karakas, C., Tahsin Yilmaz, M., A new application on fatty acid stability of fish fillets: Coating with probiotic bacteria-loaded polymer-based characterized nanofibers. *J. Food Saf.*, *38*, 12547, 2018.
50. Ceylan, Z., Meral, R., Karakaş, C.Y., Dertli, E., Yilmaz, M.T., A novel strategy for probiotic bacteria: Ensuring microbial stability of fish fillets using characterized probiotic bacteria-loaded nanofibers. *Innov. Food Sci. Emerg. Technol.*, *48*, 212–218, 2018.

51. Ceylan, Z., Unal SengOr, G.F., Yilmaz, M.T., Amino acid composition of gilthead sea bream fillets (Sparus aurata) coated with thymol-loaded chitosan nanofibers during cold storage. *J. Biotechnol.*, *256*, S28, 2017.
52. Chakdar, H. and Pabbi, S., *Algal pigments for human health and cosmeceuticals*, Elsevier B.V., Amsterdam, The Netherlands, 2017.
53. Chandika, P., Ko, S.C., Jung, W.K., Marine-derived biological macromolecule-based biomaterials for wound healing and skin tissue regeneration. *Int. J. Biol. Macromol.*, *77*, 24–35, 2015.
54. Chanthini, A.B., Balasubramani, G., Ramkumar, R., Sowmiya, R., Balakumaran, M.D., Kalaichelvan, P.T., Perumal, P., Structural characterization, antioxidant and *in vitro* cytotoxic properties of seagrass, cymodocea serrulata (R.Br.) asch. & magnus mediated silver nanoparticles. *J. Photochem. Photobiol. B Biol.*, *153*, 145–152, 2015.
55. Chen, Y., Lin, H., Li, Z., Mou, Q., The anti-allergic activity of polyphenol extracted from five marine algae. *J. Ocean Univ. China*, *14*, 681–684, 2015.
56. Chien, R.C., Yen, M.T., Mau, J.L., Antimicrobial and antitumor activities of chitosan from shiitake stipes, compared to commercial chitosan from crab shells. *Carbohydr. Polym.*, *138*, 259–264, 2016.
57. Chiu, C.Y., Chang, T.C., Liu, S.H., Chiang, M.T., The regulatory effects of fish oil and chitosan on hepatic lipogenic signals in high-fat diet-induced obese rats. *J. Food Drug Anal.*, *25*, 919–930, 2017.
58. Choulis, N.H., Miscellaneous drugs materials, medical devices, and techniques, in: *Side Effects of Drugs Annual*, vol. 33, pp. 1009–1029, Elsevier B.V., Amsterdam, The Netherlands, 2011.
59. Chung, M.J., Park, J.K., Park, Y.I., Anti-inflammatory effects of low-molecular weight chitosan oligosaccharides in IgE-antigen complex-stimulated RBL-2H3 cells and asthma model mice. *Int. Immunopharmacol.*, *12*, 453–459, 2012.
60. Ciriminna, R., Meneguzzo, F., Delisi, R., Pagliaro, M., Enhancing and improving the extraction of omega-3 from fish oil. *Sustain. Chem. Pharm.*, *5*, 54–59, 2017.
61. Ciriminna, R., Scurria, A., Avellone, G., Pagliaro, M.A., Circular economy approach to fish oil extraction. *ChemistrySelect*, *4*, 5106–5109, 2019.
62. Connor, W.E., Cefrancesco, C.A., Connor, S., N-3 fatty acids from fish oil effects on plasma lipoproteins and hypertriglyceridemic patients. *Ann. N. Y. Acad. Sci.*, *683*, 16–34, 1993.
63. Cunha, L. and Grenha, A., Sulfated seaweed polysaccharides as multifunctional materials in drug delivery applications. *Mar. Drugs*, *14*, 42, 2016.
64. Curado Borges, M., de Miranda Moura dos Santos, F., Weiss Telles, R., Melo de Andrade, M.V., Toulson Davisson Correia, M.I., Lanna, C.C.D., Omega-3 fatty acids, inflammatory status and biochemical markers of patients with systemic lupus erythematosus: A pilot study. *Rev. Bras. Reumatol.*, *57*, 526–534, 2017.
65. Custódio, C.A., Reis, R.L., Mano, J.F., Photo-cross-linked laminarin-based hydrogels for biomedical applications. *Biomacromolecules*, *17*, 1602–1609, 2016.

66. Ahire, E.D., Surana, K.R., Patil, C.D., Shah, H.S., Sonwane, G.B., Talele, S.G., Role of omega-3 fatty acids in different neurodegenerative disorders, in: *Applied Pharmaceutical Science and Microbiology*, pp. 173–194, Apple Academic Press, 2020.
67. Cutrona, K.J., Kaufman, B.A., Figueroa, D.M., Elmore, D.E., Role of arginine and lysine in the antimicrobial mechanism of histone-derived antimicrobial peptides. *FEBS Lett.*, 589, 3915–3920, 2015.
68. Das, S., Paul, B., Sengupta, J., Datta, A., Beneficial effects of fish oil to human health: A review. *Agric. Rev.*, 30, 199–205, 2009.
69. Dawczynski, C., Schubert, R., Jahreis, G., Amino acids, fatty acids, and dietary fibre in edible seaweed products. *Food Chem.*, 103, 891–899, 2007.
70. De Souza, D.R., da Silva Pieri, B.L., Comim, V.H., de Oliveira Marques, S., Luciano, T.F., Rodrigues, M.S., De Souza, C.T., Fish oil reduces subclinical inflammation, insulin resistance, and atherogenic factors in overweight/obese type 2 diabetes mellitus patients: A pre-post pilot study. *J. Diabetes Complicat.*, 34, 107553, 2020.
71. Derby, C., Cephalopod ink: Production, chemistry, functions and applications. *Mar. Drugs*, 12, 2700–2730, 2014.
72. Derby, C.D., Kicklighter, C.E., Johnson, P.M., Zhang, X., Chemical composition of inks of diverse marine molluscs suggests convergent chemical defenses. *J. Chem. Ecol.*, 33, 1105–1113, 2007.
73. Dilli, D., Soylu, H., Tekin, N., Turkish neonatal society guideline on the neonatal hemodynamics and management of hypotension in newborns. *Türk Pediatri Ars.*, 53, Suppl. 1, 65–75, 2019.
74. DiNicolantonio, J.J. and O'Keefe, J.H., Good fats versus bad fats: A comparison of fatty acids in the promotion of insulin resistance, inflammation, and obesity. *Mo. Med.*, 114, 303–307, 2017.
75. Draget, K.I. and Taylor, C., Chemical, physical and biological properties of alginates and their biomedical implications. *Food Hydrocoll.*, 25, 251–256, 2011.
76. Du, C., Abdullah, J.J., Greetham, D., Fu, D., Yu, M., Ren, L., Li, S., Lu, D., Valorization of food waste into biofertiliser and its field application. *J. Clean. Prod.*, 187, 273–284, 2018.
77. El-Naggar, M.M., Haneen, D.S.A., Mehany, A.B.M., Khalil, M.T., New synthetic chitosan hybrids bearing some heterocyclic moieties with potential activity as anticancer and apoptosis inducers. *Int. J. Biol. Macromol.*, 150, 1323–1330, 2020.
78. Emadzadeh, M., Sahebi, R., Khedmatgozar, H., Sadeghi, R., Farjami, M., Sharifan, P., Ravanshad, Y., Ferns, G.A., Ghayour-Mobarhan, M.A., Systematic review and meta-analysis of the effect of vitamin D-fortified food on glycemic indices. *BioFactors*, 46, 502–513, 2020.
79. Emerton, V. and Choi, E., *Essential guide to food additives*, Royal Society of Chemistry, Cambridge, UK, 2008.

80. Ermakova, S., Sokolova, R., Kim, S.M., Um, B.H., Isakov, V., Zvyagintseva, T., Fucoidans from brown seaweeds sargassum hornery, eclonia cava, costaria costata: Structural characteristics and anticancer activity. *Appl. Biochem. Biotechnol.*, *164*, 841–850, 2011.
81. Fahmy, S.R., Soliman, A.M., Ali, E.M., Antifungal and antihepatotoxic effects of sepia ink extract against oxidative stress as a risk factor of invasive pulmonary aspergillosis in neutropenic mice. *Afr. J. Tradit. Complement. Altern. Med.*, *11*, 148–159, 2014.
82. Fan, X., Bai, L., Mao, X., Zhang, X., Novel peptides with anti-proliferation activity from the porphyra haitanesis hydrolysate. *Process Biochem.*, *60*, 98–107, 2017.
83. Farooqui, A.A., *Beneficial effects of fish oil on human brain*, Springer, New York, NY, USA, 2009.
84. Feng, X., Tjia, J.Y.Y., Zhou, Y., Liu, Q., Fu, C., Yang, H., Effects of tocopherol nanoemulsion addition on fish sausage properties and fatty acid oxidation. *LWT*, *118*, 108737, 2020.
85. Fernando, I.P.S., Sanjeewa, K.K.A., Samarakoon, K.W., Lee, W.W., Kim, H.S., Kang, N., Ranasinghe, P., Lee, H.S., Jeon, Y.J.A., Fucoidan fraction purified from chnoospora minima; A potential inhibitor of lps-induced inflammatory responses. *Int. J. Biol. Macromol.*, *104*, 1185–1193, 2017.
86. Fertah, M., Belfkira, A., Dahmane, E.M., Taourirte, M., Brouillette, F., Extraction and characterization of sodium alginate from moroccan laminaria digitata brown seaweed. *Arab. J. Chem.*, *10*, S3707–S3714, 2017.
87. Fiore, G., Poli, A., Di Cosmo, A., D'ischia, M., Palumbo, A., Dopamine in the ink defence system of sepia officinalis: Biosynthesis, vesicular compartmentation in mature ink gland cells, nitric oxide (NO)/CGMP-induced depletion and fate in secreted ink1. *Biochem. J.*, *378*, 785–791, 2004.
88. Fitton, J.H., Stringer, D.N., Park, A.Y., Karpiniec, S.S., Therapies from fucoidan: New developments. *Mar. Drugs*, *17*, 571, 2019.
89. Fitzgerald, C., Aluko, R.E., Hossain, M., Rai, D.K., Hayes, M., Potential of a renin inhibitory peptide from the red seaweed palmaria palmata as a functional food ingredient following confirmation and characterization of a hypotensive effect in spontaneously hypertensive rats. *J. Agric. Food Chem.*, *62*, 8352–8356, 2014.
90. Flammini, L., Martuzzi, F., Vivo, V., Ghirri, A., Salomi, E., Bignetti, E., Barocelli, E., Hake fish bone as a calcium source for efficient bone mineralization. *Int. J. Food Sci. Nutr.*, *67*, 265–273, 2016.
91. Flores, E., Arévalo, S., Burnat, M., Cyanophycin and arginine metabolism in cyanobacteria. *Algal Res.*, *42*, 101577, 2019.
92. Gades, M.D. and Stern, J.S., Chitosan supplementation and fecal fat excretion in men. *Obes. Res.*, *11*, 683–688, 2003.
93. Ganesan, A.R., Tiwari, U., Rajauria, G., Seaweed nutraceuticals and their therapeutic role in disease prevention. *Food Sci. Hum. Wellness*, *8*, 252–263, 2019.

94. Giri, S.S., Sahoo, S.K., Sahu, A.K., Mukhopadhyay, P.K., Nutrient digestibility and intestinal enzyme activity of clarias batrachus (Linn.) juveniles fed on dried fish and chicken viscera incorporated diets. *Bioresour. Technol.*, *71*, 97–101, 2000.
95. Gleadall, I.G., Guerrero-Kommritz, J., Hochberg, F.G., Laptikhovsky, V.V., The inkless octopuses (Cephalopoda: Octopodidae) of the Southwest Atlantic. *Zool. Sci.*, *27*, 528, 2010.
96. Gómez-Estaca, J., Calvo, M.M., Álvarez-Acero, I., Montero, P., Gómez-Guillén, M.C., Characterization and storage stability of astaxanthin esters, fatty acid profile and α-tocopherol of lipid extract from shrimp (L. vannamei) waste with potential applications as food ingredient. *Food Chem.*, *216*, 37–44, 2017.
97. Gómez-Guzmán, M., Rodríguez-Nogales, A., Algieri, F., Gálvez, J., Potential role of seaweed polyphenols in cardiovascular-associated disorders. *Mar. Drugs*, *16*, 250, 2018.
98. Gorzelanny, C., Pöppelmann, B., Strozyk, E., Moerschbacher, B.M., Schneider, S.W., Specific interaction between chitosan and matrix metalloprotease 2 decreases the invasive activity of human melanoma cells. *Biomacromolecules*, *8*, 3035–3040, 2007.
99. Goto, M., Iohara, D., Michihara, A., Ifuku, S., Azuma, K., Kadowaki, D., Maruyama, T., Otagiri, M., Hirayama, F., Anraku, M., Effects of surface-deacetylated chitin nanofibers on non-alcoholic steatohepatitis model rats and their gut microbiota. *Int. J. Biol. Macromol.*, *164*, 659–666, 2020.
100. Graff, I.E., Øyen, J., Kjellevold, M., Frøyland, L., Gjesdal, C.G., Almås, B., Rosenlund, G., Lie, Ø., Reduced bone resorption by intake of dietary vitamin D and K from tailor-made atlantic salmon: A randomized intervention trial. *Oncotarget*, *7*, 69200–69215, 2016.
101. Guéguen, L. and Pointillart, A., The bioavailability of dietary calcium. *J. Am. Coll. Nutr.*, *19*, 119S–136S, 2000.
102. Hahn, B.H. and Kono, D.H., Animal models in lupus, in: *Dubois' Lupus Erythematosus and Related Syndromes*, D.J. Wallace, and B.H. Hahn, (Eds.), pp. 164–215, Elsevier Inc., Amsterdam, The Netherlands, 2019.
103. Haider, J., Majeed, H., Williams, P.A., Safdar, W., Zhong, F., Formation of chitosan nanoparticles to encapsulate krill oil (*Euphausia superba*) for application as a dietary supplement. *Food Hydrocoll.*, *63*, 27–34, 2017.
104. Halder, M., Petsophonsakul, P., Akbulut, A., Pavlic, A., Bohan, F., Anderson, E., Maresz, K., Kramann, R., Schurgers, L., Vitamin K: Double bonds beyond coagulation insights into differences between vitamin K1 and K2 in health and disease. *Int. J. Mol. Sci.*, *20*, 896, 2019.
105. Hamed, A.A., Abdelhamid, I.A., Saad, G.R., Elkady, N.A., Elsabee, M.Z., Synthesis, characterization and antimicrobial activity of a novel chitosan schiff bases based on heterocyclic moieties. *Int. J. Biol. Macromol.*, *153*, 492–501, 2020.

106. Hamed, I., Özogul, F., Özogul, Y., Regenstein, J.M., Marine bioactive compounds and their health benefits: A review. *Compr. Rev. Food Sci. Food Saf.*, 14, 446–465, 2015.
107. Han, M.H., Lee, D.S., Jeong, J.W., Hong, S.H., Choi, I.W., Cha, H.J., Kim, S., Kim, H.S., Park, C., Kim, G.Y. et al., Fucoidan induces ROS-dependent apoptosis in 5637 human bladder cancer cells by downregulating telomerase activity via inactivation of the PI3K/Akt signaling pathway. *Drug Dev. Res.*, 78, 37–48, 2017.
108. Hanh, N.T., Bich, P.T.N., Thao, H.T.T., Acute and subchronic oral toxicity assessment of calcium hydroxyapatite-alginate in animals. *Vietnam J. Chem.*, 57, 16–20, 2019.
109. Haq, M., Park, S.K., Kim, M.J., Cho, Y.J., Chun, B.S., Modifications of atlantic salmon by-product oil for obtaining different ω-3 polyunsaturated fatty acids concentrates: An approach to comparative analysis. *J. Food Drug Anal.*, 26, 545–556, 2018.
110. Harnedy, P.A. and FitzGerald, R.J., Bioactive peptides from marine processing waste and shellfish: A review. *J. Funct. Foods*, 4, 6–24, 2012.
111. Harnedy, P.A., O'Keeffe, M.B., FitzGerald, R.J., Fractionation and identification of antioxidant peptides from an enzymatically hydrolysed palmaria palmata protein isolate. *Food Res. Int.*, 100, 416–422, 2017.
112. Hasegawa, S., Ichiyama, T., Sonaka, I., Ohsaki, A., Okada, S., Wakiguchi, H., Kudo, K., Kittaka, S., Hara, M., Furukawa, S., Cysteine, histidine and glycine exhibit anti-inflammatory effects in human coronary arterial endothelial cells. *Clin. Exp. Immunol.*, 167, 269–274, 2012.
113. Hayashi, K. and Ito, M., Antidiabetic action of low molecular weight chitosan in genetically obese diabetic KK-Ay mice. *Biol. Pharm. Bull.*, 25, 188–192, 2002.
114. Himaya, S.W.A., Ryu, B., Ngo, D.H., Kim, S.K., Peptide isolated from japanese flounder skin gelatin protects against cellular oxidative damage. *J. Agric. Food Chem.*, 60, 9112–9119, 2012.
115. Holeček, M., Histidine in health and disease: Metabolism, physiological importance, and use as a supplement. *Nutrients*, 12, 848, 2020.
116. Holick, M.F., The vitamin D deficiency pandemic: Approaches for diagnosis, treatment and prevention. *Rev. Endocr. Metab. Disord.*, 18, 153–165, 2017.
117. Hondebrink, L., Tan, S., Hermans, E., van Kleef, R.G.D.M., Meulenbelt, J., Westerink, R.H.S., Additive inhibition of human A1β2γ2 GABAA receptors by mixtures of commonly used drugs of abuse. *Neurotoxicology*, 35, 23–29, 2013.
118. Honold, P.J., Nouard, M.L., Jacobsen, C., Fish oil extracted from fish-fillet by-products is weakly linked to the extraction temperatures but strongly linked to the omega-3 content of the raw material. *Eur. J. Lipid Sci. Technol.*, 118, 874–884, 2016.
119. Hosomi, R., Yoshida, M., Fukunaga, K., Seafood consumption and components for health. *Glob. J. Health Sci.*, 4, 72–86, 2012.

120. Hu, X., Tao, N., Wang, X., Xiao, J., Wang, M., Marine-derived bioactive compounds with anti-obesity effect: A review. *J. Funct. Foods, 21*, 372–387, 2016.
121. Huang, R., Mendis, E., Kim, S.K., Improvement of ACE inhibitory activity of chitooligosaccharides (COS) by carboxyl modification. *Bioorg. Med. Chem., 13*, 3649–3655, 2005.
122. Huang, S., Chen, J.C., Hsu, C.W., Chang, W.H., Effects of nano calcium carbonate and nano calcium citrate on toxicity in ICR mice and on bone mineral density in an ovariectomized mice model. *Nanotechnology, 20*, 375102, 2009.
123. Huang, T., Tu, Z.C., Wang, H., Liu, W., Zhang, L., Zhang, Y., ShangGuan, X.C., Comparison of rheological behaviors and nanostructure of bighead carp scales gelatin modified by different modification methods. *J. Food Sci. Technol., 54*, 1256–1265, 2017.
124. Huang, T.H., Wang, P.W., Yang, S.C., Chou, W.L., Fang, J.Y., Cosmetic and therapeutic applications of fish oil's fatty acids on the skin. *Mar. Drugs, 16*, 256, 2018.
125. Hughes, L., Black, L., Sherriff, J., Dunlop, E., Strobel, N., Lucas, R., Bornman, J., Vitamin D content of australian native food plants and australian-grown edible seaweed. *Nutrients, 10*, 876, 2018.
126. Hwang, D., Kang, M., Jo, M., Seo, Y., Park, N., Kim, G.-D., Anti-inflammatory activity of β-thymosin peptide derived from pacific oyster (Crassostrea gigas) on NO and PGE2 production by down-regulating NF-KB in LPS-induced RAW264.7 macrophage cells. *Mar. Drugs, 17*, 129, 2019.
127. Iemolo, A., De Risi, M., De Leonibus, E., Role of dopamine in memory consolidation, in: *Memory Consolidation*, Nova Science Publishers, Inc., New York, NY, USA, 2015.
128. Inanli, A.G., Tümerkan, E.T.A., El Abed, N., Regenstein, J.M., Özogul, F., The impact of chitosan on seafood quality and human health: A review. *Trends Food Sci. Technol., 97*, 404–416, 2020.
129. Indumathi, P. and Mehta, A.A., Novel anticoagulant peptide from the Nori hydrolysate. *J. Funct. Foods, 20*, 606–617, 2016.
130. Jääskeläinen, T., Itkonen, S.T., Lundqvist, A., Erkkola, M., Koskela, T., Lakkala, K., Dowling, K.G., Hull, G.L., Kröger, H., Karppinen, J. *et al.*, The positive impact of general vitamin D food fortification policy on vitamin D status in a representative adult finnish population: Evidence from an 11-y follow-up based on standardized 25-hydroxyvitamin D data. *Am. J. Clin. Nutr., 105*, 1512–1520, 2017.
131. Jahn, S., Tsalis, G., Lähteenmäki, L., How attitude towards food fortification can lead to purchase intention. *Appetite, 133*, 370–377, 2019.
132. Jamshidi, A., Cao, H., Xiao, J., Simal-Gandara, J., Advantages of techniques to fortify food products with the benefits of fish oil. *Food Res. Int., 137*, 109353, 2020.
133. Javeed, A. and Mahendrakar, N.S., Effect of different levels of molasses and salt on acid production and volume of fermenting mass during ensiling of tropical freshwater fish viscera. *J. Food Sci. Technol., 32*, 115–118, 1995.

134. Je, J.Y., Park, P.J., Kim, S.K., Radical scavenging activity of hetero-chitooligosaccharides. *Eur. Food Res. Technol.*, *219*, 60–65, 2004.
135. Jeevithan, E., Qingbo, Z., Bao, B., Wu, W., Biomedical and pharmaceutical application of fish collagen and gelatin: A review. *J. Nutr. Ther.*, 2, 4, 218–227, 2013.
136. Jismi, J., Krishnakumar, K., Dineshkumar, B., Squid ink and its pharmacological activities. *GSC Biol. Pharm. Sci.*, *2*, 017–022, 2018.
137. Jridi, M., Souissi, N., Mbarek, A., Chadeyron, G., Kammoun, M., Nasri, M., Comparative study of physico-mechanical and antioxidant properties of edible gelatin films from the skin of cuttlefish. *Int. J. Biol. Macromol.*, *61*, 17–25, 2013.
138. Ahire, E.D., Sonawane, V.N., Surana, K.R., Talele, G.S., Drug discovery, drug-likeness screening, and bioavailability: Development of drug-likeness rule for natural products, in: *Applied Pharmaceutical Practice and Nutraceuticals*, pp. 191–208, Apple Academic Press, 2021.
139. Surana, K.R., Ahire, E.D., Sonawane, V.N., Talele, S.G., Talele, G.S., Molecular modeling: Novel techniques in food and nutrition development, in: *Natural Food Products and Waste Recovery*, pp. 17–31, Apple Academic Press, 2021.
140. Muanprasat, C., Chatsudthipong, V., Chitosan oligosaccharide: Biological activities and potential therapeutic applications. *Pharmacol. Ther.*, 170, 80–97, 2017.
141. Thakur, M., Marine bioactive components: Sources, health benefits, and future prospects, in: *Technological Processes for Marine Foods, From Water to Fork*, pp. 61–72, Apple Academic Press, 2019.
142. Palumbo, A., Di Cosmo, A., Gesualdo, I., Hearing, V.J., Subcellular localization and function of melanogenic enzymes in the ink gland of Sepia Officinalis. *Biochem. J.*, 323, 749–756, 1997.
143. Pujiastuti, D.Y., Ghoyatul Amin, M.N., Alamsjah, M.A., Hsu, J.L., Marine organisms as potential sources of bioactive peptides that inhibit the activity of angiotensin I-converting enzyme: A review. *Molecules*, 24, 4, 541, 2019
144. Ngo, D.H., Vo, T.S., Ryu, B. and Kim, S.K., Angiotensin-I-converting enzyme (ACE) inhibitory peptides from Pacific cod skin gelatin using ultrafiltration membranes. *Process Biochem.*, 51, 10, 1622–1628, 2016.
145. Nam, P.V., Van Hoa, N., Anh, T.T.L. and Trung, T.S., Towards zerowaste recovery of bioactive compounds from catfish (Pangasius hypophthalmus) by-products using an enzymatic method. *Waste and Biomass Valorization*, 11, 4195–4206, 2020.
146. Naila, A., Flint, S., Fletcher, G., Bremer, P. and Meerdink, G., 2010. Control of biogenic amines in food—existing and emerging approaches. *J. Food Sci.*, 75, 7, R139–R150, 2010.

7

Nutraceutical Properties of Seaweed Vitamins

Afsar Pathan[1]*, Mahima M. Mahajan[1], Pankaj G. Jain[1], Shital P. Zambad[1], Govinda S. Bhandari[2], Anmol D. Darak[3], Eknath D. Ahire[4], Amit Kumar Rajora[5] and Khemchand R. Surana[6]

[1]*Department of Pharmacology, R.C. Patel Institute of Pharmaceutical Education and Research, Shirpur, India*
[2]*Department of Pharmaceutics, R.C. Patel Institute of Pharmaceutical Education and Research, Shirpur, India*
[3]*R.C. Patel Institute of Pharmaceutical Education and Research, Shirpur, India*
[4]*Department of Pharmaceutics, METs, Institute of Pharmacy, BKC, Affiliated to Savitribai Phule Pune University, Adgaon, Nashik, Maharashtra, India*
[5]*NanoBiotechnology Lab, School of Biotechnology, Jawaharlal Nehru University, New Mehrauli Road, New Delhi, India*
[6]*Department of Pharmaceutical Chemistry, SSS's Divine College of Pharmacy, Satana, Nashik, MH, India*

Abstract

"Nutraceuticals" is any substance that may consist of dietary food or part of a food which provides health benefits, prevention, treatment, and management of diseases. Seaweed has been ingested for generations in East Asian nations, and understanding of the health advantages of eating seaweed has recently acquired popularity in Western societies. Seaweeds include vitamins that are both water-soluble and fat-soluble; these include the fat- and water-soluble vitamins, as well as the minerals calcium, iron, iodine, magnesium, phosphorus, potassium, zinc, copper, manganese, selenium, and fluoride. Because of more nutritional and pharmaceutical constituents values, seaweeds are traditionally used dietary food or as natural medicine for treating cancer, renal disorders, psoriasis, arteriosclerosis, heart disease, type 2 diabetes mellitus, lung diseases, anti-viral, ulcers, etc. The advancement of science and technology has also provided researchers with the understanding and analytical tools necessary for better characterizing seaweed bioactive compounds in disease

---

*Corresponding author: pathanafsar5@gmail.com

Eknath D. Ahire, Raj K. Keservani, Khemchand R. Surana, Sippy Singh and Rajesh K. Kesharwani (eds.) *Vitamins as Nutraceuticals: Recent Advances and Applications*, (167–184) © 2023 Scrivener Publishing LLC

management and health benefit. The present chapter focuses on seaweed vitamins. Additionally, they have other benefits, such as decreasing blood pressure (vitamin C), preventing heart attacks, as well as biochemical functions and antioxidant activity (b-carotene), or decreasing the risk of cancer (vitamins E and C, carotenoids). Seaweeds are discussed in this chapter as potential sources of seaweed-based vitamin containing products and their therapeutic potential role.

Keywords: Diet, nutraceuticals, macroalgae, phaeophytes, rhodophytes, seaweed, vitamin

7.1 Introduction

Stephen L. Defelice introduced the term nutritional in 1989, having founded The Foundation for Innovation in Medicine in 1976 [1]. "Nutraceuticals" is any substance that may be considered a food or part of a food which provides medical or health benefits, encompassing, prevention and treatment of diseases [2]. In addition to being nutrients, nutraceuticals are also health-improving, which makes them the gray area between food and medicine? Nutritional supplements provide extra nutrition and physiological properties to foods, but they are neither food nor drugs. "Let food be your medicine, and medicine be your food," a phrase by Hippocrates, the father of medicine, expanded our investigation into the usage of marine bio resources and their impact on human health [3]. Algae are the most diverse creatures on the planet, and they also contain a great number of plant-like species. The natural polysaccharides from them can be used in the manufacture of plastics. However, they are still not well known to the plastic industry; however, they are more popular in food, biotechnology, microbiology, and even medicine. Some of these polysaccharides are agar, Carrageenan, and alginate [4]. Certain kinds of vitamins, proteins, and carbohydrates are present in seaweed. Marine algae, called seaweeds, are a group of plants that live in brackish or marine environments. There are large quantities of marine algae in the intertidal zone, in the coastal region between high and low tides, and in the sub-tidal zone down to a depth where only 0.01% of the sunlight is available [5]. Seaweeds have been used as a traditional food and supplemental medicine in many Asian countries for ten thousand years. People in China, Indonesia, the Philippines, South Korea, North Korea, Japan, and Malaysia have eaten them for many years [6]. Seaweed, on the other hand, has been used in Japanese and Chinese cuisine for generations. Due to their useful features and the introduction of Asian cuisine, they have recently gained a greater reputation in western countries and are now commonly used as food in the United States, South

America, and Europe. Seaweed's popularity has grown in recent years, making it a more flexible food item that can be used directly or indirectly in the preparation of dishes and beverages. Seaweed and its products are particularly important in the food business because of their utility as components in fertilisers, animal feed supplements, and additives for functional foods [7]. They are low in calories but high in vitamins, minerals, and vital trace elements, as well as polyunsaturated fatty acids, bioactive metabolites, proteins, polysaccharides, and dietary fiber. According to a Seafood Source report, the new products containing this new ingredient launched on the European market increased, making Europe the most innovative region globally after Asia [8]. The advantages of seaweeds have been recognized in Western nations, and they are now consumed in North America, South America, and Europe [3]. They are a varied group, with sizes ranging from a few centimeters to 100 m in length. According to their colour, they are classified into three main types: chlorophytes(green), rhodophytes (red), and pheophytes (brown) [9]. Because of high nutritional and therapeutic values, seaweeds from long time consumed as food (e.g., sea vegetables) or as herbal drug for treating diseases like stomach ailments, eczema, cancer, renal disorders, scabies, gall stones, psoriasis, asthma, arteriosclerosis, heart disease, lung diseases, etc [10]. Seaweeds are not a main source of energy although according to reports the nutritional value regarding vitamin, protein and mineral contents [11]. Seaweeds are a rich source of several water-soluble (B1, B2, B12, C) and fat-soluble (b-carotene consist of vitamin A activity, vitamin E) vitamins. People can consume foods

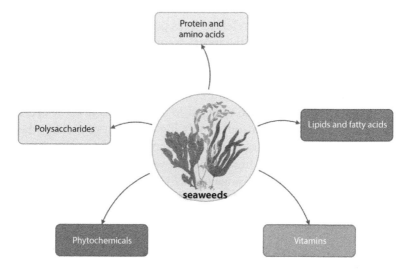

Figure 7.1 Bioactive compounds in seaweeds.

enriched with vitamins, as well as foods containing vitamins as nutraceuticals, derived from natural sources, such as seaweed to ensure they get the adequate intake of vitamins from their diets, including people on special diets, strict vegetarians, and vegans [5]. Figure 7.1 showing the bioactive compounds from the seaweed.

7.2 Bioactive Compounds from Seaweeds

7.2.1 Vitamins

Vitamins are the most important type of micronutrients since they initiate a wide variety of metabolic processes and act as a precursor for enzyme cofactors. Because higher species do not possess a metabolic pathway that can synthesis these cofactors, they are required to obtain them from an outside source. The richest source of vitamins is algae, which almost completely contains all of the essential as well as non-essential vitamins. In comparison to plants grown on land, the vitamin C content of many types of seaweed, such as *Porphyra umbilicalis*, *Himanthalia elongata*, and *Gracilaria changii*, is significantly higher. For example, the seaweed *Eisenia arborea* has a vitamin C level that is considerably higher than that of mandarin oranges, with 34.4 milligrams of vitamin C per 100 grams of dry weight [12].

7.2.2 Polysaccharides

The energy reserves and structural constituents of all creatures, including marine and higher plants, are referred to as polysaccharides. The polysaccharides found in seaweed are the most essential macromolecules, as they account for more than 80% of the total weight of the plant. Dietary fibers are refractory polysaccharides that are not digested by the body but can ferment to variable degrees due to the enzymatic activity of microbes in the gut [13]. Dietary fibers are also referred to as indigestible carbohydrates. Edible seaweeds contain an astonishingly high amount of dietary fiber in species, such as Codium, Gracilaria, Ulva, and Acanthopora, where the levels of polysaccharides are higher than in wheat bran. The dietary fiber content of edible seaweed can range from 23.5% to 64% DW (dry weight).

7.2.3 Lipids and Fatty Acids

The energy reserves and structural constituents of all creatures, including marine and higher plants, are referred to as polysaccharides.

The polysaccharides found in seaweed are the most essential macromolecules, as they account for more than 80% of the total weight of the plant. Dietary fibers are refractory polysaccharides that are not digested by the body but can ferment to variable degrees due to the enzymatic activity of microbes in the gut. Dietary fibers are also referred to as indigestible carbohydrates. Edible seaweeds contain an astonishingly high amount of dietary fiber in species, such as *Codium*, *Gracilaria*, *Ulva*, and *Acanthopora*, where the levels of polysaccharides are higher than in wheat bran. The amount of dietary fiber in edible seaweed can be anywhere from 23.5% to 64% DW (dry weight) [14].

7.2.4 Phytochemicals

In comparison to plants, seaweeds have a larger variety of secondary metabolites, which continues to pique the interest of the research community due to the potential bioactivity of these metabolites. Seaweeds are also a rich source of dietary fiber. In general, the phytochemicals in seaweeds that have received the most research attention are phlorotannins, gallic acid, quercetin, phloroglucinol, and carotenoids and its derivatives. There have been numerous reports of polyphenol compounds being found in all types of seaweed; however, it is most likely that these compounds are most abundant in brown and red seaweeds [15].

7.3 Seaweed Vitamins as Nutraceuticals

Seaweed component varies by species; however, many of them spend a significant amount of time in presence of sunlight in the an aquatic environment. As a result, seaweeds consist of a wide range of antioxidants, vitamins and protecting pigments are included. Seaweeds include vitamins that are both water-soluble and fat-soluble. These include the fat- and water-soluble vitamins A, D, E, K, C, B1, B2, B9, and B12, as well as the minerals iron, phosphorus, iodine, magnesium, potassium, zinc, calcium, copper, manganese, selenium, and fluoride [16]. 100 grammes of dried S. japonica seaweed, for instance, includes 0.57 mg carotene, 0.69 mg (vitamin B1), 0.36 mg riboflavin (vitamin B2), 1.6 mg niacin, 8.2 g protein, 0.1 g fat, 57 g polysaccharides, 9.8 g crude fibers, 12.9 g minerals, 2.25 mg calcium, and 0.15 g iron, along with 262 kcal of energy [8].

It contains a various types of phytochemicals, polyphenols, carotenoids, vitamin E, and minerals, which can act as antioxidants so as to reduce the occurrence of lipid peroxidation and LDL oxidation caused by reactive oxygen species, such as hydroxyl and superoxide anions [17]. Therefore, the edible seaweeds can be used as superfoods with lots of nutritional benefits as well as health promoting properties.

7.4 Types of Seaweed Vitamin

Figure 7.2 shows the vitamins found in seaweed as well as the many sources of those vitamins, and Table 7.1 describes the various forms of seaweed vitamins, as well as their characteristics [6, 18–22].

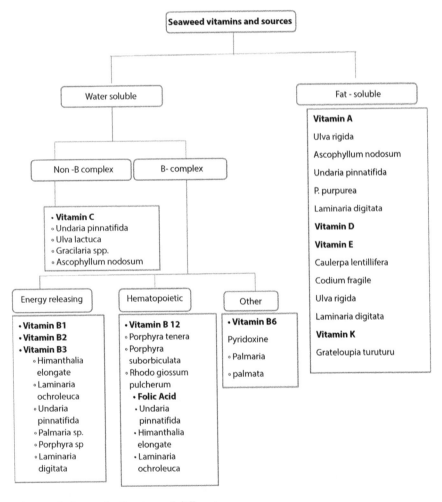

Figure 7.2 Seaweeds vitamins and different sources.

Table 7.1 Types of seaweed vitamins and their properties.

Sr. no.	Seaweed vitamin	Species of seaweed	Properties	References
1	Green Vitamin A, B1, B2, C	o *Ulva* species o *Ulva rigida* o *Gelidium pristoides* o *Monostroma nitidum*	Viscosity and thickening, suspension, caking, gelling, adhesion, encapsulation, inhibit viruses, form retention. Also used for Anticoagulant and Antithrombotic Properties.	[23, 24]
2	Red (Rhodophyta)	o *Gracilaria cervicornis* o *Porphyra tenara* o *Alaria* o *Laurencia microcladia*	Gelling, chemical reactivity, gelation, foaming, suspension, improving quality, controlling moisture. Anti-tumour effect, anti-oxidant, anti-inflammatory, antimicrobial.	[23, 25–27]
3	Brown Vit. V, E	o *Laminaria* o *Sargassum vulgare* o *Padina* o *Ecklonia cava*	Viscosity and thickening, suspension, caking, gelling, adhesion, encapsulation, inhibit viruses, form retention. Antioxidant, anticancer, immunomodulatory, antiproliferative.	[23, 28–30]

7.5 Vitamin Composition in Seaweed

Seaweeds have a complex vitamin profile influenced by factors such as algal species, season, algal growth stage, and environmental conditions, just as minerals do. Reports state that 100 grams of seaweed supply up to three times the daily recommended amount of vitamin A, B2 and B12, and two-thirds the daily recommended amount of vitamin C [18]. Seaweed is great source of vitamin c and in some species the ascorbic acid content is sufficient to cover the recommended daily intake (30 mg) for adults [19]. The vitamin C content varies from 0.41 mg (1% of RNI) in *Ascophyllum nodosum* to 9.24 mg (23% of RNI) in *Undaria pinnatifida*. The contain found in *Undaria pinnatifida* is more as compared to other species of seaweed [20]. Thiamine (B1) and riboflavin (B2) are water-soluble vitamin are carried out to the tissue but not stored in tissue. They are found in plant and animal food and some dietary supplements. Riboflavin is required for the proper development and function of the skin, lining of the digestive tract, blood cells, and many other parts of the body [21]. Vitamins of the B group, especially vitamin B1 (thiamine) and vitamin B2 (riboflavin), are found in most red and brown seaweeds B12 content was found to be more in some seaweed than beef or fish meat. The majority of seaweeds contain not only B12 analogs that are active in mammals, but also other B12 analogs [31]. Our results indicate that rhodophyta phylum (red algae), such as *Porphyra tenera, Porphyra suborbiculata* and *Rhodoglossum pulcherum*, contained B12 and its analogs at a much higher content than phaephyta phylum (brown algae) such as hijiki and kombu. Porphyra suborbiculata contained almost only B12, but akaba-gin-nansou contained exclusively analogs as detected by methods utilizing the specificity of two B12-binding proteins [6]. Some species *Undaria pinnatifida, Himanthalia elongate*, and *Laminaria ochroleuca* are rich source of vitamin (B9) Folic acid studied in all seaweed (*Himanthalia elongata, Laminaria ochroleuca, Palmaria* spp., *Undaria pinnatifida* and *Porphyra* spp. and *Saccorhiza polychides*) the single most abundant form is 5-CH3–H4-folate, except Porphyra and Himanthalia [32]. B6 (pyridoxine) is involved in the formation of a number of enzymes involved in metabolism of protein. It has been reported that nitrogen, lipid, and carbohydrate metabolism, as well as the biosynthesis of chlorophyll and ethylene, are controlled by various forms of vitamin B6 [33]. This vitamin was high in *P. palmata* during winter months, when the sporogenic tissues were at their peak [34]. Seaweed is a good source of some fat soluble (β-carotene, ergocalciferol and cholecalciferol and α-tocopherol) vitamins. Vitamins obtain from algae are very important due to their antioxidant activity, biochemical functions and other health benefits - Preventive measures of cardiovascular diseases (β-carotene), decreases the risk of developing cancer (tochopherol and carotenoids) [35] (wakame) *Undaria pinnatifida* and (nori) *Porphyra purpurea* both contain high concentration of retinal, i.e., vitamin A than *Ulva rigida, Ascophyllum nodosum, Laminaria digitata* [36, 37]. As regards the vitamin contents in seaweed, vitamin A was the most abundant, although vitamin

E and vitamin C, which are important antioxidants, were also present in large amounts. Vitamin E contain is more abundant in *Caulerpa lentillifera* than *Codium fragile, Ulva rigida, Laminaria digitate* [38]. Regarding *G. turuturu*, a chemical analysis revealed the presence of α-tocopherol and phytonadione (vitamin K1) along with phospholipid, glycolipid and ecosapenteanoic acid [39]. So, The nutrient-rich nature of seaweed makes it a highly recommended food as they are a good source of minerals, vitamins A, vitamins B1, vitamins B2, vitamins B9, vitamins B12, vitamins C, vitamins D, vitamins E, and vitamins K), and essential minerals (calcium, iron, iodine, magnesium, phosphorus, potassium, zinc, copper, manganese, selenium, and fluoride),dietary fibers [40].

7.5.1 Therapeutic Properties of Seaweed Vitamins

The bioactive compounds that present in seaweed can play a major beneficial role in disease management in humans. Vitamins, pigments, polyphenols, polysaccharides, fatty acids, and peptides have been shown to have a variety of positive biological qualities that might possibly contribute to the creation of functional foods and nutraceuticals. The bioactive analysed are evaluated for anti-inflammatory, antioxidant, anticancer, antitumor, antiviral, antitumor, antitumor and antitumor properties, both *in vitro* and *in vivo* models [14].

Type 2 Diabetes Mellitus
Type 2 diabetes mellitus, also called as adult-onset diabetes it is diet-related metabolic disorder that responds well to dietary intervention, unlike the often genetically inherited type 1 diabetes (an autoimmune disorder), that is related to beta cell destruction of the pancreas, and need insulin injections for the treatment. Drugs commonly used for the treatment of type 2 diabetes, such as the α-amylase and α-glucosidase inhibitor Acarbose, may cause gastric discomfort and diarrhoea [41]. Other type of seaweed also has anti-diabetic effect, seaweed has been shown in many animal studies and in vitro studies [42]. In clinical trials, regular intake of *Undaria pinnatifida* and *Sacchariza polyschides* (as *Gigantea bulbosa*) adjusts blood glucose levels and reduces serum triglyceride levels, and increases high-density lipoprotein cholesterol in subjects with type 2 diabetes [41].

Obesity
Various anti-obesity agents have been suggested as medical treatments of obesity. However, due to side effects, many of these agents are not approved for use. High-G alginates collected from the seaweed *Laminaria hyperborea*

inhibited pancreatic lipase substantially more than high-M alginates taken from the *Lessonia nigrescens* species. Alginate inhibits lipase present in pancreas and is being studied as an anti-obesity drug in human studies [42, 43].

Cardiovascular Diseases
CVD consist of disorders related to heart and blood vessels, which include coronary heart disorder, cerebrovascular disease, peripheral arterial disease, hypertension, dyslipidemia, atherosclerosis and thrombosis and embolism.

Dyslipidemia
Dyslipidemia are also the most common remediable risk factors for atherosclerosis, which is a main cause of the most common pathological process leading to CVDs including myocardial infarction, heart failure, and stroke [44]. The addition of seaweeds and/or extracts to the diet may have a possible protective effect. This is supported by the favourable findings of epidemiological research relating the use of seaweeds, medicinal herbs, and fruits to the prevention of hyperlipidemia in diverse culture [8].

Hypertension
In fact, the varieties within different algae Rhodophyta, Chlorophyta and Phaeophyta seaweed Macroalgae provides a diverse range of substances, such as carbohydrates, protein, and minerals, as well as a rich supply of health-promoting secondary metabolites with unique features and uses, such as the prevention and treatment of cardiovascular disease risk factors. The entire extract (aqueous or alcoholic) or fractions rich in a specific kind of chemical are most macroalgae products identified in the scientific literature as having antihypertensive and/or anti-obesity properties (e.g., fucoidans, alginates, phlorotannins) [45]. Peptide extracts of seaweeds in human cell culture, and animal *in vivo* trials, can significantly reduce blood pressure in single doses and long-term administration [46]. The antihypertensive properties of macroalgal peptides have also been studied *in vivo* models [47].

Anti-Cancer
There is a correlation between greater seaweed consumption and lower rates of diet-related disorders, including cancer [48], Several substances, including fucoxanthin, polyphenols, and other antioxidants; phlorotannins; iodine; and sulphated polysaccharides, such as fucoidan, have been

related to the numerous processes by which seaweeds trigger death in cancer cells.

Anti-Inflammatory
Brown seaweed, especially Sargassum, is known to have many health-related benefits including high inflammatory activities [49]. The activity of anti-inflammatory action are reported in animal model of ameliorating systemic inflammation and insulin resistance in high fat diet-induced obese mice model [50].

Psoriasis
Psoriasis is known as chronic inflammatory autoimmune skin disease characterized by accelerated tumour necrosis factor-α (TNF-α)/interleukin-23 (IL-23)/IL-17 axis and hyperproliferation of epidermal keratinocytes. Seaweed has been reported in psoriasis mouse model generated by a Traf3ip2 mutation, feeding a diet high in fucoidan (a seaweed fiber) alleviated symptoms of psoriasis-like dermatitis while boosting Bacteroides in the stomach [51]. In TNF receptor-associated factor 3-interacting protein 2 (Traf3ip2) mutant mice (m-Traf3ip2 mice), fucoidan administration reduced facial itching and altered the intestinal environment. In the mouse model used in this study, the Traf3ip2 mutation was linked to psoriasis [52].

Antioxidant
Natural antioxidants have a modest ability to slow oxidative processes and are quite expensive. As a result, there is a need to produce natural antioxidants that are more strong, less expensive, and safer. Recently, the antioxidant effects of some seaweed *Ecklonia cava, Sargassum micracanthum, Ecklonia stolonifera, Hizikia fusiformis, Grateloupia filicina, Chondrus ocellatus,* and *Meristotheca papulose* were investigated [53]. The antioxidant content varies from solvent to solvent.

Anti-bacterial: Antibacterial, anti-microbial, cytotoxic activity of seaweed is found in different marine algae [54]. The two brown seaweeds *Spatoglossum schmittii* and *Stoechospermum marginurn*, belonging to the family Dictyotaceae, have been the only sources from which spatane diterpenoids have antibacterial activity. It shows action against growth of *Staphylococcus aureus* bacteria [55].

Other Properties include: Seaweed also used in certain kind of sunscreen, anti-aging, anticellulite treatment and slimming, as well as having antioxidant, photoprotective, moisturizing, and whitening properties [56].

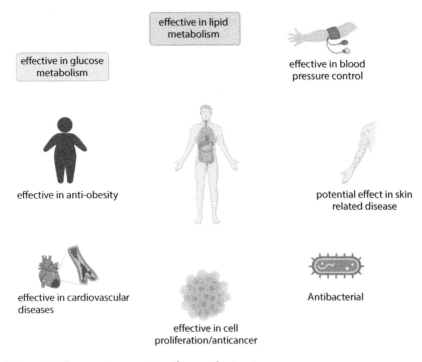

Figure 7.3 Therapeutic properties of seaweeds vitamins.

Seaweeds are primarily used as phycocolloids sources, thickening and gelling agents in a variety of industrial applications, including food [23]. Figure 7.3 indicates the therapeutic properties of seaweeds vitamins.

7.6 Future Perspectives

Seaweed is rich source of lipid, minerals, vitamins, polysaccharide, calcium, carotenoids and lactin. Since China, Japan, and Korea have experienced the benefits of seaweed; they have been using it as an important dietary component for centuries. Meanwhile, seaweeds are becoming more recognized as valuable food sources in other parts of Asia, Africa, as well as western countries, and a growing interest is developing to manufacture functional food products from seaweeds. The advancement of science and technology has also provided researchers with the understanding and analytical tools necessary for better characterizing seaweed bioactive compounds in disease management and health promotion. There has been a surge in interest in seaweeds internationally due to the phycocolloids, dried seaweeds, fucoidans, and laminarin products with the growing understanding of these seaweed compounds health-related properties, significant work have been made to discover more direct food applications using these compounds. However, despite high expectations, no commercially successful product range has yet been developed using these compounds to target optimum health and nutrition of humans [57]. Seaweed is emerging as an attractive natural source to synthesize compounds that are used in therapeutic and Nutraceuticals products. Due to their cost, feasibility, and environmentally friendly production processes, high yields of extraction and availability of biomass in natural ecosystems, seaweeds offer advantages over other sources of bioactive compounds. Some *Rhodophyta* species, like *Gracilaria gracilis, Kappaphycus alvarezii*, and *Pyropia/Porphyra* spp., are more likely to be successful. The extraction methods need to be optimized to be more eco-friendly and cost-effective, with a high purity level to support the industries that want to work with these biomolecules and to obtain more than one compound from seaweed biomass to create add-value products [58–60].

7.7 Conclusion

The change in dietary patterns in the western world has resulted in the emergence of certain chronic diseases which include diabetes, cardiovascular disease, etc. Nutraceuticals are promoted by pharmaceutical companies as preventing noncommunicable diseases. With an increased acceptance of nutraceuticals and higher expenditure on nutraceutical products per capita, these markets are nearing maturity. The worldwide burden of noncommunicable, lifestyle-related illnesses, such as type 2 diabetes, hypertension, obesity, cancer, antibiotic resistance, and heart disease exerts a significant pressure on afflicted nations' health care budgets and resources. This may be addressed by using various species of seaweed and seaweed isolates in the diet as part of a healthier lifestyle. Seaweeds are a sustainable source of bioactive compounds for human health and functional food applications. Seaweed is not known to many populations outside Asia; however, it may be promoted by intelligent product design, development, advertising, and integration with commonly used devices. Mineral constituents of seaweed are very changeable according to different factors like the environmental conditions and certain behaviour of each seaweed species. Thus, more research is required to clarify the interactions by analyzing binding sites of the certain vitamin, the affinity for specific biomolecules, the molecular docking, etc. More human intervention studies with defined health-related outcomes are required in the future to determine how chronic ingestion of whole seaweeds and their derived bioactive components impacts human health. Mechanisms of action must also be identified in order to support future health claims connected with seaweed intake and uses in the food and nutraceuticals sectors.

Acknowledgment

The authors thank R.C. Patel Institute of Pharmaceutical Education and Research Shirpur, 425405 India and MET's Institute of Pharmacy, BKC, which is affiliated with Savitribai Phule Pune University, Nashik, MH India. EDA wishes to express gratitude to the NFST/RGNF/UGC, Government of India, for providing financial assistance in the form of a fellowship (award 202021-NFST-MAH-01235).

References

1. Aronson, J.K., Defining 'nutraceuticals': Neither nutritious nor pharmaceutical. *Br. J. Clin. Pharmacol.*, 83, 1, 8–19, 2017.
2. Dudeja, P. and Gupta, R.K., Nutraceuticals, in: *Food safety in the 21st Century*, pp. 491–496, Academic Press, Elsevier Inc., 2017.
3. Tanna, B. and Mishra, A., Metabolites unravel nutraceutical potential of edible seaweeds: An emerging source of functional food. *Compr. Rev. Food Sci. Food Saf.*, 17, 6, 1613–1624, 2018.
4. Gade, R., Tulasi, M.S., Bhai, V.A., Seaweeds: A novel biomaterial. *Int. J. Pharm. Pharm. Sci.*, 5, suppl. 2, 40–44, 2013.
5. Joshi, A., Desai, A.Y., Mulye, V., Seaweed resources and utilization: An overview. *Biotech. Express*, 2, 22, 46–50, 2015.
6. Bocanegra, A., Bastida, S., Benedí, J., Ródenas, S., Sánchez-Muniz, F.J., Characteristics and nutritional and cardiovascular-health properties of seaweeds. *J. Med. Food*, 12, 2, 236–258, 2009.
7. Rajauria, G., Cornish, L., Ometto, F., Msuya, F.E., Villa, R., Identification and selection of algae for food, feed, and fuel applications, in: *Seaweed Sustainability*, pp. 315–345, Academic Press, Elsevier Inc, 2015.
8. Afonso, N.C., Catarino, M.D., Silva, A.M.S., Cardoso, S.M., Brown macroalgae as valuable food ingredients. *Antioxidants*, 8, 9, 365, 2019.
9. Lorenzo, J.M. *et al.*, Proximate composition and nutritional value of three macroalgae: Ascophyllum nodosum, fucus vesiculosus and bifurcaria bifurcata. *Mar. Drugs*, 15, 11, 1–11, 2017.

10. Peng, Y. et al., Chemical composition of seaweeds, Elsevier Inc, in: *Seaweed Sustainability: Food and Non-Food Applications*, 2015.
11. Manivanna, K., Thirumaran, G., Devi, G.K., Hemlatha, A., Ananthraman, P., Biochemical composition of seaweeds from Mandapam coastal regions along Southeast coast of India. *Am. J. Bot.*, 1, 2, 32–37, 2008.
12. Hernández-Carmona, G. et al., Monthly variation in the chemical composition of eisenia arborea J.E. areschoug. *J. Appl. Phycol.*, 21, 5, 607–616, 2009.
13. Nunraksa, N., Rattanasansri, S., Chirapart, A., Proximate composition and the production of fermentable sugars, levulinic acid, and HMF from Gracilaria fisheri and Gracilaria tenuistipitata cultivated in earthen ponds. *J. Appl. Phycol.*, 31, 1, 683–690, 2019.
14. Ganesan, A.R. and Rajauria, G., Seaweed nutraceuticals and their therapeutic role in disease prevention. *Food Sci. Hum. Wellness*, 8, 3, 252–263, 2019.
15. Abirami, R.G. and Kowsalya, S., Quantification and correlation study on derived phenols and antioxidant activity of seaweeds from gulf of mannar. *J. Herbs Spices Med. Plants*, 23, 1, 9–17, 2017.
16. Qin, Y., Applications of bioactive seaweed substances in functional food products, in: *Bioactive Seaweeds for Food Applications*, pp. 111–134, Elsevier Inc, 2018.
17. Chan, P.T., Matanjun, P., Yasir, S.M., Tan, T.S., Antioxidant and hypolipidaemic properties of red seaweed, gracilaria changii. *J. Appl. Phycol.*, 26, 2, 987–997, 2014.
18. Ortiz, J. et al., Dietary fiber, amino acid, fatty acid and tocopherol contents of the edible seaweeds ulva lactuca and durvillaea antarctica. *Food Chem.*, 99, 1, 98–104, 2006.
19. Liso, R. and Calabrese, G., Research on ascorbic acid physiology in red algae. 2. Dehydroascorbic acid compartmentation in the cell. *Phycologia*, 13, 3, 205–208, 1974.
20. Cherry, P., O'hara, C., Magee, P.J., Mcsorley, E.M., Allsopp, P.J., Risks and benefits of consuming edible seaweeds. *Nutr. Rev.*, 77, 5, 307–329, 2019.
21. Rahmani, N. and Muller, H.G., The fate of thiamin and riboflavin during the preparation of couscous. *Food Chem.*, 55, 1, 23–27, 1996.
22. Yamada, S., Sasa, M., Yamada, K., Fukuda, M., Release and uptake of vitamin B12 by Asakusanori (porphyra tenera) seaweed. *J. Nutr. Sci. Vitaminol. (Tokyo)*, 42, 6, 507–515, 1996.
23. Kumar, C.S., Ganesan, P., Suresh, P.V., Bhaskar, N., Seaweeds as asource of nutritionally beneficial compounds—A review. *J. Food Sci. Technol. (JFST)*, 45, 1–13, 2008.
24. Green, M. et al., Anticoagulant and antithrombotic properties *in vitro* and *in vivo* of a novel sulfated polysaccharide from marine green alga monostroma nitidum. *Mar. Drugs*, 17, 4, 1–21, 2019.
25. Lee, J., Hou, M., Huang, H., Chang, F., Yeh, C., Marine algal natural products with anti-oxidative, anti-inflammatory, and anti-cancer properties. *Cancer Cell Int.*, 13, 1, 1, 2013.

26. Elena, S., Sergey, B., Mikhail, S., Alexey, G., Elena, S., Antimicrobial bio-components from red algae species: A review of application and health benefits. *Steroids*, 5, 3, 85–90, 2018.
27. Campos, A., Souza, C.B., Lhullier, C., Falkenberg, M., Schenkel, E.P., Ribeiro-do-Valle, R.M., Siqueira, J.M., Anti-tumour effects of elatol, a marine derivative compound obtained from red algae Laurencia microcladia. *J. Pharm. Pharmacol. (JPP)*, 64, 8, 1146–1154, 2012.
28. Athukorala, Y., Kim, K., Jeon, Y., Antiproliferative and antioxidant properties of an enzymatic hydrolysate from brown alga, Ecklonia cava. *Food Chem. Toxicol.*, 44, 7, 1065–1074, 2006.
29. Melnikov, V.Y. and Molitoris, B.A., Improvements in the diagnosis of acute kidney injury. *Saudi J. Kidney Dis. Transplant.*, 19, 4, 537–544, 2008.
30. Zaporozhets, T. and Besednova, N., Prospects for the therapeutic application of sulfated polysaccharides of brown algae in diseases of the cardiovascular system. *Pharm. Biol.*, 54, 12, 3126–3135, 2016.
31. Yamada, S., Shibata, Y., Takayama, M., Narita, Y., Sugawara, K., Fukuda, M., Content and characteristics of vitamin B12 in some seaweeds. *J. Nutr. Sci. Vitaminol.*, 42, 6, 497–505, 1996.
32. de Quirós, A.R.B. and de Ron, C.C., Determination of folates in seaweeds by high-performance liquid chromatography. *J. Chromatog. A*, 1032, 135–139, 2004.
33. Tambasco-studart, M., Titiz, O., Raschle, T., Forster, G., Amrhein, N., Fitzpatrick, T.B., Vitamin B6 biosynthesis in higher plants. *Proc. Natl. Acad. Sci.*, 102, 38, 13687–13692, 2005.
34. Ryzhik, I.V., Klindukh, M. P., Dobychina, E. O., The b-group vitamins in the red alga Palmaria palmata (Barents sea): Composition, seasonal changes and influence of abiotic factors. *Algal Res.*, 59, 11–15, 2021.
35. Dobreva, D.A., Panayotova, V.Z., Stancheva, R.S., Stancheva, M., Simultaneous HPLC determination of fat soluble vitamins, carotenoids and cholesterol in seaweed and mussel tissue. *Bulg. Chem. Commun.*, 49, 112–117, 2017.
36. Maeda, H., Hosokawa, M., Sashima, T., Funayama, K., Miyashita, K., Fucoxanthin from edible seaweed, undaria pinnatifida, shows antiobesity effect through UCP1 expression in white adipose tissues. *Biochem. Biophys. Res. Commun.*, 332, 2, 392–397, 2005.
37. Gamero-vega, G., Palacios-Palacios, M., Quitral, V., Nutritional composition and bioactive compounds of red seaweed: A mini-review. *J. Food Nutr. Res.*, 8, 8, 431–440, 2020.
38. Ratana-Arporn, P. and Chirapart, A., Nutritional evaluation of tropical green seaweeds caulerpa lentillifera and ulva reticulata. *Agric. Nat. Res.*, 40, 6, 75–83, 2006.
39. Pereira, A.G., Fraga-Corral, M., Garcia-Oliveira, P., Lourenço-Lopes, C., Carpena, M., Prieto, M.A., Simal-Gandara, J., The use of invasive algae

species as a source of secondary metabolites and biological activities: Spain as case-study. *Mar. Drugs*, 19, 4, 178, 2021.
40. Lomartire, S., Marques, J.C., Gonçalves, A.M., An overview to the health benefits of seaweeds consumption. *Mar. Drugs*, 19, 6, 341, 2021.
41. Shannon, E. and Abu-Ghannam, N., Seaweeds as nutraceuticals for health and nutrition. *Phycologia*, 58, 5, 563–577, 2019.
42. Gabbia, D., Dall'Acqua, S., Di Gangi, I.M., Bogialli, S., Caputi, V., Albertoni, L., Marsilio, I., Paccagnella, N., Carrara, M., Giron, M.C., De Martin, S., The phytocomplex from Fucus vesiculosus and Ascophyllum nodosum controls postprandial plasma glucose levels: An *in vitro* and *in vivo* study in a mouse model of NASH. *Mar. Drugs*, 15, 2, 41, 2017.
43. Chater, P.I., Wilcox, M.D., Houghton, D., Pearson, J.P., The role of seaweed bioactives in the control of digestion: implications for obesity treatments. *Food Funct.*, 6, 11, 3420–3427, 2015.
44. Sowers, J.R., Epstein, M., Frohlich, E.D., Diabetes, hypertension, and cardiovascular disease: an update. *Hypertension*, 37, 4, 1053–1059, 2001.
45. Seca, A.M.L., Overview on the antihypertensive and anti-obesity effects of secondary metabolites from seaweeds, 2018.
46. Wijesekara, I. and Kim, S.K., Angiotensin-I-converting enzyme (ACE) inhibitors from marine resources: Prospects in the pharmaceutical industry. *Mar. Drugs*, 8, 4, 1080–1093, 2010.
47. Fitzgerald, C., Aluko, R.E., Hossain, M., Rai, D.K., Hayes, M., Potential of a renin inhibitory peptide from the red seaweed Palmaria palmata as a functional food ingredient following confirmation and characterization of a hypotensive effect in spontaneously hypertensive rats. *J. Agric. Food Chem.*, 62, 33, 8352–8356, 2014.
48. Park, Y., Dietary patterns and colorectal cancer risk in a Korean population: A case control study, 2012.
49. Giriwono, P.E., Iskandriati, D., Tan, C.P., Andarwulan, N., Sargassum seaweed as a source of anti-inflammatory substances and the potential insight of the tropical species: A review. *Mar. Drugs*, 17, 10, 590, 2019.
50. Oh, J., Kim, J., Lee, Y., Anti-inflammatory and anti-diabetic effects of brown seaweeds in high-fat diet-induced obese mice. *Nutr. Res. Pract.*, 10, 1, 42–48, 2016.
51. Kanda, N., Hoashi, T., Saeki, H., The defect in regulatory t cells in psoriasis and therapeutic approaches. *J. Clin. Med.*, 10, 17, 2021.
52. Takahashi, M. *et al.*, Improvement of psoriasis by alteration of the gut environment by oral administration of fucoidan from cladosiphon okamuranus. *Mar. Drugs*, 18, 3, 2020.
53. Cho, S. *et al.*, The antioxidant properties of brown seaweed (sargassum siliquastrum) extracts. *J. Med. Food*, 10, 3, 479–485, 2007.
54. Abirami, R.G. and Kowsalya, S., Phytochemical screening, microbial load and antimicrobial activity of underexploited seaweeds. *Int. Res. J. Microbiol.*, 3, 10, 328–332, 2012.

55. Lanka, S. and Lanka, S., Anti-bacterial activity of extracts from the brown seaweed stoechospermum marginatum. *Phytochemistry*, 21, 4, 944–945, 1982.
56. Bedoux, G., Hardouin, K., Burlot, A.S., Bioactive components from seaweeds: Cosmetic applications and future development, in: *Advances in Botanical Research*, vol. 71, pp. 345–378, Academic Press, 2014.
57. Mendis, E. and Kim, S.K., Present and future prospects of seaweeds in developing functional foods, 1st ed, in: *Advances in Food and Nutrition Research*, vol. 64, pp. 1–15, Elsevier Inc, 2011.
58. Cotas, J., Leandro, A., Pacheco, D., Gonçalves, A.M.M., Pereira, L., A comprehensive review of the nutraceutical and therapeutic applications of red seaweeds (Rhodophyta). *Life*, 10, 3, 2020.
59. Ahire, E.D., Sonawane, V.N., Surana, K.R., Talele, G.S., Drug discovery, drug-likeness screening, and bioavailability: Development of drug-likeness rule for natural products, in: *Applied Pharmaceutical Practice and Nutraceuticals*, pp. 191–208, Apple Academic Press, 2021.
60. Surana, K.R., Ahire, E.D., Sonawane, V.N., Talele, S.G., Talele, G.S., Molecular modeling: Novel techniques in food and nutrition development, in: *Natural Food Products and Waste*, pp. 17–31, Apple Academic Press, 2021.

8
Vitamins as Nutraceuticals for Pregnancy

Tushar N. Lokhande[1]*, Kshitij S. Varma[1], Shrikant M. Gharate[1], Sunil K. Mahajan[1] and Khemchand R. Surana[2]

[1]*Department of Pharmaceutical Chemistry, Mahatma Gandhi Vidyamandir's Pharmacy College, Panchavati, Nashik, Maharashtra, India*
[2]*Department of Pharmaceutical Chemistry, Shreeshakti Shaikshanik Sanstha, Divine College of Pharmacy, Satana, Nashik, Maharashtra, India*

Abstract

Maintaining excellent and sound health necessitates a well-balanced diet. A well-balanced diet is also suggested throughout pregnancy. Vitamins are necessary nutrients for our bodies to function properly. Vitamins help to improve our immune system, and many of them work as coenzymes for different processes in our bodies. As a result, a vitamin deficit can cause the immune system to malfunction or impede the operations of essential enzymes. Vitamins do not contain calories or energy, but they are essential for our health. During pregnancy, a woman must not only look after her own health but also her feed intake and overall health have a significant impact on the health of the growing fetus in her womb, as well as the baby's future health. Vitamins, such as folic acid, are regarded to be particularly important for a mother's health throughout pregnancy and for a healthy pregnancy. Other vitamins, such as A, D, and B complex, are also essential for the mother's and baby's health. Vitamins aid in the development of the fetus' immune system. Various herbal remedies as just a source of vitamins have also been discussed.

Keywords: Vitamins, nutraceutical, pregnancy

Corresponding author: tusharlokhande@hotmail.com

Eknath D. Ahire, Raj K. Keservani, Khemchand R. Surana, Sippy Singh and Rajesh K. Kesharwani (eds.) *Vitamins as Nutraceuticals: Recent Advances and Applications*, (185–204) © 2023 Scrivener Publishing LLC

8.1 Introduction

Physiological changes occur in women throughout pregnancy in order to ensure the appropriate development and health of the fetus. These changes also help the mother and baby prepare for the birth [1, 2]. Weight increase is the first change that occurs during pregnancy. According to the guidelines, a woman's gestational weight gain (GWG) should be between 11 and 16 kg for a woman of normal weight (BMI 19 to 24 kg/m^2). The placenta, uterus, amniotic fluid, mammary gland, blood, and adipose tissue all contribute to physiological GWG. Hormonal changes are also important throughout pregnancy [3]. On the one hand, preexisting hormone production primarily estrogens, progesterone, and prolactinincreases, and the main generating tissues alter (the secretion becomes placental). The placenta, on the other hand, produces particular hormones such as human chorionic gonadotropin (hCG). These hormones play a critical role in ensuring a healthy pregnancy and their concentration changes as the pregnancy progresses [4, 5]. Women's dietary needs rise during pregnancy to sustain all of these changes and to guarantee that the fetus/baby develops normally.

8.1.1 Diet and Nourishment in Pregnancy

The stages of reproduction are fundamentally those of fetal nutrition throughout pregnancy and breastfeeding after birth. The maternal reproductive system, as well as many other organs, expand and become more active in order to serve this objective. During pregnancy and breastfeeding, the mother's food intake is the source of this new build-up and increased activities. As a result, gestation and lactation meals must be sufficient and nutritious in order to nourish both the mother and her unborn child, whether in the pregnancy. During the last months of pregnancy, a pregnant woman's diet should contain 20% higher calories (300 calories extra) than a non-pregnant woman's diet. Extra protein, minerals, and vitamins should be included. Lactation diets should provide daily additional calories (700 calories) for milk production and increased activity by the mother; yet, they should be slightly more nutritious than pregnancy diets in terms of protein (70 g), minerals, and vitamin content [6].

A nutrient is a material that an organism consumes in order to grow, reproduce and survive. Macronutrients and micronutrients are the two major categories of nutrition. Macronutrients are chemicals that the body requires in big amounts, whereas micronutrients are nutrients that the body requires in little amounts. Carbohydrates, proteins, and fats are macronutrients that provide molecules for the human body's structural and metabolic functions. They are necessary for the body's correct functioning [7]. Although all nutrients are vital, the following six are particularly critical for the fetus's growth and development throughout pregnancy:

1) carbohydrates,
2) proteins,
3) fats,
4) vitamins,
5) minerals,
6) water.

Vitamins are naturally occurring essential substances that are required for survival. To function effectively, our bodies need vitamins. Most vitamins are impossible for us to generate, at least not in sufficient quantities to meet our needs. As a result, we must receive them from the food we consume. Several of the vitamins officially known performs a specialized purpose in the body, making them one of a kind and indispensable. There is no single diet that includes all of the vitamins and minerals that the body requires, and inadequate nutrient consumption leads to deficiencies. To meet the body's vitamin and mineral requirements, a diverse diet is essential.

Vitamins are divided into two categories: water-soluble and fat-soluble. Water-soluble vitamins are not well-preserved in our bodies. Water-soluble vitamins that are in excess are easily excreted from the body through urine. Fat-soluble vitamins, on the other hand, are water insoluble, and excess fat-soluble vitamins are stored in our body's fat tissues. Hypervitaminosis is a condition caused by an excess of fat-soluble vitamins in the body. Fats soluble vitamins contain vitamins A, D, E, K, and vitamins that are water-soluble contain vitamins B_1, B_2, B_3, B_6, B_7, B_9, B_{12} and Vitamins C. Dietary intake and medical supplementation of a few key vitamins are sufficient to keep both the mother and the fetus healthy during pregnancy [8, 9]. Figure 8.1 shows the different vitamins and there body function.

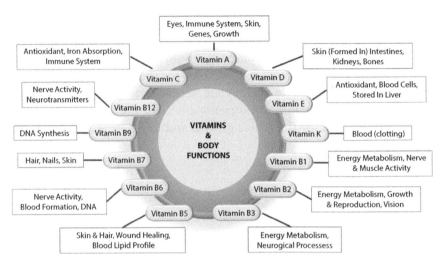

Figure 8.1 Vitamins and body functions [10, 11].

8.2 Role of Important Vitamins in Pregnancy

8.2.1 Vitamin A/Retinol

When there is an abruptly poor diet consumption of vitamin A, or there is a sustained period of dietary scarcity, or when there is a simultaneous combination of these two situations, i.e., both lengthy and severe, also with possible mediation of an underlying disease vitamin A deficiency occurs [12]. Vitamin A deficiency can cause subclinical issues like poor iron mobilization, cellular differentiation, and immune response reduction, as well as clinical issues like higher infectious morbidity, growth retardation, anemia, and xerophthalmia [13]. Vitamin A is important for both the pregnant woman and the fetus, as it is required for the advancement of other organs and the fetal skeleton, as well as the maintenance of the fetal immune system [13–16]. It is also required for the management of maternal night vision and fetal ocular health. Vitamin A molecule concentrations in the mother and infant have been linked to neonatal outcome [17]. The heart, the peripheral nervous system and its related structures, the circulatory, urogenital, and respiratory systems, as well as the skull, skeleton, and limbs, are the principal target tissues of vitamin A deficiency [18]. In infants born, vitamin A insufficiency during the second trimester was linked to a multiple increased risk to develop schizophrenia and certain other schizophrenia spectrum illnesses [19].

Toxicity: There is little basis of the recommendation on the vitamin A doses that are harmful to women of reproductive age or during various stages of pregnancy. There is a danger of teratogenicity so when dose of containing vitamin A is greater than 10,000 IU per day. There have been reports of abnormalities in infants whose mothers took high dosages of containing vitamin A (>25,000 IU/day) during pregnancy. These studies focus on urinary tract abnormalities [20]. Miscarriage and congenital abnormalities of the nervous system and cardiac systems have been related to the increase in levels of vitamin A (retinoic acid) in mother's blood within the first trimester of pregnancy [21]. Given the danger of cardiac malformation, a retinol intake of 10,000 IU per day each during pregnancy is associated with a higher risk for foetal cardiopathy (absolute risk of 1% to 2%), indicating the need for foetal echocardiography throughout the prenatal period [22].

8.2.2 Vitamin D/Calciferol

All women who have been identified as having a risk of vitamin D insufficiency during pregnancy should be screened at the time of their first visit to the physician, or at any point during the pregnancy if monitoring has been missed. Vitamin D3 supplements should be given to vitamin D deficient ladies every day for six weeks. Vitamin D levels aren't monitored on a regular basis. Vitamin D supplements must be provided to pregnant women beginning in the second trimester. The initial line of treatment should be oral supplementation. However, in addition to supplementing to cure the deficit, proper sun exposure instruction is critical. To improve vitamin D production, it is recommended that you spend at least 15-30 minutes per day in the sun [23, 24].

8.2.3 Vitamin E/Tocopherol

Vitamin E aids in the production and maintenance of red blood cells, as well as the maintenance of healthy skin and eyes, as well as the strengthening of your natural immune system. Vitamin E intake may assist to minimize the incidence of oxidative stress-related pregnancy problems. Vitamin E administration in pregnancy has to be evaluated for efficacy and safety [25]. Female infertility, miscarriage, early delivery, eclampsia, fetal intrauterine development restriction, and other pregnancy-related illnesses can all be caused by a shortage of vitamin E [26–28]. Vitamin E is important in the following situations:

1. **Infertility:** Oxidative stress is caused by an excess of reactive oxygen species produced and/or an insufficient

consumption of antioxidants. When the formation of reactive oxygen species and some other radicals surpasses the ability of antioxidants to scavenge them, cell damage can ensue. The most of reactive oxygen species are produced by the mitochondrial respiratory chain, and oxidative stress can impact female reproductive, leading to infertility [29].

2. **Endometriosis:** Endometriosis is a disorder in which endometrial tissue is seen just outside of the wall of the uterus [30].
3. **Miscarriage:** Miscarriage is a significant pregnancy problem that can be caused by a number of different factors. Dietary supplementation women with micronutrients before and during pregnancy period reduce miscarriage. Vitamin insufficiency has been associated with a higher risk of miscarriage [31].
4. **Polycystic ovary syndrome (PCOS):** In women of childbearing age, polycystic ovarian syndrome is a frequent congenital abnormality [32].
5. **Embryonic development:** The development and creation of the human embryo is referred to as human embryonic development. Even during early stages of development, it is characterized by the embryo's cell growth and cellular differentiation activities [33].
6. **Premature delivery:** Around 150 lakh new-borns (1 in 10) are born prematurely each year around the world. After pneumonia, prematurity seems to be the second biggest cause of death in neonates. Visual, auditory, and learning problems plague premature babies [34].
7. **Uterine fibroids:** Uterine fibroids, also known as myomas, are benign uterine tumours. Prolonged or heavy menstrual period, pelvic pressure or ache, and reproductive dysfunction are the most common symptoms [35].
8. **Preeclampsia:** Preeclampsia is a leading cause of new-born morbidity in both mothers and babies [36].
9. **Intrauterine growth restriction:** Intrauterine restriction (IUGR) occurs when foetuses are unable to meet their genetically based growth rate, resulting in low birth weight (LBW) offspring. It is a concern in both human and animal medicine [37].
10. **Premature rupture of membranes:** Membrane breakdown before 37 weeks' gestation in the lack of labour is known as preterm, premature rupture of membranes (PPROM) [38].

8.2.4 Vitamin B1/Thiamine

The need for thiamine, just like all the other vitamins and minerals, increases dramatically during pregnancy. The need for thiamine appears to be higher as in third trimester. The cause for this is the growing fetus's increased utilization and demand. Water-soluble vitamins, like as thiamine, are found to be 2-fold more in umbilical cords than in maternal blood, according to studies. Thiamine is a water-soluble vitamin that can be found in a variety of foods, including leafy green vegetables, cereals, eggs, and pulses. Normally, thiamine intake is not recommended for pregnant women, but in some situations, thiamine, along with other nutrients, may be given to women who are dehydrated owing to excessive vomiting during pregnancy to prevent deficiency symptoms. Thiamine aids in the conversion of carbohydrates into energy for both the mother and the infant. It is necessary for the growing bay's brain development as well as the pregnant mother's good health, including her central nervous system, muscle, and heart function [39, 40].

8.2.5 Vitamin B7/Biotin

Biotin belongs to the B-complex family of nutrients. It aids in the production of fatty acids, glucose usage, protein metabolism, and cyanocobalamin, folic acid utilization. The consequences of vitamin deficiency and excess have yet to be discovered. Green beans, egg whites, dark green veggies, kidneys, and liver are all good sources [41].

8.2.6 Vitamin B9/Folic Acid

Folic acid promotes in the prevention of miscarriage and birth problems such as neural tube defects and spina bifida. Folic acid-rich foods should be included in the diet of pregnant women. Green vegetables, cereals, and folic acid enhanced margarine are all reliable sources for folic acid in the diet. Because it is difficult to receive enough folic acid from food alone during pregnancy, supplementation is necessary. Some women are advised to take a larger dose of 5 milligrams (mg) of folic acid a day every day if they have a higher chance of having a pregnancy caused by a neural tube abnormality or are taking medication for epilepsy. Folic acid supports in development as well as in the maintenance of pregnancy. Doctors recommend taking a 400 microgram (g) folic acid tablet each day continuing until the baby is 12 weeks old [42]. Folic acid supplementation should be continued until the second or third trimester, according to some specialists. Supplementing with 400 mg of folic acid per day throughout the second or third trimester of pregnancy has been shown to improve folate status of maternal and cord blood, as well as avoid the rise in homocysteine levels that occurs later in pregnancy. More research is needed to see if these effects are useful during pregnancy [43].

8.2.7 Vitamin B12/Cobalamin/Cyanocobalamin

Cyanocobalamin is a water-soluble vitamin found in meat, dairy products, fish, and eggs, it's important to get enough of it [44]. It's required for the bone marrow's regular generation by red blood cells as well as the formation of nerve cells. Megaloblastic anemia and, through myelin degradation, neurological abnormalities (autonomic dysfunction, neuropathic) or even neuropsychiatric disorders like dementia are caused by vitamin B12 deficiency. Vitamin B12 deficiency is common in vegan diets. Megaloblastic anemia can also be caused by a lack of folate, which should be considered when determining the cause of the anemic state [45, 46].

8.2.8 Vitamin C/Ascorbic Acid

Vitamin C is a solid substance that is water soluble [47]. Although most animals and plants produce ascorbic acid, primate and living beings lack gluconolactone oxidase, a critical enzyme in the ascorbate manufacturing process. As a result, these species' daily vitamin C requirements should be met by diet. Vitamin C is found in orange, citrus, grapefruit, leafy green vegetables, and cow liver [48]. Vitamin C is essential for chronic wounds and appropriate immunological function, as well as the formation of collagen, which provides strength to connective tissues. Scurvy is a disorder in which the generated collagen is unstable. Vitamin C deprivation induces alterations in the connective tissue, due to the formation of scurvy. Muscle soreness, joint swelling, and bleeding are all indications of scurvy. Vitamin C is a powerful antioxidant and free radical scavenger that can be used topically to treat a variety of skin conditions, including those induced by photoaging [49, 50]. Vitamin C can be used to treat skin hyperpigmentation because it suppresses the activation of melanocytes, or cells associated with the manufacture of pigment [51]. Table 8.1 comprising the scientific name, source, deficiency diseases of vitamins.

Table 8.1 Scientific name, source, deficiency diseases of vitamins.

Name of vitamin	Scientific name	Sources	Deficiency disease	Reference
Vitamin A	Retinol	Dark green and yellow-colored vegetables and fruits, cod liver oil, milk, butter and other dairy products	Night blindness, dry skin, weak teeth and bones	[52]
Vitamin D	Calciferol	Sunlight, eggs, meat, fish, mushrooms	Anxiety, depression, weak immune system, rickets	[53]
Vitamin E	Tocopherol	Almonds, hazelnuts, spinach, tomatoes	Visual disturbances, general unwellness	[54]
Vitamin B1	Thiamine	Bread yeast, sprouts	Weak memory, Disturbances in sleep, feeling irritated	[55]
Vitamin B7	Biotin	Eggs, milk, vegetables, cereals, nuts (almonds, walnuts, peanuts), liver, kidney, yeast, soybeans. Other: synthesized by intestinal bacteria	Nutritional biotin deficiency	[56]

(Continued)

Table 8.1 Scientific name, source, deficiency diseases of vitamins. (*Continued*)

Name of vitamin	Scientific name	Sources	Deficiency disease	Reference
Vitamin B9	Folate	Dark green leafy vegetables, beans, lentils, asparagus, wheat germ, yeast, peanuts, oranges, strawberries	Folic acid deficiency anemia	[57]
Vitamin B12	Cobalamin	Fish, meat, raw milk, organic yogurt	Joint pains, poor dental health, chronic fatigue	[58]
Vitamin C	Ascorbic Acid	Fruits—papaya, pineapple, kiwi fruit, mango, tomatoes	Poor healing of wounds, bleeding gums, dry and scaly skin, scurvy	[59]

8.3 Concept of Nutraceuticals

The term "nutraceutical" is a combination of "nutrient" and "pharmaceutical" (a prescription drug). Nutraceuticals may contain compounds with the "natural" goal of treating or preventing disease, but which are not universally acknowledged as safe (Figure 8.2) [60].

"Let diet be the medication and medication be the diet," the Greek physician sir Hippocrates said approximately 2500 years ago, and we understand the truth of his words today. Functional foods, dietary supplements, and nutraceuticals are defined as "any ingredient that could be regarded a food or part of a food that provides health and medical advantages, particularly disease prevention and treatment." "Nutraceuticals" has to be the most appropriate term used to describe this group. This title was created by Stephen DeFelice, the chairman and chief executive of a Medicine Research Foundation located Cranford, New Jersey [61]. With these phenomena, ideas like nutraceuticals, nutritional treatment, phytonutrients, and phytotherapy have evolved [62]. These active or beneficial foods, phytonutrients, and phytomedicines have been shown to improve health and immunological function, as well as reduce adverse effects and preserve wellness [63].

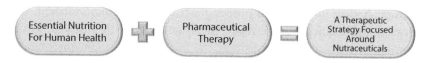

Figure 8.2 Diagrammatic representation of concept of nutraceuticals [65].

Clinical test findings from animal testing and studies are required throughout the pharmaceutical advancement process for assessment of the effects. In the past, there was no validation procedure for foods in the prevention of diseases, on the other hand. However, as the composition of food has been scientifically established to induce lifestyle-related disorders, it is becoming a cultural issue in recent years [64, 65].

Nutraceutical Advantages
Natural compounds and health products may provide a number of advantages to consumers:

1. It has the potential to improve the nutritional content of our diet.
2. It is possible that it will help us survive longer.
3. May assist us in avoiding certain medical disorders.
4. Doing something for oneself may provide a psychological advantage.
5. May be seen as being more "natural" than orthodox medication, with less negative side effects.
6. Food for special-needs populations may be presented (for example, heavy nutritious foodstuff for the older) [66].

8.4 Targeted Nutrition Foods for Pregnancy

Pregnant women have unique dietary needs due to the need to support the fetus' growth and development as well as the mother's health [67, 68]. Deficits in ferrous, folate, vitamin D, salt, and calcium, for example, can cause anemia, birth abnormalities, hyperglycemia, overweight, preeclampsia, and psychological issues in the foetus and mother while pregnancy. Many women have been observed to have an insufficient micronutrient balance during pregnancy, which could lead to negative health impacts in their children in the future. As a result, functional meals and beverages can be designed expressly for pregnant women's needs. This can be accomplished by providing a proper macronutrient, micronutrient, and nutraceutical balance. Furthermore, meals enriched with probiotic strains or probiotic bacteria may encourage the formation of a gut microbiome, which may aid in the prevention of most of these gestation health issues. The use of multicomponent-bioactive delivery systems in the production of functional meals and beverages for pregnant women may thus be advantageous. Vitamin D, for example, is oil-soluble and can be contained within the fat droplets of an oil-in-water mixture, however iron or calcium can be disseminated in a bioavailable form within the aqueous phase. Women who are vegans or vegetarians may need to supplement their diet with additional nutrients like vitamin B12, which may be deficient in their typical diet. There are a variety of vitamin-rich supplements for pregnant women on the market, as well as some treatments designed to alleviate morning sickness symptoms. Furthermore, there are several protein-rich powders that may be mixed with water to make healthy beverages for pregnant women. However, there are currently only a handful usable food and beverage goods that use modern structural design principles to improve efficacy. It will be critical for ensuring that any future goods are founded on good nutrition science, are safe, inexpensive, and efficient, and have appealing sensory characteristics [64, 65].

8.5 Concentrations of Vitamins During Pregnancy

Fats-soluble vitamins: Due to hemodilution, blood vitamin A doses decrease gradually during pregnancy, and there is evidence that inadequate nutrient vitamin A consumption can also reduce blood levels, but while concentrations are high are difficult to read as they are not a great reflection of underlying condition. During pregnancy, the active constituent of serum vitamin D (1, 25-dihydroxycholecalciferol) rises, although the inert form (25-hydroxycholecalciferol) falls. Vitamin E levels are known to rise during pregnancy, most likely due to the hyperlipidemic state that comes with it [65].

Water-soluble vitamins: During pregnancy, blood vitamin C levels drop by 50 percent, partially due to the foetus's increased absorption and partly due to hemodilution. During pregnancy, the amounts of thiamine and riboflavin in the blood decrease as well. Research indicates that serum thiamine levels fall during pregnancy while urine elimination of vitamin metabolites rises. Vitamin concentrations fall through pregnancy as a result of physiologic changes brought on by higher blood volume or by increasing demands on mass transportation all over the placenta [66]. Folate levels may drop during pregnancy due to poor intestinal absorption, insufficient intake, or rising demands [67]. During pregnancy, arterial cobalamin concentrations decrease, that may be irrespective of meals and may not indicate a decrease in maternal storage or a biochemical deficiency. Biotin levels are much lesser in gestation than in non-pregnant, non-lactating states, and they fall gradually throughout the pregnancy. Pantothenic acid levels are thought to drop during pregnancy and then rebound to normal within a week following birth [67, 68].

8.6 Role of Vitamins in the Body

Table 8.2 shows the role of vitamins in the body.

Table 8.2 Role of vitamin in body.

Role	Description	References
Release energy	Numerous B vitamins are essential constituents of linked coenzymes (enzyme-aid molecules) that help undo energy from meals.	[68]
Produce energy	In the generation of energy, B-complex, and vitamin interact.	
Build proteins and cells	Vitamins B complex and vitamin C help cells reproduce by enzymes that break down amino acid residues (the basic components of proteins).	[69]
Make protein	One of the many functions of substance is to aid in the formation of protein that knits together wounds, strengthens vessel walls, and serves as a foundation for bone and teeth.	

8.7 Herbal Sources as a Vitamin

Herbs have been utilized for the treatment of numerous diseases since ancient times, with just minor adverse effects. As noted below, a variety of plants are good sources of vitamins (Table 8.3):

Table 8.3 Common name, biological name, constituent, vitamin involved and herbs.

Common name	Biological name	Constituent	Vitamin	Reference
Onion	Dried bulb of Allium cepa Linn	Allicin and allun	Folic Acid.	[70]
Aloe	Dried juice of leaves aloe barbadensis mil	Aloe and aloesin	Vitamins A, C and E, B12, Folic Acid	[71]
Turmeric	Rhizomes of curcuma longa	Curcumin	Vitamin C	[72]
Garlic	Dried bulb of allium sativum	Allin and allicin	Vitamins B6 and C	[73]
Senna	Dried leaves of cassi	Sennosides	Vitamin C, Vitamin E	[74]
Liquorice	Dried root of glycyrrhiza glabra	Glycyrrhizin and liquirtin	Vitamin B, Vitamin E	[75, 76]
Ginger	Rhizomes of *Zingiber officinale* (zingiberaces)	Zingiberane and echinoside	Vitamin B, Vitamin C	[77–82]

8.8 Conclusion

The nutritional state of a woman has an impact on her health, as well as the outcome of her pregnancy as well as the health of her newborn infant. The nutritional needs of pregnant women differ significantly from non-pregnant women. The literature on this topic is extensive, therefore, our conclusions constituted based on substantial data. As a result, we may divide scenarios into two categories: systematic additions and unique circumstances that may justify supplementing or the treatment of maternal or fetal illnesses, either curative or preventive. The present daily recommended intakes appear to be very much from physiological realities, and so overestimate the true demands of pregnant women. Today, the data suggest that coping mechanisms enable well-nourished, healthy women with a diverse diet to bring a regular pregnancy to term without relying on resources other than their consumption of food and the spontaneous increases that occur throughout pregnancy. Nonetheless, a tailored approach to dietary modification is advocated, taking into account women's food access, socioeconomic level, gender, ethnicity, and cultural dietary choices, as well as body mass index. Furthermore, because many of the recommendations are for straightforward pregnancies, changes should be made if difficulties emerge, such as gestational diabetes.

Acknowledgment

The authors thank Mahatma Gandhi Vidyamandir's Pharmacy College, Panchavati, Nashik, Maharashtra, India.

References

1. Heidemann, B.H. and McClure, J.H., Changes in maternal physiology during pregnancy. *BJA CEPD Rev.*, 3, 65–68, 2003.
2. Soma-Pillay, P., Nelson-Piercy, C., Tolppanen, H., Mebazaa, A., Physiological changes in pregnancy. *Cardiovasc. J. Afr.*, 27, 89–94, 2016.
3. Magon, N. and Kumar, P., Hormones in pregnancy. *Niger. Med. J.*, 53, 179–183, 2012.
4. Tkachenko, O., Shchekochikhin, D., Schrier, R.W., Hormones and hemodynamics in pregnancy. *Int. J. Endocrinol. Metab.*, 12, e14098, 2014.
5. Mensink, G.B.M., Fletcher, R., Gurinovic, M., Huybrechts, I., Lafay, L., Serra-Majem, L., Szponar, L., Tetens, I., Verkaik-Kloosterman, J., Baka, A. et al., Mapping low intake of micronutrients across Europe. *Br. J. Nutr.*, 110, 755–773, 2013.
6. Derbyshire, E., Micronutrient intakes of British adults across mid-life: A secondary analysis of the UK National diet and nutrition survey. *Front Nutr.*, 05, 01–09, 2018.
7. Egbuna, C. and Dable-Tupas, G. (Eds.), *Functional Foods and Nutraceuticals*, pp. 156–179, Springer Nature, Switzerland AG, 2020.

8. Sherwin, J.C., Reacher, M.H., Dean, W.H., Ngondi, J., Epidemiology of vitamin A deficiency and xerophthalmia in at-risk populations. *Trans. R. Soc. Trop. Med. Hyg.*, 106, 205–214, 2012.
9. Sommer, A. and Davidson, F.R., Annecy accords. Assessment and control of vitamin A deficiency: The annecy accords. *J. Nutr.*, 132, Suppl. 9, 2845S–2850S, 2002.
10. Trumbo, P., Yates, A.A., Schlicker, S., Poos, M., Dietary reference intakes: Vitamin A, vitamin K, arsenic, boron, chromium, copper, iodine, iron, manganese, molybdenum, nickel, silicon, vanadium, and zinc. *J. Am. Diet. Assoc.*, 101, 294–301, 2001.
11. El-Khashab, E.K., Hamdy, A.M., Maher, K.M., Fouad, M.A., Abbas, G.Z., Effect of maternal vitamin A deficiency during pregnancy on neonatal kidney size. *J. Perinat. Med.*, 41, 199–203, 2013.
12. Downie, D., Antipatis, C., Delday, M.I., Maltin, C.A., Sneddon, A.A., Moderate maternal vitamin A deficiency alters myogenic regulatory protein expression and perinatal organ growth in the rat. *Am. J. Physiol. Regul. Integr. Comp. Physiol.*, 288, R73–R79, 2005.
13. Sommer, A. and Vyas, K.S., A global clinical view on vitamin A and carotenoids. *Am. J. Clin. Nutr.*, 96, 1204S–1206S, 2012.
14. Hanson, C., Lyden, E., Anderson-Berry, A., Kocmich, N., Rezac, A., Delair, S., Furtado, J., Van Ormer, M., Izevbigie, N., Olateju, E.K. et al., Status of retinoids and carotenoids and associations with clinical outcomes in maternal-infant pairs in Nigeria. *Nutrients*, 10, E1286, 2018.
15. Zile, M.H., Function of vitamin A in vertebrate embryonic development. *J. Nutr.*, 131, 705–708, 2001.
16. Bao, Y., Ibram, G., Blaner, W.S., Quesenberry, C.P., Shen, L., McKeague, I.W., Schaefer, C.A., Susser, E.S., Brown, A.S., Low maternal retinol as a risk factor for schizophrenia in adult offspring. *Schizophr. Res.*, 137, 159–165, 2012.
17. Chagas, M.H., Flores, H., Campos, F.A., Santana, R.A., Lins, E.C., (Vitamin A tertogenicity). *Rev. Bras. Saude Matern. Infant.*, 3, 247–252, 2003.
18. Miller, R.K., Hendrickx, A.G., Mills, J.L., Hummler, H., Wiegand, U.W., Periconceptional vitamin A use: How much is teratogenic? *Reprod. Toxicol.*, 12, 75–88, 1998.
19. Donofrio, M.T., Moon-Grady, A.J., Hornberger, L.K., Copel, J.A., Sklansky, M.S., Abuhamad, A., Cuneo, B.F., Huhta, J.C., Jonas, R.A., Krishnan, A. et al., Diagnosis and treatment of foetal cardiac disease: A scientific statement from the American heart association. *Circulation*, 129, 2183–2242, 2014.
20. Konradsen, S., Ag, H., Lindberg, F., Hexeberg, S., Jorde, R., Serum 1,25-dihydroxy vitamin D is inversely associated with body mass index. *Eur. J. Nutr.*, 47, 2, 87–91, 2008.
21. De-Regil, L.M., Palacios, C., Lombardo, L.K., Peña-Rosas, J.P., Vitamin D supplementation for women during pregnancy (review). *Cochrane Database Syst. Rev.*, 1, 1, 01–15, 2016.

22. Rumbold, A., Ota, E., Hori, H., Miyazaki, C., Crowther, C.A., Vitamin E supplementation in pregnancy. *Cochrane Database Syst. Rev.,* 9, 01–28, 2015.
23. Gagne, A., Wei, S.Q., Fraser, W.D., Julien, P., Absorption, transport, and bioavailability of vitamin e and its role in pregnant women. *J. Obstet. Gynaecol. Can.,* 31, 3, 210–7, 2009.
24. Wahid, S., Khan, R.A., Feroz, Z., Reduction in mortality and teratogenicity following simultaneous administration of folic acid and vitamin E with antiepileptic, antihypertensive and anti-allergic drugs. *J. Pharm. Bioallied Sci.,* 6, 3, 185–91, 2014.
25. Hubalek, M., Buchner, H., Mörtl, M.G., Schlembach, D., Huppertz, B., Firulovic, B., Köhler, W., Hafner, E., Dieplinger, B., Wildt, L., Dieplinger, H., The vitamin e-binding protein afamin increases in maternal serum during pregnancy. *Clin. Chim. Acta,* 434, 41, July 1, 2014.
26. Ruder, E.H., Hartman, T.J., Goldman, M.B., Impact of oxidative stress on female fertility. *Curr. Opin. Obstet. Gynecol.,* 21, 3, 219, June 2009.
27. Vitale, S.G., Capriglione, S., Peterlunger, I., La Rosa, V.L., Vitagliano, A., Noventa, M., Valenti, G., Sapia, F., Angioli, R., Lopez, S., Sarpietro, G., Rossetti, D., Zito, G., The role of oxidative stress and membrane transport systems during endometriosis: A fresh look at a busy corner. *Oxid. Med. Cell. Longev.,* 01, 01–14, 2018.
28. Rumbold, A., Middleton, P., Pan, N., Crowther, C.A., Vitamin supplementation for preventing miscarriage. *Cochrane Database Syst. Rev.,* 01, 01-38, 2011.
29. Bellver, J., Rodríguez-Tabernero, L., Robles, A., Muñoz, E., Martínez, F., Landeras, J., García-Velasco, J., Fontes, J., Álvarez, M., Álvarez, C., Acevedo, B., Polycystic ovary syndrome throughout a woman's life. *J. Assist. Reprod. Genet.,* 35, 1, 25–39, Jan. 1, 2018.
30. Siddiqui, M.A., Ahmad, U., Ali, A., Ahsan, F. and Haider, M.F., Role of Vitamin E in Pregnancy. In Vitamin E in Health and Disease-Interactions, Diseases and Health Aspects. *IntechOpen.,* 01, 01-22, 2021.
31. Nour, N.M., Premature delivery and the millennium development goal. *Rev. Obstet. Gynecol.,* 5, 2, 100, 2012.
32. Stewart, E.A., Uterine fibroids. *Lancet,* 357, 9252, 293–8, Jan. 27, 2001.
33. Akyol, D., Mungan, T., Görkemli, H., Nuhoglu, G., Maternal levels of vitamin E in normal and preeclamptic pregnancy. *Arch. Gynecol. Obstet.,* 263, 4, 151–5, Apr. 1, 2000.
34. Brodsky, D. and Christou, H., Current concepts in intrauterine growth restriction. *J. Intensive Care Med.,* 19, 6, 307–19, Nov. 2004.
35. Shubert, P.J., Diss, E., Iams, J.D., Etiology of preterm premature rupture of membranes. *Obstet. Genecol. Clin. North Am.,* 19, 2, 251–63, Jun. 1, 1992.
36. Butterworth, R.F., Maternal thiamine deficiency: Still a problem in some world communities. *Am. J. Clin. Nutr.,* 74, 6, 712–713, 2001.
37. Baker, H., Frank, O., Thompson, A.D. *et al.,* Vitamin profile of 174 mothers and newborns at parturition. *Am. J. Clin. Nutr.,* 28, 59–65, 1975.

38. Hsu, S.-M., Raine, L., Fanger, H., A comparative study of the peroxidase-antiperoxidase method and an avidin-biotin complex method for studying polypeptide hormones with radioimmunoassay antibodies. *Am. J. Clin. Pathol.*, 75, 5, 734–738, 2016.
39. Egbuna, C. and Dable-Tupas, G. (Eds.), *Functional Foods and Nutraceuticals*, pp. 156–179, Springer Nature, Switzerland AG, 2020.
40. McNulty, B., McNulty, H., Marshall, B., Ward, M., Molloy, A.M., Scott, J.M., Dornan, J., Pentieva, K., Impact of continuing folic acid after the first trimester of pregnancy: Findings of a randomized trial of folic acid supplementation in the second and third trimesters. *Am. J. Clin. Nutr.*, 98, 92–98, 2013.
41. Hariz, A. and Bhattacharya, P.T., Megaloblastic anemia, in: *StatPearls (Internet)*, StatPearls Publishing, Treasure Island (FL, 2019, Available from: https://www.ncbi.nlm.nih.gov/books/NBK537254.
42. Lykstad, J. and Sharma, S., Biochemistry, water soluble vitamins, in: *StatPearls (Internet)*, pp. 53–58, StatPearls Publishing, Treasure Island (FL, 2019.
43. Ankar, A. and Kumar, A., Vitamin B12 deficiency (cobalamin), in: *StatPearls (Internet)*, pp. –52, StatPearls Publishing, Treasure Island (FL, 2019.
44. Halliwell, B., Vitamin C and genomic stability. *Mutat. Res. Fundam. Mol. Mech. Mutagen.*, 475, 1, 29–35, 2001.
45. Ferraro, P.M., Curhan, G.C., Gambaro, G., Taylor, E.N., Total, dietary, and supplemental vitamin C intake and risk of incident kidney stones. *Am. J. Kidney Dis.*, 67, 3, 400–407, 2016.
46. Sorice, A., Guerriero, E., Capone, F., Colonna, G., Castello, G., Costantini, S., Ascorbic acid: Its role in immune system and chronic inflammation diseases. *Mini Rev. Med. Chem.*, 14, 5, 444–452, 2014.
47. Gomez, L.A., Tchekalarova, J.D., Atanasova, M., da Conceição Machado, K., de Sousa Rios, M.A., Paz, M.F.C.J. *et al.*, Anticonvulsant effect of anacardic acid in murine models: Putative role of GABAergic and antioxidant mechanisms. *Biomed. Pharmacother.*, 106, 1686–1695, 2018.
48. Telang, P.S., Vitamin C in dermatology. *Indian Dermatol. Online J.*, 4, 2, 143–145, 2013.
49. Ross, S., Functional foods: The food and drug administration perspective. *Am. J. Clin. Nutr.*, 71, 6, 1735S–1738S, 2000.
50. Biesalski, H.K., Nutraceuticals: The link between nutrition and medicine. *Oxid. Stress Dis.*, 6, 1–26, 2001.
51. Berger, M.M. and Shenkin, A., Vitamins and trace elements: Practical aspects of supplementation. *Nutrition*, 22, 9, 952–955, 2006.
52. Ramaa, C.S., Shirode, A.R., Mundada, A.S., Kadam, V.J., Nutraceuticals-an emerging era in the treatment and prevention of cardiovascular diseases. *Curr. Pharm. Biotechnol.*, 7, 1, 15–23, 2006.
53. Chintale, A.G., Kadam, V.S., Sakhare, R.S., Birajdar, G.O., Nalwad, D.N., Role of nutraceuticals in various diseases: A comprehensive review. *IJRPC*, 3, 2, 2231–2781, 2013.

54. Milman, N., Paszkowski, T., Cetin, I., Castelo-Branco, C., Supplementation during pregnancy: Beliefs and science. *Gynecol. Endocrinol.*, 32, 509–516, 2016.
55. Parisi, F., di Bartolo, I., Savasi, V.M., Cetin, I., Micronutrient supplementation in pregnancy: Who, what and how much? *Obstet. Med.*, 12, 5–13, 2019.
56. Cetin, I., Buhling, K., Demir, C. et al., Impact of micronutrient status during pregnancy on early nutrition programming. *Ann. Nutr. Metab.*, 74, 269–278, 2019.
57. Akkerman, R., Faas, M.M., de Vos, P., Non-digestible carbohydrates in 1029 infant formula as substitution for human milk oligosaccharide functions: Effects on microbiota and gut maturation. *Crit. Rev. Food Sci. Nutr.*, 59, 1486–1497, 20192019.
58. Cavdar, G., Papich, T., Ryan, E.P., Microbiome, breastfeeding and public health policy in the United States: The case for dietary fiber. *Nutr. Metab. Insights*, 12, 01–10, 2019.
59. Wallingford, J.C. and Underwood, B.A., Vitamin a deficiency in pregnancy, lactation, and the nursing child, in: *Vitamin A Deficiency and Its Control*, J.C. Bauernfeind, (Ed.), pp. 101–52, Academic Press, New York, 1986.
60. Underwood, B.A., Maternal vitamin A status and its importance in infancy and early childhood. *Am. J. Clin. Nutr.*, 59, suppl, 517S–24S, 1994.
61. Moghissi, K.S., Risks and benefits of nutritional supplements during pregnancy. *Obstet. Gynecol.*, 58, 685–785, 1981.
62. Wickens, D., Wilkins, M.H., Lyne, C.J. et al., Free radical oxidation (peroxidation) products in plasma in normal and abnormal pregnancy. *Ann. Clin. Biochem.*, 18, 158–62, 1981.
63. Drife, J. and MacNab, G., Mineral and vitamin supplements. *Clin. Obstet. Gynaecol.*, 13, 253–67, 1986.
64. Ahire, E.D., Sonawane, V.N., Surana, K.R., Talele, G.S., Drug discovery, drug-likeness screening, and bioavailability: Development of drug-likeness rule for natural products, in: *Applied Pharmaceutical Practice and Nutraceuticals Natural Product Development*, 01, 191–208, Apple Academic Press, Inc., USA, 2021.
65. Surana, K.R., Ahire, E.D., Sonawane, V.N., Talele, S.G., Talele, G.S., Molecular modeling: Novel techniques in food and nutrition development, in: *Natural Food Products and Waste Recovery*, pp. 17–31, Apple Academic Press, Inc., USA, 2021.
66. Kazzi, G.M., Gross, C.L., Bork, M.D., Moses, D., Vitamins and minerals, in: *Principles of Medical Therapy in Pregnancy*, 3rd ed, N. Gleicher, and L. Buttin, (Eds.), pp. 311–9, Appleton and Lange, Old Tappan, NJ, 1998.
67. Hytten, F.E., Nutrition, in: *Clinical Physiology in Obstetrics*, F. Hytten, and G. Chamberlain, (Eds.), pp. 163–92, Blackwell Scientific Publications, Oxford, United Kingdom, 1980.
68. Czeizel, A.B., Folic acid in the prevention of neural tube defects. *J. Pediatr. Gastroenterol. Nutr.*, 20, 4–16, 1995.

69. Metz, J., McGrath, K., Bennett, M., Hyland, K., Bottinglieri, T., Biochemical indices of vitamin B12 nutrition in pregnant patients with subnormal serum vitamin B12 levels. *Am. J. Hematol.*, 48, 251–5, 1995.
70. Csapó, J., Albert, C., Prokisch, J., The role of vitamins in the diet of the elderly II. Water solublevitamins. *Acta Univ. Sapientiae Alimentaria*, 10, 1, 146–66, 2017.
71. Ball, G.F., *Water-Soluble Vitamin Assays in Human Nutrition*, Springer, Science Business Media, B.V., 2012.
72. Cardelle-Cobas, A., Soria, A.C., Corzo, N., Villamiel, M., A comprehensive survey of garlic functionality, *Nova Science Publishers Inc.*, 01, 1–60, 2010.
73. Bhattacharya, M., Malik, S., Singh, A., Aloe vera barbadensis: A review on its ethanopharmacological value. *J. Pharm. Res.*, 4, 4507–10, 2011.
74. Kumar, N. and Sakhya, S.K., Ethnopharmacological properties of Curcuma longa: A review. *Int. J. Pharm. Sci. Res.*, 4, 1, 103, Jan 2013.
75. Rizwani, G.H. and Shareef, H., Genus allium: The potential nutritive and therapeutic source. *J. Pharm. Nutr. Sci.*, 1, 158–63, 2011.
76. Kamagaté, M., Koffi, C., Kouamé, N.M., Akoubet, A., Alain, N., Yao, R., Die, H.M., Ethnobotany, phytochemistry, pharmacology and toxicology profiles of cassia siamea lam. *J. Phytopharm.*, 3, 1, 57–76, 2014.
77. Damle, M., Glycyrrhiza glabra (liquorice)-a potent medicinal herb. *Int. J. Herb. Med.*, 2, 2, 132-6, 2014.
78. Sharma, Y., Ginger (zingiber officinale)-an elixir of life a review. *Pharma Innov.*, 6, 11, 22, 2017.
79. Keservani, R.K., Kesharwani, R.K., Vyas, N., Jain, S., Raghuvanshi, R., Sharma, A.K., Nutraceutical and functional food as future food: A review. *Der. Pharm. Lett.*, 2, 1, 106–116, 2010a.
80. Keservani, R.K., Kesharwani, R.K., Sharma, A.K., Vyas, N., Chadoker, A., Nutritional supplements: An overview. *Int. J. Curr. Pharm. Rev. Res.*, 1, 1, 59–75, 2010b.
81. Keservani, R.K., Sharma, A.K., Kesharwani, R.K., An overview and therapeutic applications of nutraceutical and functional foods, in: *Recent Advances in Drug Delivery Technology*, pp. 160–201, 2017.
82. Keservani, R.K., Sharma, A.K., Kesharwani, R.K. (Eds.), Nutraceuticals and Dietary Supplements: *Applications in Health Improvement and Disease Management*, Apple Academic Press, New York, 01, 01–54, 2020.

54. Milman, N., Paszkowski, T., Cetin, I., Castelo-Branco, C., Supplementation during pregnancy: Beliefs and science. *Gynecol. Endocrinol.*, 32, 509–516, 2016.
55. Parisi, F., di Bartolo, I., Savasi, V.M., Cetin, I., Micronutrient supplementation in pregnancy: Who, what and how much? *Obstet. Med.*, 12, 5–13, 2019.
56. Cetin, I., Buhling, K., Demir, C. et al., Impact of micronutrient status during pregnancy on early nutrition programming. *Ann. Nutr. Metab.*, 74, 269–278, 2019.
57. Akkerman, R., Faas, M.M., de Vos, P., Non-digestible carbohydrates in 1029 infant formula as substitution for human milk oligosaccharide functions: Effects on microbiota and gut maturation. *Crit. Rev. Food Sci. Nutr.*, 59, 1486–1497, 20192019.
58. Cavdar, G., Papich, T., Ryan, E.P., Microbiome, breastfeeding and public health policy in the United States: The case for dietary fiber. *Nutr. Metab. Insights*, 12, 01–10, 2019.
59. Wallingford, J.C. and Underwood, B.A., Vitamin a deficiency in pregnancy, lactation, and the nursing child, in: *Vitamin A Deficiency and Its Control*, J.C. Bauernfeind, (Ed.), pp. 101–52, Academic Press, New York, 1986.
60. Underwood, B.A., Maternal vitamin A status and its importance in infancy and early childhood. *Am. J. Clin. Nutr.*, 59, suppl, 517S–24S, 1994.
61. Moghissi, K.S., Risks and benefits of nutritional supplements during pregnancy. *Obstet. Gynecol.*, 58, 685–785, 1981.
62. Wickens, D., Wilkins, M.H., Lyne, C.J. et al., Free radical oxidation (peroxidation) products in plasma in normal and abnormal pregnancy. *Ann. Clin. Biochem.*, 18, 158–62, 1981.
63. Drife, J. and MacNab, G., Mineral and vitamin supplements. *Clin. Obstet. Gynaecol.*, 13, 253–67, 1986.
64. Ahire, E.D., Sonawane, V.N., Surana, K.R., Talele, G.S., Drug discovery, drug-likeness screening, and bioavailability: Development of drug-likeness rule for natural products, in: *Applied Pharmaceutical Practice and Nutraceuticals Natural Product Development*, 01, 191–208, Apple Academic Press, Inc., USA, 2021.
65. Surana, K.R., Ahire, E.D., Sonawane, V.N., Talele, S.G., Talele, G.S., Molecular modeling: Novel techniques in food and nutrition development, in: *Natural Food Products and Waste Recovery*, pp. 17–31, Apple Academic Press, Inc., USA, 2021.
66. Kazzi, G.M., Gross, C.L., Bork, M.D., Moses, D., Vitamins and minerals, in: *Principles of Medical Therapy in Pregnancy*, 3rd ed, N. Gleicher, and L. Buttin, (Eds.), pp. 311–9, Appleton and Lange, Old Tappan, NJ, 1998.
67. Hytten, F.E., Nutrition, in: *Clinical Physiology in Obstetrics*, F. Hytten, and G. Chamberlain, (Eds.), pp. 163–92, Blackwell Scientific Publications, Oxford, United Kingdom, 1980.
68. Czeizel, A.B., Folic acid in the prevention of neural tube defects. *J. Pediatr. Gastroenterol. Nutr.*, 20, 4–16, 1995.

69. Metz, J., McGrath, K., Bennett, M., Hyland, K., Bottinglieri, T., Biochemical indices of vitamin B12 nutrition in pregnant patients with subnormal serum vitamin B12 levels. *Am. J. Hematol.*, 48, 251–5, 1995.
70. Csapó, J., Albert, C., Prokisch, J., The role of vitamins in the diet of the elderly II. Water solublevitamins. *Acta Univ. Sapientiae Alimentaria*, 10, 1, 146–66, 2017.
71. Ball, G.F., *Water-Soluble Vitamin Assays in Human Nutrition*, Springer, Science Business Media, B.V., 2012.
72. Cardelle-Cobas, A., Soria, A.C., Corzo, N., Villamiel, M., A comprehensive survey of garlic functionality, *Nova Science Publichers Inc.*, 01, 1–60, 2010.
73. Bhattacharya, M., Malik, S., Singh, A., Aloe vera barbadensis: A review on its ethanopharmacological value. *J. Pharm. Res.*, 4, 4507–10, 2011.
74. Kumar, N. and Sakhya, S.K., Ethnopharmacological properties of Curcuma longa: A review. *Int. J. Pharm. Sci. Res.*, 4, 1, 103, Jan 2013.
75. Rizwani, G.H. and Shareef, H., Genus allium: The potential nutritive and therapeutic source. *J. Pharm. Nutr. Sci.*, 1, 158–63, 2011.
76. Kamagaté, M., Koffi, C., Kouamé, N.M., Akoubet, A., Alain, N., Yao, R., Die, H.M., Ethnobotany, phytochemistry, pharmacology and toxicology profiles of cassia siamea lam. *J. Phytopharm.*, 3, 1, 57–76, 2014.
77. Damle, M., Glycyrrhiza glabra (liquorice)-a potent medicinal herb. *Int. J. Herb. Med.*, 2, 2, 132-6, 2014.
78. Sharma, Y., Ginger (zingiber officinale)-an elixir of life a review. *Pharma Innov.*, 6, 11, 22, 2017.
79. Keservani, R.K., Kesharwani, R.K., Vyas, N., Jain, S., Raghuvanshi, R., Sharma, A.K., Nutraceutical and functional food as future food: A review. *Der. Pharm. Lett.*, 2, 1, 106–116, 2010a.
80. Keservani, R.K., Kesharwani, R.K., Sharma, A.K., Vyas, N., Chadoker, A., Nutritional supplements: An overview. *Int. J. Curr. Pharm. Rev. Res.*, 1, 1, 59–75, 2010b.
81. Keservani, R.K., Sharma, A.K., Kesharwani, R.K., An overview and therapeutic applications of nutraceutical and functional foods, in: *Recent Advances in Drug Delivery Technology*, pp. 160–201, 2017.
82. Keservani, R.K., Sharma, A.K., Kesharwani, R.K. (Eds.), Nutraceuticals and Dietary Supplements: *Applications in Health Improvement and Disease Management*, Apple Academic Press, New York, 01, 01–54, 2020.

9
Role of Vitamins in Metabolic Diseases

Simona D'souza[1], Pavan Udavant[1], Jayesh Kadam[1], Shubham Khairnar[1], Eknath D. Ahire[2]* and Rahul Sable[1]

[1]Department of Pharmacology, MET's Institute of Pharmacy, Bhujbal Knowledge City, Adgaon, Nashik, Maharashtra, India
[2]Department of Pharmaceutics, MET's Institute of Pharmacy, Bhujbal Knowledge City, Adgaon, Nashik, Maharashtra, India

Abstract

Metabolic disease has become more common and is still the main cause of death around the world. The etiology of these disorders is based on interactions between genetic, environmental, and dietary variables, resulting in a complex phenotype. In this sense, the deficiency of vitamins seen in the general population are frequent due to a variety of circumstances. Vitamin deficiencies are diseases-causing micronutrients that are essential for cellular metabolism. In parallel to their nutritional functions, vitamins are increasingly being identified as key modulators of expression of genes and signal transduction when consumed in therapeutic doses. Vitamin supplementation has been examined to treat and prevent metabolic diseases in different types of randomized nonclinical and clinical trials. However, there is debate about its effectiveness in the treatment and prevention of certain diseases; for example, some studies demonstrate that vitamin C can help reduce the occurrence of cancer, while others show that it can also cause cancer owing to a response. In this chapter, we will look at how vitamins can help avoid metabolic diseases like diabetes, obesity, cardiovascular disease, stroke, renal disease, cancer, and others, as well as how they can cause metabolic disease in some situations.

Keywords: Vitamins, metabolic diseases, function, role

---

*Corresponding author: eknathahire05@gmail.com; eknatha_iop@bkc.met.edu

Eknath D. Ahire, Raj K. Keservani, Khemchand R. Surana, Sippy Singh and Rajesh K. Kesharwani (eds.) *Vitamins as Nutraceuticals: Recent Advances and Applications*, (205–234) © 2023 Scrivener Publishing LLC

Abbreviations

AGEs	Advanced Glycation End Products
AI	Adequate intake
AMD	Age-related Macular Degeneration
CKD	chronic kidney disease
CKD-MBD	chronic kidney disease–Mineral Bone Disorder
CoA	coenzyme A
CVD	cardiovascular disease
DBP	Diastolic Blood Pressure
DRIs	Dietary Reference Intakes
EAR	Estimated Average Requirement
EMD	Ectopic Mineralization Disorders
FAD	Flavin Adenine Dinucleotide
FAO	Food and Agriculture Organization
FGF-23	fibroblast growth factor-23
FMN	Flavin Mononucleotide
GAS6	Growth Arrest Specific Protein 6
GD	Graves' disease
GGCX	Gamma-Glutamyl Carboxylase
Gla	Gamma-Carboxyglutamic Acid
Glu	Glutamic Acid
GRP	Gla-Rich Protein
HCC	Hepatocellular Carcinoma
Hcy	Homocysteine
HOMA-IR	Homeostatic Model Assessment for Insulin Resistance
HT	Hashimoto's thyroiditis
IDDM	Insulin Dependent Diabetes Mellitus
LDL	Low-Density Lipoprotein
MGP	Matrix Gla Protein
NAFLD	Non-Alcoholic Fatty Liver Disease
NASEM	National Academies of Sciences, Engineering, and Medicine
NASH	Non-Alcoholic Steatohepatitis
NIDDM	Non-Insulin Dependent Diabetic Mellitus
PABA	Para-Aminobenzoic Acid
PLP	Pyridoxal 50-Phosphate
PMP	Pyridoxamine 50-Phosphate
PNP	Pyridoxine 50-Phosphate
PPAR	Peroxisome Proliferator Activated Receptor
PXE	Pseudoxanthoma Elasticum

RAE	Retinol Activity Equivalents
RA	Retinoic Acid
RBP4	Retinol Binding Protein
ROS	Reactive Oxygen Species
SBP	Systolic Blood Pressure
T2DM	Type 2 DM
TCTs	Tocotrienols
TOCs	Tocopherols
UL	Tolerable Upper Intake Level
VDR	Vitamin D Receptor
VKDP	Vitamin K-Dependent Proteins
WHO	World Health Organization

9.1 Introduction

Vitamins are a family of chemical compounds that the human body cannot produce but that are required for the normal functioning of the body's basic processes. Vitamins are required for metabolism, development, and normal physiological function. The body produces only vitamin D; all other vitamins must be received through food. Metabolic diseases are caused by enzyme deficits that are essential for the transformation of one chemical to another. There are two categories of metabolic disorders: inherited metabolic disorders and acquired metabolic illnesses. Evidence reveals that the human lifestyle is connected to an inherited epigenetic pattern that affects gene expression and protein function, resulting in metabolic diseases and disorders. Diseases that interfere with the conversion of food (here vitamins) into energy are defined to as metabolic diseases. Inherited metabolic illnesses affect not more than one in every three thousand infants, making them extremely rare.

9.1.1 Introduction to Vitamins

Vitamins, with the exception of vitamin D, are a category of chemical substances that are required for optimal cell function, physiological processes, growth, and development and must be received through the diet. Four fat-soluble vitamins (vitamin A, vitamin D, vitamin E, and vitamin K) and nine water-soluble vitamins (B1, B2, B3, B5, B6, B7, B9, B12, and C) are required by different species, and humans require four fat-soluble vitamins (vitamin A, vitamin D, vitamin E, and vitamin K) and nine water-soluble vitamins (vitamins B1, B2, B3, B5, B6, B7, B9, B12, and C) [1]. They are

Table 9.1 Vitamins and their food sources.

Vitamins	Food sources
Vitamin B1	Sunflower seeds, watermelon, tomato, spinach, soy milk, ham, pork chops.
Vitamin B2	Eggs, liver, fish, beef, spinach, broccoli, mushroom, and milk.
Vitamin B3	Grains, dairy products, almonds, chicken, spinach, potatoes, tomato, meat, fish.
Vitamin B5	Mushrooms, avocados, whole grains, chicken, tomato, and broccoli.
Vitamin B6	Beans, almonds, red meat, fish, eggs, spinach, lentils, potatoes, bananas, and watermelon.
Vitamin B8	Soybeans, whole grains, and fish yolks.
Vitamin B9	Tomatoes, broccoli, spinach, legumes, fortified cereals, asparagus, green beans, and orange juice black-eyed peas.
Vitamin B12	Meat, fish, milk, eggs, chicken, cheese, and fortified soy milk.
Vitamin C	Citrus fruits, strawberries, kiwis, broccoli, spinach, potatoes, tomatoes, snow peas, and bell peppers.
Vitamin A	Carrots, mangoes, squash, spinach, pumpkin, turnip greens, broccoli, beef, liver, eggs, shrimp, fish, fortified milk, cheese, carrots, mangoes, squash, spinach, pumpkin, turnip greens, broccoli.
Vitamin D	Fortified milk and margarine, fatty fish, egg yolk, liver.
Vitamin E	Polyunsaturated plant oils, avocados, margarine, whole grains, nuts, wheat, sunflower seeds, shrimp, tofu.
Vitamin K	Cabbage, spinach, broccoli, liver, eggs, milk.

ingested into the human body, but some of them (in small amounts) can be created endogenously. Hypovitaminosis, also called as vitamin deficiency, is caused by a shortage of vitamins in the body, whereas hypervitaminosis is caused by an overabundance of vitamins (applicable mainly to fat-soluble vitamins). Avitaminosis is now extremely rare, and it may be due to hypovitaminosis, which may be because of lack of vitamin(s) in the diet, poor absorption in the gastrointestinal tract, or an increase in the body's demand. Almost all vitamins are necessary for the human body's optimal growth and development. Furthermore, the recommended vitamin intake is dependent on a number of characteristics, including age, gender, and health. A diet rich in vitamin natural components can protect us from significant health problems. Table 9.1 shows the Vitamins and their food sources.

9.1.1.1 Fat-Soluble Vitamins

Vitamins that are fat-soluble are apolar compounds that are hydrophobic isoprene derivatives. They are not generated in significant quantities in the body; thus, they must be consumed as food. The appropriate absorption of lipids is necessary for the smooth absorption of these vitamins. The transport of these vitamins through the bloodstream is aided by certain lipoproteins or carrier proteins.

9.1.1.2 Water-Soluble Vitamins

B vitamins play a pivotal role in enzymatic reactions as cofactors. They are water-soluble, and any unnecessary is excreted in the form of urine. Thiamine (vitamin B1), riboflavin (vitamin B2), niacin (nicotinic acid, nicotinic acid amide, vitamin B3), pantothenic acid (vitamin B5), vitamin B6 (pyridoxine, pyridoxal, pyridoxamine), biotin (vitamin B7), folic acid (pteroylglutamic acid, vitamin B9), and cobalamin (vitamin B12). B vitamins are required for the digestion of carbohydrates and lipids for energy production, therefore higher levels of B complex vitamins are required in conjunction with greater physical activity. And, therefore, their importance in athletes is heightened, and it is critical to their performances (Table 9.2) [2].

Table 9.2 Water-soluble and fat-soluble vitamins.

Water-soluble vitamins	Fat-soluble vitamins
• Vitamin B Complex Groups 1) Vitamin B1 (Thiamine) 2) Vitamin B2 (Riboflavin) 3) Vitamin B3 (Nicotinamide) 4) Vitamin B5 (Pantothenic Acid) 5) Vitamin B6 (Pyridoxine) 6) Vitamin B8 (Biotin) 7) Vitamin B9 (Folic Acid or Folate) 8) Vitamin B12 (Cobalamins) • Vitamin C (Ascorbic Acid or Ascorbate)	• Vitamin A (Retinoid) • Vitamin D (Cholecalciferol or Ergocalciferol) • Vitamin E (Tocopherols) • Vitamin K (Phylloquinone or Menaquinones)

9.2 Metabolic Diseases

All disorders that interfere with the conversion of food into energy are termed to as metabolic diseases. Inherited metabolic illnesses are known as inborn errors of metabolism; however, they can also be acquired over time. Inherited metabolic illnesses affect not more than one in every three thousand infants, making them extremely rare. Gaucher's disease, for example, affects 1/60,000 of the world's population and is caused by a deficiency of an enzyme called glucocerebrosidase, which is engaged in the metabolism of a fatty substance known as cerebroside [3].

Metabolic illnesses are a huge health burden for people all over the world. Although a substantial number of Mendelian metabolic illnesses have been identified, the majority of metabolic illness burden is accounted for by complex disorders like diabetes mellitus, which have both heritable genetic and environmental components [4].

Metabolic diseases are caused by enzyme deficits that are required for the conversion of one metabolite to another. The anomalies or symptoms of metabolic illnesses are caused by the accumulation of high amounts of any one or more metabolites, or by a metabolite deficit. Inherited metabolic disorders and acquired metabolic disorders. Inherited metabolic disorders are caused by inborn metabolic mistakes caused by genetic flaws, which result in limitations in enzyme production or abnormalities in enzyme activity. Inherited metabolic disorders, such as Tay-Sachs disease, Hurler syndrome, Gaucher's disease, and Fabry disease, are caused by anomalous metabolic physiology of humans. Other inherited metabolic disorders include peroxisomal disorders (Zellweger syndrome and adrenoleukodystrophy), and Lysosomal Storage Disorders (Tay-Sachs disease, Hurler syndrome, Gaucher's disease, and Fabry disease). Acquired metabolic disorders are associated with like unhealthy lifestyle along with little physical activity and excessive caloric intake. Evidence suggests that the human lifestyle is linked to an inherited epigenetic pattern that influences gene expression and protein function, resulting in the emergence of metabolic diseases and disorders. The most common metabolic disease linked to the global obesity and diabetes epidemic is metabolic syndrome [5].

9.2.1 Role of Fat-Soluble Vitamins in Metabolic Diseases

9.2.1.1 Vitamin A

Vitamin A refers to a class of fat-soluble retinoids that includes retinol (retinol is the parent compound of all bioactive retinoids but it is retinoic acid (RA) that is the active metabolite of vitamin A) and retinyl esters. Vitamin A is an essential micronutrient, along with other vitamins, minerals, and other substances. This means that our bodies are unable to produce it and that it must be consumed through our diet.

Preformed vitamin A, which is also called as retinol (the "active" form of vitamin A), is present in animal-based foods such as dairy, fish, eggs, and organ meats. Provitamin A or vitamin A (or vitamin A carotenoids) is found in plant sources in the form of carotenoids, which must be converted to retinol (the "active" form of vitamin A) in the intestine. Also, the carotenoids are the pigments that give plants their green color and some fruits and vegetables their red or orange color. Actual provitamin A carotenoid constituent in the diet is beta-carotene, alpha-carotene, and beta-cryptoxanthin. Other carotenoids in foods, such as lutein, lycopene and zeaxanthin, are not converted to vitamin A by the body and are termed to as non-provitamin A carotenoids.

Vitamin A is essential for cellular communication, immunological function, growth, and development, as well as male and female reproduction. Because it promotes cell growth and differentiation, vitamin A is essential for the proper development and maintenance of the eyes, heart, lungs, and many other organs. Vitamin A is particularly important for vision because it is one among the most important components of rhodopsin, which is a light-sensitive protein present in the retina that responds to light which enters the eye, and it helps the conjunctival membranes and cornea differentiate and operate normally. Also, vitamin A is required for a variety of physiological activities, including the integrity and function of all surface tissues (epithelia), such as the skin, respiratory tract lining, gut, bladder, inner ear, and eye (https://ods.od.nih.gov/factsheets/VitaminA-HealthProfessional/) [6, 7].

Recommended Intake (Table 9.3)
The DRIs produced by the NASEM give vitamin A and other nutrient intake guidelines. DRIs are a collection of reference standards, which are needed to plan and track the dietary intakes of healthy persons (https://ods.od.nih.gov/factsheets/VitaminA-HealthProfessional/).

Table 9.3 Recommended dietary allowances (RDAs) for vitamin A.

Age	Male	Female
Birth to 6 Months	400 mcg RAE	400 mcg RAE
7–12 months	500 mcg RAE	500 mcg RAE
1–3 years	300 mcg RAE	300 mcg RAE
4–8 years	400 mcg RAE	400 mcg RAE
9–13 years	600 mcg RAE	600 mcg RAE
14–18 years	900 mcg RAE	700 mcg RAE
19–50 years	900 mcg RAE	700 mcg RAE
51+ years	900 mcg RAE	700 mcg RAE

Table adapted from ((https://ods.od.nih.gov/factsheets/VitaminA-HealthProfessional/)).

1) The Recommended Dietary Allowance: It is the amount of food that the WHO recommends to fulfil the needs of nearly all healthy people (97–98%).
2) Adequate intake: When there is insufficient data to define an RDA, intake at this amount is presumed to ensure nutritional adequacy.
3) Estimated Average Requirement: A daily consumption level calculated to meet the needs of half of all healthy people. Typically used to measure nutrient consumption of groups of people and to develop nutritionally suitable diets for them.
4) Tolerable Upper Intake Level: The maximum daily intake is unlikely to be harmful to one's health.

To account for the varied bioactivities of retinol and provitamin a carotenoids, which are all metabolized by the body into retinol, RDAs for vitamin A are reported as RAE.

    1 mcg RAE is equivalent to;
    1 mcg retinol,
    2 mcg supplemental beta-carotene,
    12 mcg dietary beta-carotene, or
    24 mcg dietary alpha-carotene or beta-cryptoxanthin

Role of Vitamin A in Metabolic Diseases
It should be mentioned that many investigators and readers believe that the activity of vitamin A–related proteins reported to be used in metabolic disorder, such as RBP4 and ALDH1A1, involve impacts on the levels and signalling of vitamin A. Changes in RBP4 levels, for example, that impact vitamin delivery to tissues, are frequently considered to affect vitamin A effects in these tissues. However, the majority of research linking RBP4 levels to metabolic disorder do not include retinol, retinyl esters, or retinoic acid levels [8].

Following section focuses on diseases and disorders in which vitamin A or carotenoids might play a role:

1) Age-Related Macular Degeneration
The major cause of substantial vision loss in elderly persons is degeneration AMD. The etiology of AMD is more complicated, involving intricate interplay between genetic vulnerability, environmental variables (including oxidative stress), and normal ageing. Because oxidative stress involved in AMD pathogenesis, supplements containing antioxidant-rich carotenoids like beta-carotene, lutein, and zeaxanthin may be beneficial in preventing or treating the disease. Lutein and zeaxanthin (which are not precursors to vitamin A) accumulate in the retina, which is the damaged tissue in the eye caused by AMD (https://ods.od.nih.gov/factsheets/VitaminA-HealthProfessional/).

2) Measles
Measles killed more than 207,500 people worldwide in 2019, largely minors under the age of 5 in low-income nations. Deficiency of vitamin A is a major risk factor for severe measles. To avoid morbidity and death, including from measles, the WHO recommends large oral doses of vitamin A for children living in countries where deficiency of vitamin A is common (https://ods.od.nih.gov/factsheets/VitaminA-HealthProfessional/).

3) Type 2 Diabetes
Several studies have linked type 2 diabetes to higher levels of circulating vitamin A or serum RBP4 (a protein required for retinol transport in the blood). Early reports of elevated serum RBP4 and/or urine RBP4 levels in type 2 diabetes patients failed to find a reason or a downstream effect. B.B. Kahn's laboratory was the first to describe a role for high RBP4 serum levels in 2005. RBP4 expression was seen to be higher in the fatty tissue of mice with impaired insulin action in the muscle and liver *in vivo*.

In numerous genetic and diet-induced models of obesity and type 2 diabetes, increased levels of this adipokine (a term used to describe hormones or paracrine substances produced by adipose tissue) were linked to insulin resistance [9, 10].

4) Vitamin A, Vitamin A–Related Proteins and Liver Disease
Vitamin A signaling and metabolism defects have been linked to NAFLD and NASH, as well as later stage liver disease like Fibrosis, Cirrhosis, and HCC in the literature. However, the fundamental mechanisms responsible for this are still unknown. NAFLD is a catch-all name for a number of disorders defined by an excessive buildup of fat within hepatocytes, and it is a major cause of late-stage liver damage. NAFLD is found in nearly 90% of morbidly obese adults, and the illness can range from mild hepatic steatosis to the more severe NASH. If not treated, these early stages of the illness might proceed to fibrosis & cirrhosis [11].

5) Obesity
Obese rats receiving vitamin A supplementation (129 mg vitamin A/kg diet for 2 months) demonstrated a reduction in their adiposity index and retroperitoneal adipose tissue weight, but lean rats showed only a minor reduction. However, in lean rats, this treatment leads to an increase in the retroperitoneal adipose tissue apoptotic index, with anti-apoptotic protein under expression and pro-apoptotic protein overexpression (proteins Bcl2 and Bax, respectively). Vitamin A supplementation affects adipose tissue mass in lean and obese rats via distinct pathways, according to the authors.

Differences in dietary fruit, vegetable, and energy intakes among both obese and non-obese participants could be one explanation underlying the inverse relationships found between blood carotenoids and adiposity. Obese people may consume in excess amount of energy meals, yet they may not be getting all of their micronutrients. Furthermore, a person with a higher fat mass would absorb a larger proportion of ingested carotene via fat tissue than a lean person, resulting in lower serum carotenoid concentrations as compared to lean people [12, 13].

9.2.1.2 Vitamin D

Vitamin D is a fat-soluble prohormone that is involved in calcium and phosphorus metabolism and skeletal homeostasis also plays a crucial role in bone mineral metabolism. The most prevalent type of vitamin D is cholecalciferol, also called as vitamin D3, which is made from

7-dehydrocholesterol, a precursor to cholesterol, and is created by sunlight on the skin. It can also be obtained from animal (cholecalciferol-D3) and vegetable (ergocalciferol-D2) sources in the diet. Being biologically active, two hydroxylations are required for vitamin D in the body, the first in the liver while the second in the kidney, results in the form known as 1,25(OH)2 vitamin D or calcitriol [14].

Vitamin D possesses pleiotropic effects in numerous cell types in many life forms, additionally play a role in calcium and bone metabolism. These include a possible role in insulin action and the development of obesity. As a result, hypovitaminosis D has been associated to hypertension, atherogenic dyslipidemia, and an elevated risk of cardiovascular disease. Nonalcoholic fatty liver disease has also been linked to metabolic syndrome, regardless of the traits that define the syndrome. Most tissues and cells in the body include the vitamin D receptor (VDR). Vitamin D is primarily responsible for bone metabolism and homeostasis of calcium and phosphorus. Recent data suggests that vitamin D insufficiency, which is ubiquitous worldwide, may play a role in autoimmune illnesses, malignancies, metabolic syndromes, cardiovascular disease, infection, and all-cause mortality, in addition to skeletal effects. Low vitamin D levels have also been associated to an autoimmune thyroid disorder as Hashimoto's thyroiditis and Graves' disease. Both lifestyle changes and supplements can help with hypovitaminosis D [15, 16].

Role of Vitamin D in Metabolic Diseases

1) Type 2 Diabetes
Type 2 diabetes is caused by impaired beta-cell activity, increased resistance to insulin, and systemic inflammation, and there is indication that vitamin D modulates these pathways.

Insulin secretion
Vitamin D appears to play a role in insulin secretion regulation, beta-cell survival, and calcium flux within beta-cells, according to preclinical investigations. According to a series of studies, vitamin D deficiency decreases glucose-mediated insulin production in rat pancreatic beta cells, while vitamin D supplementation appears to recover such glucose-stimulated insulin secretion. The 25(OH) D-1-hydroxylase enzyme (CYP27B1) activates vitamin D within the pancreatic beta cell, allowing for a significant paracrine effect of circulating 25-hydroxyvitamin D. The modulation of extracellular calcium concentration and passage through the beta cell is another function of vitamin D in the pancreatic beta cell. The secretion of

insulin is a calcium-dependent mechanism, changes in the flux of calcium could influence insulin secretion [17].

Insulin sensitivity

Vitamin D can influence insulin sensitivity in many ways. Insulin receptor expression appears to be stimulated by 1,25 (OH)2D, which affects insulin sensitivity. By activating PPAR-delta, a transcription factor that affects the metabolism of fatty acid in skeletal muscle and adipose tissue, 1,25 (OH)2D may enhance insulin sensitivity. Vitamin D also shows increase in oxidative phosphorylation in muscles following exercise. Insulin sensitivity may also be influenced by 1,25 (OH)2D's function to regulate the concentration of extracellular calcium and flow across cell membranes [18].

Inflammation

The relationship between t2DM and systemic inflammation is now extensively acknowledged. Although increased cytokines have been associated with insulin resistance, they may also play a beta-cell dysfunction by active beta-cell apoptosis. Vitamin D may enhance the sensitivity of insulin and boost beta-cell survival by directly altering the synthesis and cytokine effects [19].

2) Hepatic Steatosis

Long-term sufferers of metabolic syndrome are thought to be at a higher risk of developing hepatic steatosis. A hypothesis of two or three hits has been offered. The harm produced by fatty infiltration linked with insulin resistance and obesity is considered the initial hit. Hepatic injury resulting from mechanisms connected to oxidative stress and delayed cellular regeneration is assumed to be the cause of the second and third hits. We would expect a link involving hypovitaminosis D and nonalcoholic fatty liver disease because it is linked to metabolic syndrome. Vitamin D levels were shown to be lower among people with non-alcoholic fatty liver disease identified by liver biopsy, according to research. Changes in the control of inflammatory and anti-oxidant pathways have been associated to hypovitaminosis D, and also impacting the metabolic syndrome phenotype; all of these findings have been connected to the etiology of steatosis. There is currently no compelling proof about vitamin D administration improving hepatic steatosis clinically. Treatment with ursodeoxycholic acid, which raises vitamin D levels, has demonstrated some improvement in nonalcoholic steatohepatitis when alanine transaminase levels were utilised as the result [20].

3) Cancer

Dialysis patients appear to have a greater cancer risk. In recent animal and preclinical investigations, activated vitamin D has shown to suppress proliferation, limit invasiveness and angiogenesis, induce apoptosis, and impede differentiation. Chemotherapy and radiation have been found to have a synergistic impact. However, to produce antineoplastic effects, exceptionally large dosages of calcitriol are necessary, resulting in hypercalcemia and hyperphosphatemia. The molecular mechanism appears to be influenced by the interaction between calcitriol and the retinoid X receptor heterodimer, which influences genes downstream. Although studies on cancer prevention and reduction in the dialysis population are scarce, it is possible that this medicine and the newer vitamin D receptor activators may have favorable effects on cancer prevention and progression [21].

4) Chronic Kidney Disease

The klotho gene and FGF-23 have recently been identified as important regulators of vitamin D. Klotho is mostly expressed in the kidney's distal tubule. It can function as a hormone or as a circulating form. It aids in the activation of the FGF-23 receptor by performing the role of a cofactor. A klotho gene mutation causes a condition that resembles CKD but with alterations that are generally linked with accelerated ageing. Hypercalcemia, hyperphosphatemia, and increased calcitriol are other symptoms of the syndrome. FGF-23 regulates renal sodium-dependent phosphate co-transporters, which modulates renal phosphate excretion (NaPi2a and NaPi2c). Klotho binds to FGF-23 receptors and acts as a cofactor, allowing diverse cells to respond to FGF-23. FGF-23 is a vitamin D counter-regulatory hormone. FGF-23 levels rise after vitamin D delivery, lowering calcitriol synthesis in the kidney by inhibiting the 1-hydroxylase gene [22].

9.2.1.3 *Vitamin E*

Evans and Bishop discovered and defined vitamin E in 1922; it comes in eight natural forms (α, β, γ, δ, tocopherols and tocotrienols) and can be present in a number of items containing fats of both vegetable and animal origin, such as olive or almond oil, hazelnuts, and egg yolk, as well as in the liver [23]. Vitamin E can be found in many foods and plants, ranging from edible oils to nuts, and is made up of TOCs and TCTs. Wheat, rice bran, oat, palm, barley, coconut, and annatto are examples of vitamin E-rich foods. Rye, poppy, maize, amaranth, walnut, hazelnut, sunflower, and grape and pumpkin seeds are among the other sources. Human milk and palm dates have also been found to contain vitamin E derivatives (Phoenix canariensis). Rice bran, palm oil, and annatto oil have been regarded as the highest sources of TCTs among the several vitamin E sources [24].

Vitamin E is a powerful anti-inflammatory chemical because it affects a variety of components that affect the immune system, either directly or indirectly. Platelet aggregation suppression is also aided by vitamin E by blocking enzymes like PKC, which is a crucial signal transduction pathway in a number of cell types. Because of its free-radical scavenging and anti-inflammatory capabilities, α-tocopherol has a dermatological benefit: it protects the skin from UV radiation and speeds wound healing after injuries such as ulcers or burns. It also has a long list of advantages, ranging from anti-cancer properties to illness prevention and improved quality of life in the elderly [25].

Role of Vitamin E in Metabolic Diseases

1) Cardiovascular disease
Numerous research has looked at the health advantages of vitamin E, and many of them have found that supplementing with vitamin E lowers the relative risk of CVD. The LDL oxidation theory has fueled research into vitamin E and other antioxidants as potential CVD preventatives. Morel *et al.*, presented the LDL oxidation hypothesis, which is now widely regarded as a plausible explanation for the development of atherosclerosis, an age-related process that is a major source of morbidity and mortality from CVD in Western countries.

Particles of LDL oxidation in the wall of the artery is thought to start a complicated chain of events that leads to the formation of fatty streaks and atherosclerotic plaques, constriction of the arteries, plaque rupture, and heart attack. Polyunsaturated fatty acids in LDL particles are prone to oxidation. The principal fat-soluble antioxidant found in LDL particles is vitamin E, specifically a-tocopherol. Each LDL particle carries between five and nine vitamin E molecules, which protect the LDL from the damage of oxidation. Increased vitamin E content in LDL particles, as a result of increased vitamin E intake through supplements, boosts LDL resistance to oxidation and lowers macrophage absorption, according to *in vitro* studies. As a result, it's thought that vitamin E's *in vitro* protection of LDL from oxidation could be a viable mechanism for vitamin E's *in vivo* action in lowering CVD risk, as observed in various observational studies [26].

9.2.1.4 Vitamin K

Vitamin K, commonly known as naphthoquinone, is a group of fat-soluble molecules with a ring structure of 2-methyl-1,4-naphthoquinone but differ in origin and function. Vitamin K1 (phylloquinone), vitamin K2 (menaquinone), and vitamin K3 (menadione) are the three major forms now known, which differ in the side chains connected to the 2-methyl-1,4-naphthoquinone ring at position 3 [27, 28].

Functions of Vitamin K

1) As a cofactor for the catalyses the conversion of Glu residues to gamma-carboxyglutamic acid (Gla) in VKDPs via vitamin K-dependent gamma-glutamyl carboxylase, which is located in the endoplasmic reticulum of cells in all mammalian organs. Convert the protein-bound glutamate into carboxy-glutamate.
2) Needed for II, VII, IX, and X coagulation cascade factors.
3) Important for the natural anticoagulants proteins S and C.
4) Has a significant impact on osteogenesis, vascular protection, metabolic, hepatic, and renal diseases.

Vitamin K1 is mostly found in flowering or leafy vegetables (spinach, cabbage, broccoli lettuce, Brussels sprouts), although it can also be found in chickpeas, soya, peas, beef liver, green tea, eggs and pork [29, 30].

Recommendation

> The WHO and the FAO recommend the Vitamin K as;
> 65 micrograms per day for males, and
> 55 micrograms per day for women,
> Based on a 1 microgram per kilogram of body weight need computed. The SINU recommends a vitamin K consumption of
> 140 mcg/day for those aged 18–59, and
> 170 mcg/day for people aged >60 [31]

Role of Vitamin K in Metabolic Diseases

1) Chronic Kidney Disease
Patients with CKD have low vitamin K levels. Vitamin K reserves in CKD patients can be affected by a variety of reasons, the most common

of which are food restriction, uraemia-associated dysbiosis, and medications. Furthermore, deficiency is exacerbated by dietary restrictions caused by the high potassium content of most vitamin K-rich green vegetables. The "Vitamin K cycle," which contains vitamin K epoxide reductase, DT-diaphorase, and g-glutamyl carboxylase, recycles vitamin K in addition to dietary intake. Vitamin K recycling was discovered to be reduced in rats with CKD, which was likely caused by lower activity of g-glutamylcarboxylase, which works in a similar way to coumarins.

Patients with CKD are more prone to develop vascular calcification (VC) and bone fractures, contributing to their greater morbidity and death rates [32].

2) Chronic Kidney Disease–Mineral Bone Disorder

CKD-MBD describes the loss of bone quality as a result of compromised kidney function, and also the resulting development of bone and mineral metabolism problems. As a result, CKD patients, especially those on haemodialysis, are at a higher risk of fracture than the general population.

Bone remodelling is a continuous dynamic process primarily involving two antagonistically acting cells: osteoblasts, which control bone creation, and osteoclasts, which control bone resorption. Vitamin K is directly implicated in bone metabolism, according to several publications (both *in vivo* and *in vitro*). Some of them showed that vitamin K2 reduces bone resorption, which is likely related to a decrease in the production of bone resorbing chemicals such prostaglandin E2 and interleukin 6. *In vitro* studies have shown that vitamin K increases human osteoblast-induced bone mineralization, as well as to prevent bone loss in steroid-treated or ovariectomized rats. Vitamin K2 is also a cofactor for osteocalcin, a protein involved in bone mineralization (bone Gla protein or BGP) and MGP. BGP is a tiny protein with 49 amino acids that is synthesized in bone by osteoblasts and secreted into the circulation in minute amounts.

MGP is a 10.6-kDa protein of 84 amino acids that is water insoluble. The majority of it is produced by smooth muscle cells and chondrocytes, which is then secreted into the extracellular matrix. It prevents calcification and only becomes active after carboxylation and phosphorylation. Vitamin K plays a role as a cofactor, allowing -glutamyl carboxylase to carboxylate 5 glutamic acid residues at positions 2, 37, 41, 48, and 52; in addition, casein kinase phosphorylates 3 serine residues at locations 3, 6, and 9. The method for suppressing vascular calcification would be the attachment of calcium ions to carboxyl groups.

GRP is a 74-amino-acid protein having molecular weight as 10.2 kDa. GRP, like many other matrix proteins, requires vitamin K to function and prevents vascular calcification by binding and sequestering calcium ions, similar to the matrix Gla protein.

GAS6 is a protein of 75 kDa that is triggered by a carboxylation mechanism involving vitamin K. GAS6 is largely involved in cell formation and proliferation regulation, and osteoblasts deposit it into the bone matrix. GAS6, not like the other VKDPs, has been demonstrated to promote bone resorption by increasing osteoclast activity [33].

3) Ectopic Mineralization Disorders
Two separate discoveries suggest that vitamin K and associated substances may have a role in the etiology of ectopic mineralization disorders:

> I) GGCX mutations cause a calcification which is a rare phenotype similar to PXE, but with deficiencies in vitamin K dependent clotting factors; and
> II) Patients with PXE have substantially lower vitamin K serum levels than the normal population.

Keutel syndrome is characterized by aberrant cartilage calcification, peripheral pulmonary stenosis, and midfacial hypoplasia in individuals due to homozygous mutations in the MGP gene. Surprisingly, in babies suffering from warfarin-induced embryopathy, produced by maternal usage of the coumarin derivative warfarin between weeks 6 and 9, a clinically indistinguishable condition might be found. The fundamental etiology of this illness has thus been postulated to be dysfunctional-glutamyl carboxylation of MGP caused by warfarin-mediated suppression of the vitamin K cycle [34].

4) Obesity
Vitamin K which a fat-soluble vitamin, Obesity causes some fat-soluble nutrients to be stored in the body. As a result, high levels of vitamin K are found in adipose tissue, and a rise in obesity was connected to lower levels of vitamin K in older persons. Vitamin K is essential for bone metabolism, as previously stated. Obesity has been linked to the progress of osteoporosis. Kim and colleagues explored the role of vitamin K1 and K2 supplementation on bone turnover and morphology of structure in an obese mouse model, they discovered that vitamin K supplementation reversed the bone deterioration caused by obesity (induced by a high-fat diet) by modulating the activities of both osteoblasts and osteoclasts.

Although the levels of osteocalcin were identical in both groups, in obese patients, Razni *et al.* discovered a significantly lower amount of carboxylated osteocalcin (Gla-OC) than in nonobese controls. They discovered no correlations with leptin and osteocalcin in obese participants, nor between leptin, adiponectin, and resistin [35].

5) Diabetes

Insulin binds to osteoblasts, causing osteocalcin to be secreted, which increases pancreatic beta-cell proliferation. The undercarboxylated variant of osteocalcin has indeed been revealed to be an active hormone that regulates glucose metabolism in conjunction to being a biomarker for vitamin K. Diabetes has also been connected to it. When Hussein *et al.* used the vitamin K2 analog menaquinone-4 (MK-4, menaterenone) on diabetic rats, they noticed a dose-dependent reduction in glucose test (FPG), HbA1c, and HOMA-IR when compared to the untreated diabetic rat group. In the three treated groups, there was a dose-dependent increase in fasting insulin and homeostatic model assessment for -cell function (HOMA-B) levels. Their findings revealed that when vitamin K2 was given, osteocalcin expression was induced in a dose-dependent manner. In type 2 diabetic rats, vitamin K2 supplementation resulted in an increase in total osteocalcin levels, this has been linked to decrease in insulin resistance and an increase in insulin sensitivity [36].

9.2.2 Role of Water-Soluble Vitamins in Metabolic Diseases

9.2.2.1 Vitamin B3

Vitamin B3 or niacin, has a role in energy production, normal enzyme function, digestion, fostering a healthy appetite, and maintaining healthy skin and nerves. Liver, fish, poultry, meat, peanuts, whole, and grain products are also good sources. Adult males need 16 milligrams of niacin per day, whereas adult females need 14 milligrams. It has, however, been associated to drunkenness, protein malnutrition, low-calorie diets, and high-refined-carbohydrate diets. Pellagra is a condition that develops due to significant lack of niacin. Cramps, nausea, skin problems and mental confusion are some of the symptoms [37].

Role of Vitamin B3 in Metabolic Disease

1) Diabetes Mellitus

Many anti-diabetic statin medicines are available on the market, but their long-term usage causes a slew of health issues. The goal of our current research is to improve the system's antioxidant potential in order to counteract the disease's consequences. Because of its low toxicity and significant antioxidant properties, niacin is a good choice for this purpose. Apart from its antioxidant properties, niacin is frequently used to treat irregularities in plasma lipid and lipoprotein metabolism, and has been utilized as a cholesterol-lowering medication for many years. Niacin has been used to treat dyslipidaemia for more than half a century [38].

9.2.2.2 Vitamin B5

Pantothenic acid contributes in the creation of hormones and the metabolism of lipids, proteins, and carbs obtained from meals. Liver, kidney, meats, egg yolk, whole grains, and legumes are all good sources. Intestinal bacteria also produce pantothenic acid. Pantothenic Acid's AI for both adult males and females is 5 mg per day [39].

Role of Vitamin B5 in Metabolic Disease

1) Huntington's Disease
An enlarged CAG repeats in exon 1 of the HTT gene causes HD, a neurological condition. The loss of GABAergic projection neurons from the striatum, after that by progressive atrophy of the putamen and other brain regions, is prevalent in mid-life, although the genetics and neurodegeneration remain unknown. A case-control study was conducted, researchers discovered widespread vitamin B5 deficiency, a necessary component of CoA for proper intermediate metabolism.

Deficiency of cerebral pantothenate is a recently found metabolic defect in people with HD that can lead to:

(i) Impairs the biosynthesis of neuronal CoA;
(ii) Stimulate the activity of polyol-pathway;
(iii) Impair TCA & Glycolysis; and
(iv) Metabolise Brain-urea.

Pantothenate insufficiency in HD could lead to neurodegeneration/dementia, which could be prevented by vitamin B5 medication.

Vitamin B5 (pantothenic acid), a major important precursor in the biosynthesis route for CoA, was found to be the most abundant metabolite in HD human brains when compared to controls. Vitamin B5 is a trace nutrient found in high amounts in the brain, up to 50 times higher than in plasma [40].

9.2.2.3 Vitamin B6

Vitamin B6 is made up of six different types of vitamers, including pyridoxine (PN), pyridoxal (PL), pyridoxamine (PM), and their 50-phosphate derivatives (PNP, PLP, and PMP). The biologically active form, pyridoxal 50-phosphate (PLP), catalyzes about 150 different enzymatic activities that catalyze important metabolic reactions like amine and amino acid synthesis, transformation, and degradation, supply of one-carbon units, trans-sulfuration, Tetrapyrrolic substances (including heme) and polyamines are synthesized, and neurotransmitter biosynthesis and degradation. Vitamin B6 recommended dietary allowance is 1.3 mg day-1 for adults; since it is found in a variety of foods such as meat, fish, poultry, vegetables, and fruits, a serious lack of this vitamin in any diet is unusual in industrialized countries [41].

Role of Vitamin B6 in Metabolic Disease

1) Diabetes Mellitus
Vitamin B6 is associated to diabetes and its consequences, according to a lot of data. PLP (Pyridoxal 50-Phosphate) levels in diabetic control vs. healthy subjects have been compared in certain population screens; in addition, several researches looked at the impact of vitamin B6 on diabetes complications, while others looked at whether it may be used as a preventative drug. Vitamin B6 levels are frequently tested by measuring plasma pyridoxal 50-phosphate (PLP) concentration, and a concentration below the cut-off level of 30 nmol/L is generally linked with an inadequate vitamin B6 status. Other ways include measuring plasma pyridoxal or total vitamin B6 and urinary 4-pyridoxic acid, and the proportion between PLP and PL [42].

Relationships between vitamin B6 and diabetes:

  a. Leklem and Hollenbeck presented the first evidence that diabetes can lower PLP levels by showing that healthy persons with diabetes had lower PLP levels after consuming glucose.
  b. The study of Toyota *et al.* [43], who showed that pyridoxine shortage can affect insulin release in rats, revealed a cause-effect relationship between low levels of PLP and diabetes. Furthermore, the authors discovered that pyridoxine depletion impairs the secretion of insulin and glucagon using *in vitro* pancreas perfusion tests [44].

2) Cancer

Diabetic patients (induced previously by vitamin B6) are more prone to develop a variety of tumors, including liver, pancreas, colorectal, and lung cancers, but the underlying mechanisms are unknown. Hyperinsulinemia and hyperglycemia were expected to perform a role in mediating this link, primarily through encouraging cell proliferation. Hyperglycemia, on the contrary, is hypothesized to have an impact on cancer by causing DNA damage through the development of AGEs and ROS [45].

9.2.2.4   Vitamin B2

Vitamin B2, often referred to as riboflavin, is the least water-soluble of the B vitamins. It is the precursor of two coenzymes known as FMN and FAD, which are directly implicated in tissue breathing, tryptophan to niacin (vitamin B3) conversion, pyridoxine activation, fat, carbohydrate, and protein metabolism, and glutathione. Grain items, cereals, bread, protein sources, chicken, eggs, fish, nuts, some fruits, legumes, dairy products, and cheese are rich in riboflavin. Riboflavin is somewhat abundant in leafy vegetables, mushrooms, and turnips [46].

9.2.2.5   Vitamin B9

Vitamin B9, also called as folic acid, is a water-soluble vitamin that is made up of a PABA of its amino ends and a carboxyl group connected to the a-amino group of glutamic acid to form an amide bond. The form of folic acid that the human body converts to folate is called folate. Folate is involved in DNA synthesis, DNA and RNA alterations, the metabolism of amino acids needed for cell division, and a sequence of biological events defined as folate-mediated one-carbon metabolism, including amino acid and nucleic acid synthesis [47].

9.2.2.6   Vitamin B12

Vitamin B12, also known as cobalamin, is a tetrapyrrolic cofactor in which four equatorial nitrogen ligands given by the corrin ring's pyrroles A-D coordinate the central cobalt atom. Whipple, Minot, and Murphy characterized it as an anti-pernicious anaemia factor in 1925. Cobalamin is involved in fatty acid and amino acid metabolism in numerous cells. Vitamin B12 is needed for the correct working of the nervous system, and the maturation of new red blood cells present in the bone marrow and DNA synthesis. It's also involved in the production of myelin, a lipid-rich coating that protects nerve cells' axons. Vitamin B12 deficiency causes demyelination, a condition in which the myelin sheath is destroyed, disrupting nerve conduction transmission and causing a variety of neurological issues [48].

Role of Vitamin B9 and B12 in Metabolic Disease

1) Stroke

B2, B6, B9, and B12 vitamins are linked to Hcy through their involvement in Met metabolism, regeneration, and homocysteine breakdown. Hcy an amino acid that has sulfur but is not found in proteins. It is produced in a multistep process in the Hcy-methionine cycle as part of the intermediate metabolism [49]. Vitamin B9, vitamin B12, and, to a lesser extent, vitamin B6 and vitamin B2 are all involved in Hcy metabolism and turnover. A number of epidemiological studies have looked into the link between high Hcy levels and a reduced risk of stroke while taking B vitamins. There are numerous publications linking vitamin B9, vitamin B12, and vitamin B6 levels to stroke, albeit not all of them are totally consistent. A single study indicated that stroke patients had lower vitamin B2 levels than controls, contradicting prior findings.

Platelet abnormalities and cigarette smoking are two major factors that influence folate's ability to prevent stroke. After adjusting for confounders, a recent study indicated that Hcy levels have a strong association with antiplatelet medication in recurrent stroke in female subjects (p 1/4 0.010) rather than male subjects (p 1/4 0.595). According to this evidence a thorough investigation of the role of B vitamin supplementation and the Hcy marker in stroke should take into account the age and gender distribution [50].

2) Cancer

When considering the mechanisms of cancer in the context of vitamin function, i.e., Vitamins appear to have a substantial impact in the early stages of carcinogenesis due to their regulation of and involvement in metabolic pathways in the cell., due to their antioxidant properties, i.e., by removing carcinogenic reactive oxygen species, and their participation in one-carbon metabolism, and thus in DNA methylation- basic epigenetic. The importance of antioxidant supplementation is extensively discussed in scientific literature. The main focus of papers dealing with the association between vitamins and malignancies is dealing with the qualitative composition of mineral mixes and vitamin, which involves the flagship antioxidants such as tocopherol, ascorbic acid, retinol, and –carotene [51].

9.2.2.7 Vitamin C

One among the most important water-soluble vitamins is ascorbic acid. It is needed for the manufacture of collagen, carnitine, and neurotransmitters. For their own needs, most animals and plants generate ascorbic acid. However, due to a deficiency of the enzyme gulonolactone oxidase, apes and humans are unable to produce ascorbic acid. As a result, ascorbic acid must be obtained mostly from fruits, vegetables, and tablets. For adults, the current RDA for ascorbic acid in the United States is 100 to 120 mg per day. Ascorbic acid has many health benefits, including antioxidant, anti-atherogenic, anti-carcinogenic, immunomodulator, and cold prevention [52].

One among the most important water-soluble vitamins is ascorbic acid. Collagen, carnitine, and neurotransmitters are all made possible by it. For their own needs, most animals and plants synthesize ascorbic acid. Apes and humans, on the contrary, are unable to produce ascorbic acid due to a lack of the enzyme gulonolactone oxidase. Consequently, the majority of ascorbic acid comes from fruits, vegetables, and tablets. In the United States, the current RDI for ascorbic acid is 100 to 120 mg per day for adults. Antioxidant, anti-atherogenic, anti-carcinogenic, immunomodulator, and cold prevention are just a few of the health benefits of ascorbic acid [53].

Role of Vitamin C in Metabolic Diseases

1) Blood Pressure

Because of its ability to donate an electron, vitamin C is a reducing agent or antioxidant, and this activity may probably be attributed to all of its metabolic functions. Antioxidants destroy free radicals and protect cells from injury by delivering one or two electrons. Antioxidant intake in the diet has been demonstrated in studies to be inversely related to hypertension. In mild-to-moderate hypertension individuals, ascorbic acid administration dramatically reduced SBP and DBP. Vitamin C, alone or in conjunction with vitamin E, enhanced nitric oxide production and decreased blood pressure in hypertension models in the lab. Furthermore, an antioxidant-rich diet has been demonstrated to lower blood pressure and minimize the infilteration of renal immune cell [54].

2) Non–Insulin-Dependent Diabetes Mellitus

Exaggerated free radical generation and a decrease in scavenger systems have been seen in non–insulin-dependent (type II) diabetic (NIDDM) patients. Antioxidants like glutathione and vitamin E are effective at lowering plasma free radical levels and improving insulin action. Vitamin C has anti-oxidant properties whose plasma concentrations in diabetics are lower than in healthy people. In healthy volunteers and NIDDM patients, an acute rise in plasma vitamin C concentrations has been demonstrated to improve insulin action. Chronic vitamin C supplementation, on the contrary, has been demonstrated to lower plasma lipid levels in healthy persons and many types of oxidative stress patients. To our information, no research has looked into the potential metabolic benefits of prolonged pharmacological vitamin C delivery in NIDDM patients over the age of 60. Aging, hyperglycemia, and higher plasma free radical levels all contribute to the progress of diabetic problems in these patients, increasing oxidative stress [55].

3) Cancer

A flurry of epidemiological research has been carried out to determine the link between ascorbic acid and cancers such breast, lungs, pancreatic, esophageal, gastric, colorectal, prostate, cervical, and ovarian cancer. With the exception of stomach cancer, the results were determined to be inconclusive. The link between a high consumption of ascorbic acid or vitamin C-rich foods and a lower risk of stomach cancer is one of the most reliable epidemiological findings on vitamin C. According to biochemical and physiological research, ascorbic acid acts as a free radical scavenger in the stomach, inhibiting the formation of cancer-causing N-nitroso compounds from nitrates and nitrite, and thereby protects against stomach cancer.

Low consumption of ascorbic acid and also other vitamins was connected to an elevated risk of cervical cancer in two of the three studies analyzed. This link requires additional investigation since the findings show that other nutrients such as vitamin E, carotenoids, and retinoic acid, either alone or in combination with ascorbic acid, may provide protection against certain malignancies. According to current research vitamin C alone will not be enough to treat most active cancers, as it seems to be more preventative than therapeutic. Vitamin C supplementation, on the contrary, has been demonstrated to improve quality of life and lengthen survival in cancer patients, thus it could be used as an adjuvant in cancer treatment [56].

9.3 Can Ascorbic Acid Lead to Cancer?

Recently, it was discovered that lipid hydroperoxide can react with ascorbic acid to produce DNA-damaging compounds, implying that lipid hydroperoxides can produce genotoxic metabolites, implying that ascorbic acid can increase mutagenesis and cancer risk. However, a variety of enzymes rapidly convert the hydroperoxides generated during the lipid peroxidation event to aldehydes. Furthermore, ascorbic acid, being a powerful antioxidant, significantly prevents the development of lipid peroxides in human plasma, as it is the first line of antioxidant defense. Lipid hydroperoxides are formed only after ascorbic acid has been depleted. Consequently, the interaction of ascorbic acid and hydroperoxide in human plasma is unlikely. High intracellular vitamin C levels have recently been found to protect human cells against oxidation-induced mutations. As a result, *in vivo* experiments are required to establish the physiological implications of these findings [57–62].

9.4 Conclusion

Vitamins are extremely beneficial to human health. Many physiological functions in human body require it. Vitamins can be obtained from a large number of food sources as well as through supplements. However, it is critical to take these vitamins in the precise proportions. An overabundance of vitamins in the body causes hypervitaminosis, whereas hypovitaminosis is caused by an insufficient number of vitamins. As a result, taking vitamins in suitable proportions is advised. Because a metabolic imbalance can lead to a variety of diseases. Vitamins in the right amounts can assist to prevent a variety of metabolic illnesses. Vitamin deficiency appears to be linked to the various components that comprise metabolic disease, according to the several studies reviewed. Similarly, vitamin supplementation may be an effective therapy technique.

Acknowledgment

The authors thank MET's Institute of Pharmacy, BKC, which is affiliated with Savitribai Phule Pune University, Nashik, MH, India. EDA wishes to express gratitude to the NFST/RGNF/UGC, Government of India, for providing financial assistance in the form of a fellowship (Award No - 202021-NFST-MAH-01235).

References

1. Abdullah, K.M., Alam, M.M., Iqbal, Z., Naseem, I., Therapeutic effect of vitamin B3 on hyperglycemia, oxidative stress and DNA damage in alloxan induced diabetic rat model. *Biomed. Pharmacother.*, 105, 1223–1231, 2018.

2. Al-Suhaimi, E.A. and Al-Jafary, M.A., Endocrine roles of vitamin K-dependent-osteocalcin in the relation between bone metabolism and metabolic disorders. *Rev. Endocr. Metab. Disord.*, 21, 1, 117–125, 2020.
3. Baj, T. and Sieniawska, E., Chapter 13-Vitamins, in: *Pharmacognosy: Fundamentals, Applications and Strategies*, 2017.
4. Bellone, F., Cinquegrani, M., Nicotera, R., Carullo, N., Casarella, A., Presta, P., Andreucci, M., Squadrito, G., Mandraffino, G., Prunestì, M., Vocca, C., Role of vitamin K in chronic kidney disease: A focus on bone and cardiovascular health. *Int. J. Mol. Sci.*, 23, 9, 5282, 2022.
5. Bellows, L., Moore, R., Anderson, J., Young, L., Water-soluble vitamins: B-Complex and Vitamin C. *Food Nutr. Series. Health; no. 9.312.*, 2012.
6. Bjørklund, G., Peana, M., Dadar, M., Lozynska, I., Chirumbolo, S., Lysiuk, R., Lenchyk, L., Upyr, T., Severin, B., The role of B vitamins in stroke prevention. *Crit. Rev. Food Sci. Nutr.*, 62, 1–14, 2021.
7. Blaner, W.S., Vitamin A signaling and homeostasis in obesity, diabetes, and metabolic disorders. *Pharmacol. Ther.*, 197, 153–178, 2019.
8. Chambial, S., Dwivedi, S., Shukla, K.K., John, P.J., Sharma, P., Vitamin C in disease prevention and cure: An overview. *Indian J. Clin. Biochem.*, 28, 4, 314–328, 2013.
9. Ellulu, M.S., Obesity, cardiovascular disease, and role of vitamin C on inflammation: A review of facts and underlying mechanisms. *Inflammopharmacology*, 25, 3, 313–328, 2017.
10. Gamna, F. and Spriano, S., Vitamin E: A review of its application and methods of detection when combined with implant biomaterials. *Materials*, 14, 13, 3691, 2021.
11. Gilbert, C., What is vitamin A and why do we need it? *Community Eye Health*, 26, 84, 65, 2013.
12. Gruber, B.M., B-group vitamins: Chemoprevention? *Adv. Clin. Exp. Med.*, 25, 3, 561–568, 2016.
13. Herrmann, W. and Herrmann, M., The controversial role of HCY and vitamin B deficiency in cardiovascular diseases. *Nutrients*, 14, 7, 1412, 2022.
14. Kennedy, D.O. and Haskell, C.F., Vitamins and cognition. *Drugs*, 71, 15, 1957–1971, 2011.
15. Kim, D., The role of vitamin D in thyroid diseases. *Int. J. Mol. Sci.*, 18, 9, 1949, 2017.
16. Mascolo, E. and Vernì, F., Vitamin B6 and diabetes: Relationship and molecular mechanisms. *Int. J. Mol. Sci.*, 21, 10, 3669, 2020.
17. Melguizo-Rodríguez, L., Costela-Ruiz, V.J., García-Recio, E., Luna-Bertos, D., Ruiz, C., Illescas-Montes, R., Role of vitamin d in the metabolic syndrome. *Nutrients*, 13, 3, 830, 2021.
18. Meydani, M., Vitamin E and prevention of heart disease in high-risk patients. *Nutr. Rev.*, 58, 9, 278–281, 2000.
19. Mody, N., Alterations in vitamin A/retinoic acid homeostasis in diet-induced obesity and insulin resistance. *Proc. Nutr. Soc.*, 76, 4, 597–602, 2017.

20. Mohd Mutalip, S.S., Ab-Rahim, S., Rajikin, M.H., Vitamin E as an antioxidant in female reproductive health. *Antioxidants*, 7, 2, p.22, 2018.
21. Nagamani, S., Sahoo, R., Muneeswaran, G., Sastry, G.N., Data science driven drug repurposing for metabolic disorders, in: *In Silico Drug Design*, pp. 191–227, Academic Press, USA, 2019.
22. Naidu, K.A., Vitamin C in human health and disease is still a mystery? An overview. *Nutr. J.*, 2, 1, 1–10, 2003.
23. Nollet, L., Van Gils, M., Verschuere, S., Vanakker, O., The role of and its related compounds in mendelian and acquired ectopic mineralization disorders. *Int. J. Mol. Sci.*, 20, 9, 2142, 2019.
24. Paolisso, G., Balbi, V., Volpe, C., Varricchio, G., Gambardella, A., Saccomanno, F., Ammendola, S., Varricchio, M., D'Onofrio, F., Metabolic benefits deriving from chronic vitamin C supplementation in aged non-insulin dependent diabetics. *J. Am. Coll. Nutr.*, 14, 4, 387–392, 1995.
25. Patassini, S., Begley, P., Xu, J., Church, S.J., Kureishy, N., Reid, S.J., Waldvogel, H.J., Faull, R.L., Snell, R.G., Unwin, R.D., Cooper, G.J., Cerebral vitamin B5 (D-pantothenic acid) deficiency as a potential cause of metabolic perturbation and neurodegeneration in Huntington's disease. *Metabolites*, 9, 6, 113, 2019.
26. Patel, T.V. and Singh, A.K., Role of vitamin D in chronic kidney disease. *Semin. Nephrol. WB Saunders*, 29, 2, 113–121, March 2009.
27. Pittas, A.G., Chung, M., Trikalinos, T., Mitri, J., Brendel, M., Patel, K., Lichtenstein, A.H., Lau, J., Balk, E.M., , and cardiometabolic outcomes: A systematic review. *Ann. Intern. Med.*, 152, 5, 307, 2010.
28. Pittas, A.G., Lau, J., Hu, F.B., Dawson-Hughes, B., The role of vitamin D and calcium in type 2 diabetes. A systematic review and meta-analysis. *J. Clin. Endocrinol. Metab.*, 92, 6, 2017–2029, 2007.
29. Rando, O.J. and Simmons, R.A., *Developmental Epigenetics and the Contribution of Parental Diet to Offspring Outcomes*, Elsevier, USA, 2019.
30. Strange, R.C., Shipman, K.E., Ramachandran, S., Metabolic syndrome: A review of the role of vitamin D in mediating susceptibility and outcome. *World J. Diabetes*, 6, 7, 896, 2015.
31. Thomas-Valdés, S., Tostes, M.D.G.V., Anunciação, P.C., da Silva, B.P., Sant'Ana, H.M.P., Association between vitamin deficiency and metabolic disorders related to obesity. *Crit. Rev. Food Sci. Nutr.*, 57, 15, 3332–3343, 2017.
32. Turan, S., Farruggio, A.P., Srifa, W., Day, J.W., Calos, M.P., Precise correction of disease mutations in induced pluripotent stem cells derived from patients with limb girdle muscular dystrophy. *Mol. Ther.*, 24, 4, 685–696, 2016.
33. National Institutes of Health. Office of Dietary Supplements, Vitamin D, fact sheet for health professionals, *NIH*, 1, 3–26, 2017. Available online: https://ods. od. nih. gov/factsheets/VitaminC-HealthProfessional.
34. Zhang, Y., Wang, T., Hu, X., Chen, G., Vitamin A and diabetes. *J. Med. Food*, 24, 8, 775–785, 2021.

35. García, O.P., Ronquillo, D., Caamaño, M.D.C., Martínez, G., Camacho, M., López, V., Rosado, J.L., Zinc, iron and vitamins A, C and E are associated with obesity, inflammation, lipid profile and insulin resistance in Mexican school-aged children. *Nutrients*, 5, 12, 5012–5030, 2013.
36. Valdés-Ramos, R., Martínez-Carrillo, B.E., Benítez-Arciniega, A.D., Vitamins and type 2 diabetes mellitus. *Endocr. Metab. Immune Disord. Drug Targets*, 15, 1, 54–63, 2015.
37. Deshmukh, S.V., Prabhakar, B., Kulkarni, Y.A., Water soluble vitamins and their role in diabetes and its complications. *Curr. Diabetes Rev.*, 16, 7, 649–656, 2020.
38. Sauve, A.A., NAD+ and vitamin B3: From metabolism to therapies. *J. Pharmacol. Exp. Ther.*, 324, 3, 883–893, 2008.
39. Aguilera-Méndez, A., Boone-Villa, D., Nieto-Aguilar, R., Villafaña-Rauda, S., Molina, A.S., Sobrevilla, J.V., Role of vitamins in the metabolic syndrome and cardiovascular disease. *Pflüg. Arch. Eur. J. Physiol.*, 10, 1–24, 2021.
40. Gheita, A.A., Gheita, T.A., Kenawy, S.A., The potential role of B5: A stitch in time and switch in cytokine. *Phytother. Res.*, 34, 2, 306–314, 2020.
41. Wilson, M.P., Plecko, B., Mills, P.B., Clayton, P.T., Disorders affecting vitamin B6 metabolism. *Inherit. Metab. Dis.*, 42, 4, 629–646, 2019.
42. Mascolo, E. and Vernì, F., Vitamin B6 and diabetes: Relationship and molecular mechanisms. *Int. J. Mol. Sci.*, 21, 10, 3669, 2020.
43. Snell, E.E. and Haskell, B.E., The metabolism of vitamin B6, in: *Comprehensive Biochemistry*, vol. 21, pp. 47–71, Elsevier, USA, 1970.
44. Friso, S., Lotto, V., Corrocher, R., Choi, S.W., Vitamin B6 and cardiovascular disease, in: *Water Soluble Vitamins*, pp. 265–290, 2012.
45. Merigliano, C., Mascolo, E., Burla, R., Saggio, I., Vernì, F., The relationship between vitamin B6, diabetes and cancer. *Front. Genet.*, 9, 388, 2018.
46. Powers, H.J., Riboflavin (vitamin B-2) and health. *Am. J. Clin. Nutr.*, 77, 6, 1352–1360, 2003.
47. Fenech, M., Folate (vitamin B9) and vitamin B12 and their function in the maintenance of nuclear and mitochondrial genome integrity. *Mutat. Res./Fundam. Mol. Mech. Mutagen.*, 733, 1-2, 21–33, 2012.
48. Thomas-Valdés, S., Tostes, M.D.G.V., Anunciação, P.C., da Silva, B.P., Sant'Ana, H.M.P., Association between vitamin deficiency and metabolic disorders related to obesity. *Crit. Rev. Food Sci. Nutr.*, 57, 15, 3332–3343, 2017.
49. Yahn, G.B., Abato, J.E., Jadavji, N.M., Role of vitamin B12 deficiency in ischemic stroke risk and outcome. *Neural Regen. Res.*, 16, 3, 470, 2021.
50. Spence, J.D., Bang, H., Chambless, L.E., Stampfer, M.J., Vitamin intervention for stroke prevention trial: An efficacy analysis. *Stroke*, 36, 11, 2404–2409, 2005.
51. Hultdin, J., Van Guelpen, B., Bergh, A., Hallmans, G., Stattin, P., Plasma folate, vitamin B12, and homocysteine and prostate cancer risk: A prospective study. *Int. J. Cancer*, 113, 5, 819–824, 2005.

52. Schlueter, A.K. and Johnston, C.S., Vitamin C: Overview and update. *J. Evid. Based Complementary Altern. Med.*, 16, 1, 49–57, 2011.
53. Evans, W.J., Vitamin E, vitamin C, and exercise. *Am. J. Clin. Nutr.*, 72, 2, 647S–652S, 2000.
54. Darko, D., Dornhorst, A., Kelly, F.J., Ritter, J.M., Chowienczyk, P.J., Lack of effect of oral vitamin C on blood pressure, oxidative stress and endothelial function in Type II diabetes. *Clin. Sci.*, 103, 4, 339–344, 2002.
55. Ting, H.H., Timimi, F.K., Boles, K.S., Creager, S.J., Ganz, P., Creager, M.A., Vitamin C improves endothelium-dependent vasodilation in patients with non-insulin-dependent diabetes mellitus. *J. Clin. Investig.*, 97, 1, 22–28, 1996.
56. Cameron, E. and Pauling, L.C., *Cancer and Vitamin C: A Discussion of the Nature, Causes, Prevention, and Treatment of Cancer with Special Reference to the Value of Vitamin C*, Linus Pauling Institute of Science and Medicine, Rome, Italy, 1979.
57. Du, J., Cullen, J.J., Buettner, G.R., Ascorbic acid: chemistry, biology and the treatment of cancer. *Biochim. Biophys. Acta Rev. Cancer*, 1826, 2, 443–457, 2012.
58. Surana, K.R., Ahire, E.D., Sonawane, V.N., Talele, S.G., Talele, G.S., Molecular modeling: Novel techniques in food and nutrition development, in: *Natural Food Products and Waste Recovery*, pp. 17–31, Apple Academic Press, New Jersey and Canada, 2021.
59. Keservani, R.K., Kesharwani, R.K., Vyas, N., Jain, S., Raghuvanshi, R., Sharma, A.K., Nutraceutical and functional food as future food: A review. *Der. Pharm. Lett.*, 2, 1, 106–116, 2010a.
60. Keservani, R.K., Kesharwani, R.K., Sharma, A.K., Vyas, N., Chadoker, A., Nutritional supplements: An overview. *Int. J. Curr. Pharm. Rev. Res.*, 1, 1, 59–75, 2010b.
61. Keservani, R.K., Sharma, A.K., Kesharwani, R.K., An overview and therapeutic applications of nutraceutical and functional foods, in: *Recent Advances in Drug Delivery Technology*, pp. 160–201, 2017.
62. Keservani, R.K., Sharma, A.K., Kesharwani, R.K. (Eds.), *Nutraceuticals and Dietary Supplements: Applications in Health Improvement and Disease Management*, CRC Press, New Jersey and Canada, 2020.

10
Beneficial Effects of Water-Soluble Vitamins in Nutrition and Health Promotion

Afsar S. Pathan[1], Pankaj G. Jain[1]*, Ashwini B. Mahajan[2], Vivek S. Kumawat[1], Eknath D. Ahire[3], Khemchand R. Surana[4], Amit K. Rajora[5] and Manju Amit Kumar Rajora[6]

[1]*Department of Pharmacology, R.C. Patel Institute of Pharmaceutical Education and Research, Shirpur, India*
[2]*Department of Drug Regulatory Affair, R.C. Patel Institute of Pharmaceutical Education and Research, Shirpur, India*
[3]*Department of Pharmaceutics, METs, Institute of Pharmacy, BKC, Adgaon, Nashik, MH, India,*
[4]*Department of Pharmaceutical Chemistry, SSS's Divine College of Pharmacy, Satana, Nashik, MH, India*
[5]*NanoBiotechnology Lab, School of Biotechnology, Jawaharlal Nehru University, New Delhi, India*
[6]*College of Nursing, All India Institute of Medical Sciences, New Delhi, India*

Abstract

Vitamins are the essential micronutrients that play an important role in the performance of normal body functions. Vitamins are considered part of the organic group. They are also important for essential human nutrition because dietary supplements such as vitamins and minerals are required to prevent metabolic disorders because they are organic compounds that humans cannot synthesize on their own. Vitamins are unique in that they can act as "external" or dietary regulatory agents in the body. This chapter includes the structure and functions of vitamins along with their biological importance and prospective. Water-soluble vitamins play a crucial role in the maintenance of the body and they are eliminated from the body, so we can take water-soluble vitamins on a daily basis in our diet. Along with this, vitamin deficiency leads to suffering from many harsh diseases, so to

---

*Corresponding author: pgjain@yahoo.com

Eknath D. Ahire, Raj K. Keservani, Khemchand R. Surana, Sippy Singh and Rajesh K. Kesharwani (eds.) *Vitamins as Nutraceuticals: Recent Advances and Applications,* (235–252) © 2023 Scrivener Publishing LLC

overcome the deficiency of vitamins, dietary supplements are provided to maintain the proper amount of vitamins in the body for overall better performance of the body.

Keywords: Vitamins, nutraceutical, water-soluble, health, promotion

10.1 Introduction

Vitamins are essential organic components that the body needs in the little amounts for metabolism, protection, health maintenance, and optimal growth of the human body [1]. Vitamins are vital nutrients that may be found in diet. The necessities are basic, yet they provide particular and important functions that are crucial for health maintenance. Vitamins are grouped into two categories based on the materials in which they will dissolve [2]. B-complex vitamins and vitamin C are water-soluble vitamins that cannot be stored in the body and therefore should be replenished on a daily basis. During food storage and preparation, these vitamins are readily lost or washed away from the body [2]. Vitamin loss may be reduced by properly storing and preparing meals. Refrigerate fresh food, keep milk and cereals away from bright light, and use vegetable cooking water to make soups to avoid vitamin loss [3]. Vitamin deficiency results in the development of pathological processes, such as specific hypovitaminosis and avitaminosis [4]. Figure 10.1 shows the solubility of vitamins.

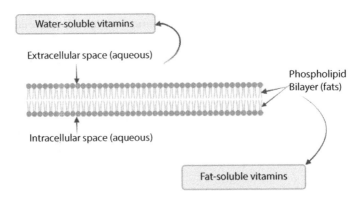

Figure 10.1 Solubility of vitamins.

10.1.1 Vitamin and Its Types

There are two types of vitamins on the basis of solubility in water and fat.

10.1.1.1 Water-Soluble Vitamins

Water-soluble vitamins dissolve quickly in water and are often eliminated readily by the body, e.g., vitamin C and vitamin B complex (thiamine, riboflavin, niacin, pantothenic acid, pyridoxine, biotin, folate, and cobalamin). There are nine water-soluble vitamins (Figure 10.2) (vitamin B-complex and vitamin C) out of which all the vitamins are required for certain cellular functions and body need. Every vitamin has its own assigned functions to perform in the body and prevent the body from disease, which arises from the deficiency of the vitamins [5].

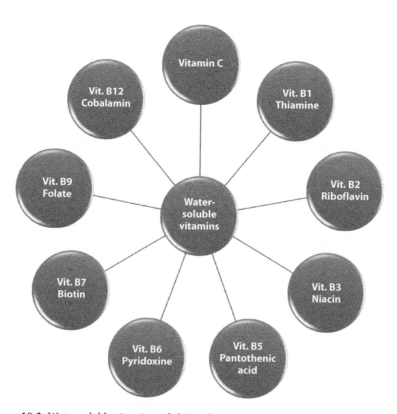

Figure 10.2 Water-soluble vitamin and their subtypes.

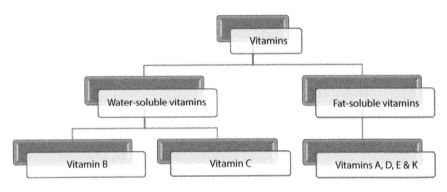

Figure 10.3 Classification of vitamin according to their solubility.

10.1.1.2 *Fat-Soluble Vitamins*

Vitamins that are fat soluble are stored in the body fats like in liver, adipose (fat) tissue, and skeletal muscle. As an outcome, the likelihood of a deficit is minimal with a well-balanced diet. e.g., Vitamins A, D, E, and K are fat-soluble. Figure 10.2 showing the water-soluble vitamin and their subtypes. Figure 10.3 shows the classifications of vitamins as per their solubility.

10.1.2 History of Vitamins

Casimir Funk (Scientist) isolates an amine-containing extract from rice polishing which effectively cures beriberi in an experimental animal in 1911 and labels it "vitamin" for "vital amine." This was eventually discovered to be thiamine (Vitamin B1) [6]. Funk introduced the vitamin hypothesis in 1912, which included antiberiberi, antirickets, antiscurvy, and antipellagra vitamins (Figure 10.4) [6].

Biological Importance of Vitamins

1. Vitamins regulate metabolic reactions in comparison with other food nutrients.
2. Vitamins are necessary for various cellular processes which carried out in human body.
3. They conduct specialized and significant roles in a range of physiological systems and are essential for sustaining good health.
4. They act as coenzymes, assisting the body in obtaining energy from meals [7].

Nutrition and Health Benefits of Water-Soluble Vitamins 239

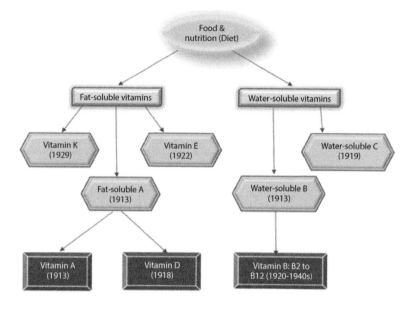

Figure 10.4 Flowchart for discovery of vitamins.

The categorization of vitamins into distinct chemical groupings is influenced by both chemical properties and functions. Every vitamin has its own curative factors to defeat the disease [8].

Below is Table 10.1, which includes name of water-soluble vitamin and its type with example and source.

10.1.2.1 Vitamin B-Complex

1. Vitamin B1: [Thiamine]

Vitamin B1 is one of the B vitamins, which are comprised of eight different types. Since its discovery, it has gone by a variety of names, including aneurin and, as of the year 2000, thiamin (thiamine) [10]. The fact that thiamin can only be stored in the body for a short time period before being excreted means that it is necessary to consume thiamin on a regular basis in order to maintain proper blood levels. Vitamin B1 is a water-soluble vitamin that is soaked up directly into the bloodstream from the gastrointestinal tract, like all other B vitamins. As soon as thiamin is sucked up into the bloodstream, it can circulate freely throughout the body without the need for carrier proteins in plasma and red blood cells until it is excreted

Table 10.1 Vitamins and their sources [9].

Sr. no.	Type of vitamin	Vitamin	Name of vitamin	Source
1.	Vitamin B-complex	Vitamin B1	Thiamine	Milk, green vegetables, cereals, pork
2.		Vitamin B2	Riboflavin	Meat & fortified foods, green vegetables
3.		Vitamin B3	Niacin	Meat, fish, poultry, cereals, liver & kidney
4.		Vitamin B5	Pantothenic acid	Meat, fish, mushroom, avocado, egg yolk
5.		Vitamin B6	Pyridoxine	Milk, meat, cereals, whole grains, egg
6.		Vitamin B7	Biotin	Liver, kidney, milk, egg yolk
7.		Vitamin B9	Folate	Egg, meat, beet root, leafy vegetables
8.		Vitamin B12	Cobalamin	Egg, meat, fish
9.	Vitamin C	Vitamin C	Ascorbic acid	Citrus fruits (orange, lemon, etc.)

in the urine. While being in the body, this can be stored in the liver for a maximum of eighteen days, after which, it is excreted. It has the ability to cross the blood-brain barrier [11]. Thiamine deficiency is the most severe of the water-soluble vitamins, and it has the greatest potential to cause the most severe clinical manifestations. In carbohydrate metabolism, thiamine is an essential coenzyme for the conversion of pyruvate to acetyl coenzyme A, which is required for the breakdown of glucose. Acute thiamine deficiency results in the accumulation of pyruvate, which is then metabolized to lactate without the presence of acidosis [7].

1. Vitamin B1: [Thiamine]

Structure	Function
	1. Aids in the release of energy from meals. 2. Encourage better appetite. 3. Crucial in nervous system function [12–14].

2. Vitamin B2: [Riboflavin]

Structure	Function
	1. Aids in the release of energy from meals. 2. Boost optimal vision and skin health [15, 16].

3. Vitamin B3: [Niacin]

Structure	Function
	1. Food-based energy generation. 2. Helps digestion and stimulates appetite. 3. Enhance skin and nerve health [17].

4. Vitamin B5: [Pantothenic acid]

Structure	Function
(structure of pantothenic acid)	1. Function as a starting point for the production of CoA and ACP. 2. Assisting in the breakdown of lipids and crabs for energy [18].

5. Vitamin B6: [Pyridoxine]

B6 is required for nucleic acid and protein biosynthesis because it provides one-carbon units that are used in the production of purines and deoxythymidylate, which affect DNA and mRNA synthesis. B6 is also required for cellular respiration. A vitamin B 6 influence on immune function is therefore logical, given that antibodies and cytokines are produced from amino acids and require vitamin B 6 to function properly as a coenzyme in their metabolism.

Structure	Function
(structure of pyridoxine)	1. Assists in protein metabolism, absorption 2. Promotes red blood cell production [19, 20].

6. Vitamin B7: [Biotin]

Structure	Function
(structure of biotin)	1. Synthesis of saturated fats (lipids) and amino acids (the building blocks of protein). 2. Promote the metabolism of protein/amino acids in root of the hair and fingernail cells [21].

7. Vitamin B9: [Folate]

Structure	Function
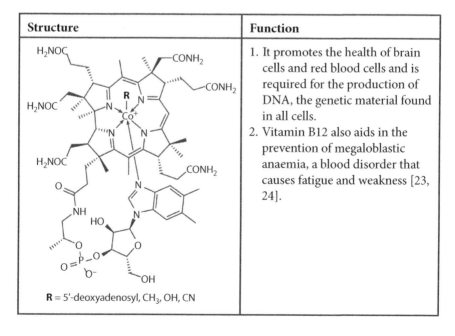	1. Regulate (together with vitamins B6 and B12) blood levels of the amino acid homocysteine, which has been linked to some chronic illnesses such as heart disease. 2. Support fast cell development during childhood, adolescence, and pregnancy [22].

8. Vitamin B12: [Cobalamin]

Structure	Function
(Structure of cobalamin with R = 5'-deoxyadenosyl, CH_3, OH, CN)	1. It promotes the health of brain cells and red blood cells and is required for the production of DNA, the genetic material found in all cells. 2. Vitamin B12 also aids in the prevention of megaloblastic anaemia, a blood disorder that causes fatigue and weakness [23, 24].

9. Vitamin C [Ascorbic acid]

Structure	Function
(chemical structure of ascorbic acid)	1. It is commonly used as a food ingredient, where it improves the nutritional value. 2. The role of vitamin C in various enzymatic processes is well established [25, 26].

10.2 Beneficial Effects of Vitamins on Nutrition

Individual B vitamin supplements for each vitamin are given the following basic numbers or names: Thiamine (B1), riboflavin (B2), niacin (B3), and so on. Niacin, pantothenic acid, biotin, and Folate are known by their names rather than their quantities. Each B vitamin functions as a cofactor (typically as a coenzyme) or as a precursor to important metabolic pathways [9].

1. Vitamin B1
All plant and animal meals include vitamin B1. Thiamine is very abundant in cereals' outer coats of seeds. Wheat milling reduces the thiamine concentration. Milk contains thiamine as well, but in little levels. It is known as anti-beriberi factor because of its ability to cure beriberi. It is also known as heat labile factor or antineuritic factor [27], e.g., thiamine is widely added to wheat flour, maize flour, and rice [28].

2. Vitamin B2
The effectiveness of the immune system is strongly dependent on the individual's dietary state. Inadequate intake of macronutrients and/or micronutrients can impair innate immune host defence. However, not all illnesses are affected similarly by nutrition [29].

3. Vitamin B3
Niacin can be produced by the amino acid tryptophan, which is required for its production. The intake of dietary tryptophan, despite the fact that this process is inefficient, appears to be critical for the body's overall niacin status. Niacin deficiency can be caused by problems with the absorption of niacin or tryptophan, which are both essential nutrients. Isoniazid (Laniazid, Nydrazid) treatment for tuberculosis is associated

with an increased risk of niacin deficiency. Digestive disorders and long-term treatment with Isoniazid (Laniazid, Nydrazid) are also risk factors. Additionally, alcoholism is considered to be the most common contributing factor to this problem. Patients with Crohn's disease have also been found to have niacin deficiency, according to recent research [30].

4. Vitamin B5

A precursor to the biosynthesis of coenzyme A (CoA) and proteins containing a phosphopantetheine prosthetic group, pantothenate is a vitamin B5 that is essential for healthy skin. Phosphopantetheine is a moiety that is donated to these proteins by CoA and is used to shuttle intermediates between the active sites of enzymes involved in fatty acid, nonribosomal peptide, and polyketide synthesis, among other processes. In addition to being a critical cofactor for cell growth, CoA participates in a wide range of metabolic reactions, including the synthesis of phospholipids, the synthesis and degradation of fatty acids, and the operation of the tricarboxylic acid cycle, among others.

5. Vitamin B6

Pyridoxal, pyridoxine, and pyridoxamine are the three different forms of vitamin B6, which can all be phosphorylated. Vitamin B6 is also known as piroxin and can be found in three different forms. The pyridoxal 5'-phosphate (PLP) form of vitamin B6 is the biologically active form of the vitamin and serves as a cofactor for more than 140 enzymes in the body. The PLP is capable of converting tryptophan into niacin, which is essential for vitamin B3 synthesis.

6. Vitamin B7

Because mammals are unable to synthesize biotin, they must obtain it through their diets from plant and microbial sources. Plant cells, as well as microorganisms, such as yeast and certain bacteria, are capable of producing biotin on their own. The water-soluble vitamin biotin can be found in a variety of foods, but at a lower concentration than the other water-soluble vitamins. Eight biotin-dense foods include liver, kidneys, heart, pancreas, egg yolk, poultry, yeast, and cow's milk, to name a few. Plants, particularly seeds, contain smaller amounts of the substance [31].

7. Vitamin B9

It is also involved in amino acid metabolism and is a key component in the formation of new cells, including red blood cells, as well as the repair of damaged cells and tissues. Because increased physical activity causes muscle tissue damage, the need for folates may increase. Folic acid, along with vitamins B12 and B6, plays an important role in methionine metabolism (an essential amino acid). If any of these essential vitamins is deficient, the level of homocysteine, an indirect metabolite in methionine metabolism, rises [32].

8. Vitamin B12

Vitamin B12 aids in DNA synthesis, is required for red blood cell formation, and its deficiency results in megaloblastic anaemia. Cobalamin absorption may be impaired due to factors, such as gene mutations or atrophic gastritis, both of which contribute to decreased secretion of Castle's intrinsic factor. Cobalamin is required for proper nervous system function. It protects nerve cells by forming layers that protect them from damage, which can lead to impaired nerve impulse transmission and neurological problems [32].

9. Vitamin C

In recent years, advances in our understanding of the mechanisms of vitamin C transport, as well as the discovery of new physiological roles for the

Table 10.2 Vitamins and related deficiencies.

Sr. no.	Vitamins	Names of vitamins	Deficiency leads diseases or disorder
1.	Vitamin B1	Thiamine	Weak memory, sleep disturbance
2.	Vitamin B2	Riboflavin	Amnesia, skin inflammation
3.	Vitamin B3	Niacin	Depression, pellagra
4.	Vitamin B5	Pantothenic acid	Fatigue, gastrointestinal problems
5.	Vitamin B6	Pyridoxine	Confusion, mood swings
6.	Vitamin B7	Biotin	Dermatitis, redness & itching of skin
7.	Vitamin B9	Folate	Megaloblastic anaemia
8.	Vitamin B12	Cobalamin	Pain of joints, poor health of teeth
9.	Vitamin C	Ascorbic acid	Poor healing of wounds, scurvy

vitamin and the potential involvement of vitamin C in cancer and heart disease, have prompted calls for revisions to the current recommendations for vitamin C intake [33].

Vitamin Deficiency

Generally speaking, a balanced diet is one that contains a variety of foods in sufficient quantities and proportions to ensure that calorie, energy, and other requirements are adequately met while also making a small provision for extra nutrients to help the body cope with illness for a short period [34]. But due to malnutrition which leads to the development of vitamin deficiency in human beings leads to various diseases and disorder (Table 10.2).

10.3 Beneficial Effects of Water-Soluble Vitamins in Health Promotion

10.3.1 Vitamin B1

Nutritional deficiency in alcoholism is associated with malnutrition and decreased absorption of vitamins, particularly vitamin B1 or thiamine, as a result of the direct effects of alcohol on the metabolism of thiamine, as well as other factors. The combination of these two factors, chronic alcoholism and thiamine deficiency (TD), in humans, can result in Wernicke's encephalopathy, an acute neurological disorder characterised by seizures and coma (WE). Weakness in the absence of alcohol is observed in non-alcoholic patients with a variety of conditions, including gastro enteric resection, chronic wasting disease, hyperemesis, and AIDS-related wasting syndrome. Furthermore, TD leads to the development of the Korsakoff syndrome [35].

10.3.2 Vitamin C

In addition to vitamin E and carotenoid, micronutrient antioxidants, such as ascorbic acid and vitamin C help to neutralize free radicals, which may play a role in the development of prostate cancer by causing oxidative damage to DNA, lipid membranes and proteins [36]. The daily recommendations for vitamins B and C is presented in Table 10.3.

Table 10.3 Recommended dietary intake of water soluble vitamins in mg/d [7].

Sr. no.	Vitamins	Age groups					
1	(mg/d)	Infants	Children	Males	Females	Pregnant	Lactation
2	Vitamin B1	0.2	0.5	0.9	0.9	1.4	1.4
3	Vitamin B2	0.3	0.5	0.9	0.9	1.4	1.6
4	Vitamin B3	2	6	12	12	18	17
5	Vitamin B5	1.7	2	4	4	6	7
6	Vitamin B6	0.1	0.5	1.0	1.0	1.9	2.0
7	Vitamin B7	5	8	20	20	30	35
8	Vitamin B9	65	150	300	300	600	500
9	Vitamin B12	0.4	0.9	1.8	1.8	2.6	2.8
10	Vitamin C	40	15	45	45	80	115

10.4 Future Prospective of Water-Soluble Vitamins

The increasing demand of vitamins as Neutraceuticals due to world largely move toward the ayurvedic and neutraceuticals market due to their less side effect on human body, many of water-soluble vitamins which cannot be synthesize in body and also which is necessary for the immune system so this types of vitamins are give major impact on daily lifestyle. For further advantage, it is necessary that work on vitamins use in daily life and how we add this types of vitamins in our daily diet.

10.5 Conclusion

Vitamins are essential organic components that the body needs in little amounts for metabolism, protection, health maintenance, and optimal growth of the human body. To avoid side effect and make healthier immune system, it is necessary to consume daily require amount of vitamins through different diet and from various neutraceuticals product. We can take water-soluble vitamins every day in our diet because they are essential for the body's maintenance and are excreted by the body. Additionally, a lack of vitamins puts a person at risk for developing a number of serious illnesses. To combat this, dietary supplements are offered to keep the body's vitamin levels balanced for improved health overall.

Acknowledgment

The authors thank R. C. Patel Institute of Pharmaceutical Education and Research Shirpur, India and MET's Institute of Pharmacy, BKC, which is affiliated with Savitribai Phule Pune University, Nashik, MH, India. EDA wishes to express gratitude to the NFST/RGNF/UGC, Government of India, for providing financial assistance in the form of a fellowship (award 202021-NFST-MAH-01235).

References

1. Rasaq, N.O., *Vitamamins: Structure and Functions*.
2. National Research Council, Water-soluble vitamins. In Recommended Dietary Allowances: 10th Edition. National Academies Press (US), 1989.
3. Said, H.M., Water-soluble vitamins. *Nutrition for the Primary Care Provider*, 111, pp. 30–37, 2015.
4. Krisanova, N.V., Ivanchenko, D.G., Rudko, N.P., Ministry of Health of Ukraine. *Gen. Med.*, 16, 1–73, 2016.
5. Schellack, G., Harirari, P., Schellack, N., B-complex vitamin deficiency and supplementation. *SA Pharm. J.*, 83, 4, 14–19, 2016.
6. Chen, G., Ni, Y., Nagata, N., Xu, L. and Ota, T., Micronutrient antioxidants and nonalcoholic fatty liver disease. *Int. J. Molecular Sci.*, 17, 9, 1379, 2016.
7. Moore, R., Water-soluble vitamins: B-complex and vitamin C. *Colorado State Univ.*, Fact Sheet, 9, 5, 2012.
8. Steinberg, F. and Rucker, R.B., The water-soluble vitamins, *Food Sci. Technol.*, New York, Marcel Dekker, 149, 1, 10 December, 2005,

9. Rafeeq, H. et al., Biochemistry of water soluble vitamins, sources, biochemical functions and toxicity. *Sch. Int. J. Biochem.*, 3, 10, 215–220, 2020.
10. Martel, J.L., Kerndt, C.C., Doshi, H. et al. *Vitamin B1 (Thiamine)* [Updated 2022 Aug 27]. In: *StatPearls [Internet]*. Treasure Island (FL): StatPearls Publishing, 2022 Jan-. Available from: https://www.ncbi.nlm.nih.gov/books/NBK482360/
11. Gibson, G.E., Hirsch, J.A., Fonzetti, P., Jordan, B.D., Cirio, R.T. and Elder, J., Vitamin B1 (thiamine) and dementia. Annals of the New York Academy of Sciences, 1367, 1, 21–30, 2016.
12. Makarchikov, A.F., Vitamin B1: Metabolism and functions. *Biochem. Suppl. Ser. B Biomed. Chem.*, 3, 2, 116–128, 2009.
13. Fattal-Valevski, A., Thiamine (vitamin B1). *Complement. Health Pract. Rev.*, 16, 1, 12–20, 2011.
14. Jurgenson, C.T., Begley, T.P., Ealick, S.E., The structural and biochemical foundations of thiamin biosynthesis. *Annu. Rev. Biochem.*, 78, 569–603, 2009.
15. Suwannasom, N., Kao, I., Pruß, A., Georgieva, R., Bäumler, H., Riboflavin: The health benefits of a forgotten natural vitamin. *Int. J. Mol. Sci.*, 21, 3, 950, 2020.
16. Pinto, J.T. and Zempleni, J., Riboflavin. *Adv Nutr.*, 7, 5, 973–975, 2016. https://doi.org/10.3945/an.116.012716
17. Lawrance, P., *Niacin (Vitamin B3)-A Review of Analytical Methods for Use in Food*, pp. 1–9, Government Chemist Programme Report, March 2015.
18. Miller, J.W. and Rucker, R.B., Pantothenic acid, in: *Present Knowledge in Nutrition Ed.*, pp. 375–390, June 2012.
19. Stach, K., Stach, W., Augoff, K., Vitamin B6 in health and disease. *Nutrients*, 13, 9, 3229, 2021.
20. Institute of Medicine (US) Standing Committee on the Scientific Evaluation of Dietary Reference Intakes, Vitamin B6. Dietary reference intakes for thiamin, riboflavin, niacin, vitamin B6, folate, vitamin B12, pantothenic acid, biotin, and choline, 1988.
21. Akram, M., Munir, N., Daniyal, M., Egbuna, C., Găman, M.A., Onyekere, P.F. and Olatunde, A., Vitamins and Minerals: Types, sources and their functions. *Functional Foods and Nutraceuticals: Bioactive Components, Formulations and Innovations*, 149–172, 2020.
22. Sobczyńska-Malefora, A. and Harrington, D.J., Laboratory assessment of folate (vitamin B9) status. *J. Clinic. Pathol.*, 71, 11, 949–956, 2018.
23. Departement of Health & Human Services, *Vitamin B12 Fact Sheet for Consumers*, pp. 1–78, National Institutes of Health, 2016.
24. National Institutes of Health, Vitamin B12 factsheet, in: *Vitamins*, pp. 3–4.
25. Davies, M.B., Austin, J. and Partridge, D.A., Biochemistry and chemistry of ascorbic acid. *Motiv. Emot.*, V-1, p. 176, 1991.
26. Doseděl, M. et al., Vitamin C—Sources, physiological role, kinetics, deficiency, use, toxicity, and determination. *Nutrients*, 13, 2, 1–36, 2021.

27. Williams, R.R., The chemistry of thiamin (vitamin B1). *J. Am. Med. Assoc.*, 110, 10, 727–732, 1938
28. Hrubša, M., Siatka, T., Nejmanová, I., Vopršalová, M., Kujovská Krčmová, L., Matoušová, K., Javorská, L., Macáková, K., Mercolini, L., Remião, F., Máťuš, M., Biological properties of vitamins of the B-complex, part 1: Vitamins B1, B2, B3, and B5. *Nutrients*, 14, 3, 484, 2022.
29. Alpert, P.T., The role of vitamins and minerals on the immune system. *Home Health Care Manage. Pract.*, 29, 3, 199–202, 2017.
30. Ilkhani, F., Hosseini, B. and Saedisomeolia, A., Niacin and oxidative stress: A mini-review. *J. Nutr. Med. Diet Care*, 2, 1, 014, 2016.
31. Carling, R.S. and Turner, C., Methods for assessment of biotin (vitamin B7), Elsevier Inc, Cambridge, Mass., USA, 2018.
32. Szczuko, M. *et al.*, Role of water soluble vitamins in the reduction diet of an amateur sportsman. *Open Life Sci.*, 13, 1, 163–173, 2018.
33. Li, Y. and Schellhorn, H.E., New developments and novel therapeutic perspectives for vitamin C. *J. Nutr.*, 137, 10, 2171–2184, 2007.
34. Alkerwi, A.A., Diet quality concept. *Nutrition*, 30, 6, 613–618, 2014.
35. Arts, N.J., Walvoort, S.J. and Kessels, R.P., Korsakoff's syndrome: A critical review. *Neuropsychiatr. Dis. Treat.*, 2875–2890, 2017.
36. Kirsh, V.A., Hayes, R.B., Mayne, S.T., Chatterjee, N., Subar, A.F., Dixon, L.B., Albanes, D., Andriole, G.L., Urban, D.A., Peters, U., Supplemental and dietary vitamin E, β-carotene, and vitamin C intakes and prostate cancer risk. *J. Nat. Cancer Institute*, 98, 4, 245–254, 2006.

11
Vitamins as Nutraceuticals for Anemia

Snehal D. Pawar[1*], Shubham D. Deore[1], Nikita P. Bairagi[1], Vaishnavi B. Deshmukh[1], Tushar N. Lokhande[2] and Khemchand R. Surana[3]

[1]M.G.V.'s Samajshri Prashant Dada Hiray, College of Pharmacy, Malegaon Nashik, India
[2]Mahatma Gandhi Vidyamandir Pharmacy College Panchavati, Nashik, India
[3]Shreeshakti Shaikshanik Sanstha's, Divine College of Pharmacy, Satana, Nashik, India

Abstract

Anemia is the severe chronic universal public health problem related with increase risk of the mortality. Anemia is a condition where adequate red blood cells are not carrying sufficient amount of oxygen to body and tissues, the body requires RBCs to survive and transport Haemoglobin, it is a complex protein that binds to the iron molecule. Further, this iron molecule carries oxygen from lungs to all body parts. It is high-risk majority associated with the pregnant women and young children. It is a disease that has multiple reasons associated with nutrition, as well as non-nutrition. Iron deficiency, destruction in the RBCs, blood loss, sickle cell formation are among the major results of vitamin deficiency. Vitamins can play a vital role in the prevention or treatment of anemia. The need for vitamins is fulfilled by nutraceutical. Nutraceuticals are the products that have various physiological benefits, and these protect against different chronic diseases. Nutraceutical is the bridge between nutrition and pharmaceutical. Nutraceutical means any nontoxic food substance that has evidence-based health benefits. The various examples of functional food are used as nutraceutical, such as spinach, broccoli, dark chocolate cashews are rich in iron. Meat, egg, sweet potato, fruit like mango papaya are rich in the vitamin A. Vegetables like cabbage, cauliflower, oil and fat like sunflower oil, soyabean oil are rich in the vitamin C and E and various sources of folate and riboflavin help in prevention of anemia.

Keywords: Nutraceuticals, functional food, vitamins, anemia, etc.

---

*Corresponding author: snehal.pawar152295@gmail.com

Eknath D. Ahire, Raj K. Keservani, Khemchand R. Surana, Sippy Singh and Rajesh K. Kesharwani (eds.) Vitamins as Nutraceuticals: Recent Advances and Applications, (253–280) © 2023 Scrivener Publishing LLC

11.1 Introduction

Dr. Stephen Defelice in 1989 discovered the term nutraceuticals. It is the combination or bridge between two words "nutrition" and "pharmaceuticals." Nutraceuticals are used for prevention of chronic disease. It consists of vitamins, minerals, herbs, amino acids, and dietary substances [1], as shown in Table 11.1. The nation of nutraceuticals pulls away from 3000 years ago. Hippocrates (460–377 B.C.) said that "let the food be the medicine and medicine be the food." Food manufacturers in the United States, in the early years of 1900's, started the addition of small amount of iodine into the salt to prevent goiter (Cranford, New Jersey in 2001). Dr. Stephen DeFelice stated that nutraceutical is a part of food or nutrient, which, in addition to its nutrient value, provides medical and health benefits, including promotion of health and prevention of chronic diseases. In countries like Japan, England or other, nutraceuticals are already becoming a part of dietary lifestyle [2].

In Germany, France, and United Kingdom the important factor of their lifestyle is diet more than the exercise, this a hereditary factor to achieve good health goals. Canada defined nutraceutical in a way that these are the products of foods but sold as drug administration, which is under authority of the Federal Food Drug and Cosmetics Act [3]. In the form of powders, pills, and other medicinal forms, they are not normally associated with food. In India, nutraceutical is seen as a food production made up of herbal raw material, which is used to prevent or treat diseases, like different types of acute and chronic maladies [4]. Nowadays nutraceutical is one of the fastest multiplying industry with having expected 7.5% compound annual growth rate. Nutraceuticals are maintained by Food and Drug Administration (FDA). The global nutraceutical market is approximately increase from $241 billion market in 2019 to $373 billion in 2025. The definite use of nutraceuticals is that it has achieved the high therapeutic outcomes with fewer side effects. In nutritionally induced acute and chronic diseases, herbal nutraceutical plays a vital role to sustain health and contribute by upgrading optimal health, longevity, and quality of life [5, 6]. Table 11.1 shows the classification of Nutraceuticals.

11.1.1 Classification of Nutraceuticals

Table 11.1 Classification of nutraceuticals [7].

Food availability	Classification of the nutraceuticals based on the chemical nature	Classification of nutraceuticals based on the mechanism of action

1. Traditional
  a. Probiotics
  b. Chemical constituent
  c. Nutraceutical enzyme
  d. Chemical constituents
  e. Nutrient
  f. Herbal
  g. Phytochemical
2. Non-traditional
  a. Fortified nutraceuticals
  b. Recombinant nutraceuticals
	1. Fatty acid
	2. Collagen hydrolysate
	3. Dietary fibers
	4. Fatty acids
	5. Flavonoids
	6. Glucosinolates
	7. Phenols
	8. Plant steroid
	9. Prebiotics
	10. Saponins
	11. Soy Proteins
	12. Phytoestrogens
	13. Sulfides
	14. Tannins
		1. Anticancer
		2. Positive impact of the lipid
		3. Antioxidant activity
		4. Anti-inflammatory activity
		5. Osteogenetic

11.2 Anemia

It is a chronic disease in which blood does not contain enough amount of red blood cells, which means low iron level in the body. Different vitamins play major roles, such as vitamin A, vitamin B12, vitamin C, vitamin E, folic acid, and riboflavin. With the help of vitamin nutraceuticals, we can control anemia [8]. According to the World Health Organization, an adult is identified as anemic if the concentration of the blood Hb falls below 13.0 g/dl. In nonpregnant women, haemoglobin concentration below the lower limit of normal are found to be a common reason in laboratory results [9]. Table 11.2 comprises types and causes of anemia.

11.2.1 Types of Anemia

Figure 11.1 comprising different types of anemia.
Types of anemia [11]

1. **Based on the Hb level**
   I. When the level of Hb is less than the 7, it is known as severe anemia.
   II. When the level of the Hb is 7 to 10 g/dl, it is known as moderate level.
2. **Based on the RBC morphology**
   I. Normochromic and normocytic anemias are due to
      a. Anemia of acute blood loss
      b. Increase hemolysis
      c. Chronic diseases causing anemia
   II. Hypochromic and microcytic anemias are due to:
      a. Due to decrease in iron level
      b. Thalassemia
   III. Normochromic and macrocytic anemias are due to:
      a. Decrease in vitamin B_{12}
      b. Insufficient folate

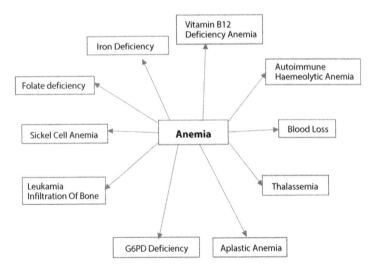

Figure 11.1 Types of anemia.

3. **Based on physiological abnormality:**
   I. Defective in the formation of RBCs
   II. Hemolytic anemia where is the increased breakdown of the RBCs.
   III. Imperfection because of an expansion in RBC forerunners when contrasted with the level of pallor.
4. **Based on etiology:**
   I. Expanded RBCs obliteration due to intra or additional red platelet abandons.
   II. Expanded blood misfortune, which might be intense or ongoing.
   III. Deficient RBCs arrangement because of Lake of elements important for erythropoiesis.
5. **Based on the category:**
   I. Increased erythrocytopenia.
   II. Blood loss anemia (nonimmune).
   III. Immune hemolysis anemia.
   IV. Related with the blood loss in the haemorrhage.
   V. Nutritional deficiency occurs due to decrease in the vitamin B_{12} and folate.
   VI. Toxicity due to drugs.
   VII. Infections.
   VIII. Infiltration of the bone marrow by the cancer cells.
   IX. Hematopoietic stem cell arrest or damage.
   X. Idiopathic.
6. **Based on RBC indices:**
   I. Normocytic:
      a. MCV is 80 to 100 fl (femtoliter).
      b. MCHC = 32% to 36%.
   II. Macrocytic:
      a. MCV = >100 fl.
   III. Microcytic and hypochromic.
      a. MCV = <80 fl.
      b. MCHC = <32%.

11.2.2 Causes of Anemia [12]

Table 11.2 Causes of anemia in intensive care.

Types of anemia	Causes of anemia
Blood Loss	Phlebotomy, Gastrointestinal Bleeding, Trauma, Surgery.
Erythropoietin Deficiencies	Inflammatory cytokines, Renal insufficiency Drugs, Decrease Bone Marrow response.
Nutritional Deficiencies	Low iron level, Low Folate Level, Low vitamin B level.
Hemolysis	Drugs Reactions, Toxins.
Coagulation Abnormalities	Sepsis syndrome, Thrombocytopenia, Liver Disease, Viral Infection, Splenomegaly.

11.3 Role of Vitamins in Nutraceuticals for Anemia

Anemia is the disorder cause mostly by deficiency of vitamins. Neutraceuticals enriched in vitamins can cure or prevent anemia. Vitamins play a vital role in anemia. The cause of anemia is iron deficiency and nutritional deficiency. According to the World Health Organization 30% world population affects anemia [13]. Vitamins deficiency in anemia leads to the lack of RBC, vitamins, such as iron, vitamin A, vitamin C, vitamin E, vitamin B_{12}, folate, and riboflavin, help cure or prevent anemia. Nowadays, doctors also recommend nutraceutical for anemia. Table 11.3 shows the types of vitamins and their roles [14]. Table 11.4 shows the Structures of Vitamins.

11.3.1 Role of Iron in Anemia as Nutraceutical

Iron is a mineral that is produced by red blood corpuscles that help to carry the oxygen in all body parts. When there is a decrease in the level of iron, it causes iron deficiency anemia, which results to fall down of oxygen supply in our body. With the help of iron, nutraceuticals play a vital role in managing iron deficiency anemia. Due to this, overall doctors suggest patients to take iron nutraceuticals. Eating foods that are rich in the iron also enhances iron level [15].

Administration of Iron
The administration of iron nutraceuticals is both orally as well as intravenously. Administration of iron through the oral route is effective in both

Table 11.3 Types of vitamins and their roles.

Sr. no.	Vitamin types	Possible role in anemia
1.	Vitamin A	Improve hematological iron
2.	Folic Acid	Cure megaloblastic anemia
3.	Vitamin B_{12}	Cure megaloblastic anemia
4.	Riboflavin	Enhance hematoligical response
5.	Vitamin C	Enhance absorption of dietary iron
6.	Vitamin E	Improve hemolytic anemia

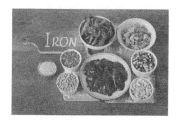

Figure 11.2 Sources of iron.

mild as well as moderate deficiency. On a daily basis, 100 to 200 mg iron is given. In severe cases, if oral fails, then iron is provided intravenously [16].

Sources of Iron
Most common sources of iron include spinach, lentils, broccoli, leafy greens, pumpkin seed, peas, legume, kidney beans, tofu, beef, egg, oysters, dark chocolate, sardine, navy beans; fruits, like tomato, cashews, are good sources of iron. Figure 11.2 shows the sources of iron [17].

11.3.2 Vitamin A

Vitamin A includes retinal, retinol, retinoic acid, and provitamin A carotenoids. Retinoic acid mostly found in animal tissues and is derived from the oxidation of retinol. In decrease of iron, neutraceuticals containing vitamin A enhance the absorption of iron in the stomach, beta carotene also helps in the increase absorption of iron [18, 19].

Vitamin A increases the growth of erythrocytes which is critical in the treatment of anemia. Vitamin A and beta carotene forms a complex with

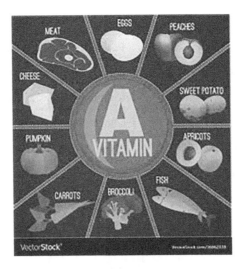

Figure 11.3 Sources of vitamin A.

an iron. Polyphenol and phytates affect the absorption of iron, it is also reduced by vitamin A and Beta carotene [20].

Sources of Vitamin A
Most common sources of vitamin A are carrot, sweet potato, liver, spinach, egg, cantaloupe, red ball paper, broccoli. Fruits, like mango, papaya, apricots, and grapefruits [10]. Enriched source of vitamin A is milk, oil containing source of vitamin a is cod liver oil, other vegetables containing rich source of vitamin A is pumpkin, kale, bitternut squash, salmon, most common rich source of vitamin A is egg yolk. Figure 11.3 shows vitamin A sources (Figure 11.3) [21].

11.3.3 Vitamin C

Iron from food is absorbed in intestinal mucosa 12 two ways. Iron consists of two parts hame and non-hame. Hame pare is absorbed easily but the non-hame part of iron is affected by diet. Here, vitamin C can improve the absorption of non-hame part of the iron. Vitamin C also suppresses the action of calcium and phosphate, which reduces absorption of non-hame part [22].

Ascorbic acid, which is vitamin C, forms a chelate with the ferric iron and enhances the absorption of the iron. Therefore taking vitamin C in the food and nutraceutical helps to treat or cure anemia [23].

Sources of Vitamin C
Most common sources of vitamin C include citrus fruits, like lemons and limes, peppers (red and green), oranges, kale, berries, sweet potatoes

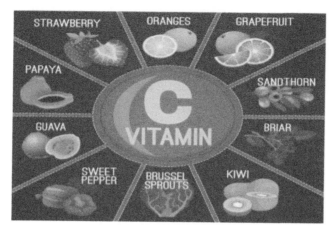

Figure 11.4 Sources of vitamin C.

vegetables, broccoli, tomato, Brussels sprouts, cauliflower, cabbage and raw and cooked leafy greens. Other fruits like strawberries, watermelon, papaya, grapes, kiwi, mango, and pineapple contain higher concentrations of vitamin C. Figure 11.4 shows sources of vitamin C [24].

11.3.4 Vitamin E

Vitamin E is a group of organic compounds that includes tocopherols and tocotrienols. Vitamin E exists in eight forms as a natural source like α, β, γ, and δ-tocopherols and α, β, γ, and δ-tocotrienols. The two common forms of vitamin E in the American diet are γ- and β-tocopherol. α-Tocopherol is mostly found in wheat germ and sunflower oil. γ-Tocopherol is mostly found in corn, soybean oil, and margarine [25].

Vitamin E is noted as an essential erythropoietic factor. Vitamin E enhances the erythropoiesis and Hb level, which is needed in the anemic condition. The need of vitamin E is fulfilled by nutraceuticals. Vitamin E reduces the oxidative stress which main cause of various types of anemia [26]. Vitamin E is a highly fat-soluble vitamin, has a property of cell membrane-stabilizing antioxidant and also works in the nonoxidant functioning. Vitamin E prevents the oxidation of the polyunsaturated fatty acid in the red blood cells [27].

Sources of Vitamin E

Most common sources (Figure 11.5) of vitamin E consist of spinach, almond, broccoli, peanuts, avocado, hazelnuts, wheat germ oil, and

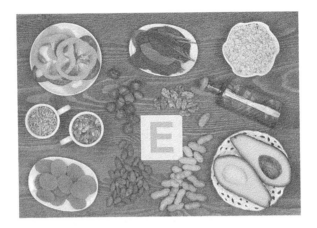

Figure 11.5 Sources of vitamin E.

sunflower seed. Fruits containing vitamin E, such as kiwifruit, mango, strawberry, pine nuts, oil containing vitamin E are olive oil, safflower oil, sunflower oil, and so on. Figure 11.5 shows sources of vitamin E [28].

11.3.5 Folate

We know that if there is not enough red blood corpuscles to transport oxygen in body tissue. There are chances of occurring anemia. Deficiency of hemoglobin leads to decreased amount of red blood carpusuls. Hemoglobin is a protein in RBC that carries oxygen. Folic acid helps to improve anemic condition by taking healthy diet, such as green leafy vegetables, breads, cereals and fruits. Folic acid works by forming new RBC that carries oxygen [29–32].

If a pregnant woman suffers from folic acid anemia, the baby born should cause serious defect like spina bifida in which the baby's spinal cord defected. Colon cancer and heart diseases are also cured by folic acid [33–36].

Sources of Folate
The good sources (Figure 11.6) of folate consist of broccoli, Brussels sprouts, leafy green vegetables, cabbage, kale, spring green, spinach, peas, chickpeas, kidney beans, peas, liver, breakfast cereals fortified with folic acid, and so on. Figure 11.6 shows sources of folate [37–40].

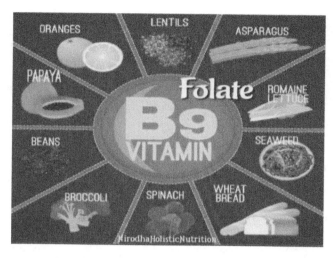

Figure 11.6 Sources of folate.

11.3.6 Vitamin B12

Vitamin B_{12} deficiency causes pernicious anemia. In this type of anemia, the body cannot make enough red blood cells due to the deficiency of vitamin B_{12}. Our body cannot make vitamin B_{12}, so there is a need to get vitamin B_{12} from food. Nutraceuticals help in supplying vitamin B_{12} and help to reduce anemic condition [41–43].

Sources of Vitamin B_{12}

Sources of vitamin B_{12} (Figure 11.7) includes liver, beef, chicken, clams, cereals, chicken breast, vegetables consist of broccoli, barley, fruits consist of banana, Brussels sprouts, other sources consist of asparagus, avocado, milk contains much amount of vitamin B_{12}. Figure 11.7 shows the sources of vitamin B_{12} [44–47].

11.3.7 Riboflavin

Riboflavin is required for many metabolic pathways. Riboflavin deficiency is common in areas where intakes of dairy products and meat are low and school children are a group at high risk for riboflavin deficiency. It appears that riboflavin deficiency, in addition to its other symptoms, may impair erythropoiesis [48–50].

Sources of Riboflavin

Large amount of riboflavin is found in milk, eggs, fortified breakfast cereals, plain yoghurt, and so on. Figure 11.8 shows the sources of riboflavin [51, 52–56].

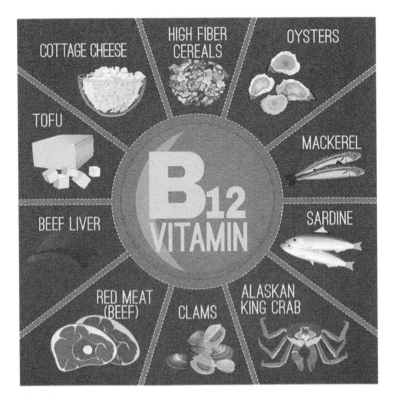

Figure 11.7 Sources of vitamin B_{12}.

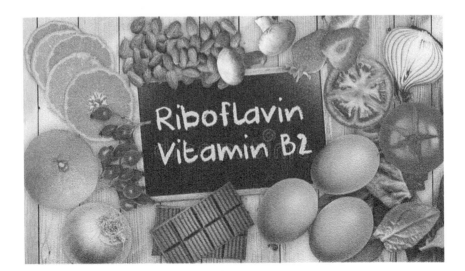

Figure 11.8 Sources of riboflavin.

11.4 Structure of Vitamins

Table 11.4 Name of vitamins with their structure.

Name of the vitamin	Structure of vitamins
Vitamin A 1. Retinol	
2. Retinal	
3. Retinoic acid	
4. Beta-carotene	

(Continued)

Table 11.4 Name of vitamins with their structure. (*Continued*)

Name of the vitamin	Structure of vitamins
Vitamin B-complex 1. Vitamin B_1 (Thiamine)	(structure)
2. Vitamin B_2 (Riboflavin)	(structure)
3. Vitamin B_3 (Niacine amide)	(structure)

(*Continued*)

Table 11.4 Name of vitamins with their structure. (*Continued*)

Name of the vitamin	Structure of vitamins
4. Vitamin B_5 (Pantothenic acid)	
5. Vitamin B_6 (Pyridoxine)	

(*Continued*)

Table 11.4 Name of vitamins with their structure. (*Continued*)

Name of the vitamin	Structure of vitamins
6. Vitamin B_7 (Biotin)	
7. Vitamin B_9 (Folic acid)	

(*Continued*)

Table 11.4 Name of vitamins with their structure. (*Continued*)

Name of the vitamin	Structure of vitamins
8. Vitamin B_{12} (Cobalamin)	
Vitamin C (Ascorbic acid)	

(*Continued*)

Table 11.4 Name of vitamins with their structure. (*Continued*)

Name of the vitamin	Structure of vitamins
Vitamin D 1. Vitamin D_2 (Ergocalciferol)	
2. Vitamin D_3 (Cholecalciferol)	

(*Continued*)

Table 11.4 Name of vitamins with their structure. (*Continued*)

Name of the vitamin	Structure of vitamins
Vitamin E 1. Alpha-Tocopherol	(chemical structure of alpha-tocopherol)
2. Beta-Tocopherol	(chemical structure of beta-tocopherol)
3. Gamma-Tocopherol	(chemical structure of gamma-tocopherol)

(*Continued*)

Table 11.4 Name of vitamins with their structure. (*Continued*)

Name of the vitamin	Structure of vitamins
4. Delta-Tocopherol	(structure)
5. Alpha-Tocotrienol	(structure)
6. Beta-Tocotrienol	(structure)
7. Gamma-Tocotrienol	(structure)

(*Continued*)

Table 11.4 Name of vitamins with their structure. (*Continued*)

Name of the vitamin	Structure of vitamins
8. Delta-Tocotrienol	
Vitamin K	
1. Vitamin K_1 (Phylloquinone)	
2. Vitamin K_2 (Menaquinone)	

(*Continued*)

Table 11.4 Name of vitamins with their structure. (*Continued*)

Name of the vitamin	Structure of vitamins
3. Vitamin K_3 (Menadione)	![structure of menadione: 1,4-naphthoquinone with CH₃ at position 2]

11.5 Conclusion

Nutritional deficiency anemia is a usual complication. It can happen when the body does not compell sufficient iron folate or vitamin B12 from diet. Vitamins as a nutraceutical plays vital role in preventing the different types of anemia. They help to improve iron level in blood. Folate and vitamin B12 prevent megaloblastic anemia. Riboflavin amplifies the hematological response to iron, and its deficiency may account for notable proportion of anemia in many people. The presented chapter helps us to know in detail about the vitamins. The chapter gives us brief idea about the nutraceuticals. Overview of anemia is also discussed in this chapter. The role of vitamins as a nutraceutical on anemia or anemic condition is reported.

Acknowledgment

The authors thank M.G.V's Samajshri Prashant Dada Hiray, College of Pharmacy, Malegaon Nashik, India.

References

1. Defelice, S.L., The nutraceutical evolution:s Its impact on food industry R and D. *Trends Food Sci. Technol.*, 6, 59–61, 1995.
2. The role of vitamins in prevention and control of anemia. *Public Health Nutr.*, 3, 2, 125–50, 2000.
3. Debra, S., Lights, V., Schulman, J.S., Medically Review, 2021.
4. Raman, D., Nutraceuticals for healthy life. *Indian J. Pharm. Educ. Res.*, 51, 3, 148–151, 2017.
5. Nutraceutical: New era's. *Pharmaceutical's J. Pharm. Res.*, 3, 1243–1247.
6. Bhat, S.G., Ascorbic acid: New role of an age-old micronutrient in the management of periodontal disease in older adults. *Geriatr. Gerontol. Int.*, 15, 241–254, 2015.
7. Nazanin, A., Richard, H., Roya, K., Review on iron and its importance for human health, 2014.
8. Shu, E.N. and Ogbodo, S.O., Role of ascorbic acid I the prevention of iron deficiency anaemia in pregnancy. *Biomed. Res.*, 16, 1, 40–44, 2005.
9. Sommer, A. and West, K.P., *Vitamin A Deficiency: Health, Survival and Vision*, Oxford University Press, New York, 1996.
10. Mejia, L.A. and Arroyave, G., The effect of vitamin A fortification of sugar on iron metabolism in preschool children in Guatemala. *Am. J. Clin. Nutr.*, 36, 87–93, 1982.

11. Koefler, H.P. and Amatruda, T.T., The effect of retinoids on haemopoiesis clinical and laboratory studies, in: *Retinoids, Differentiation, and Disease*, Pitman (Ed.), pp. 252–73, Ciba Foundation Symposium, London, 1985.
12. Amatruda, T.T. and Koefler, H.P., Retinoids and cells of the hematopoietic system, in: *Retinoids and Cell Differentiation*, M.I. Sherman, (Ed.), pp. 80–103, CRC Press, Boca Raton, Florida, 1986.
13. Jelkmann, W., Pagel, H., Hellwig, T., Fandrey, J., Effects of antioxidant vitamins on renal and hepatic erythropoietin production. *Kidney Int.*, 51, 497–501, 1997.
14. Mejia, L.A., Hodges, R.E., Rucker, R.B., Role of vitamin A in the absorption, retention, and distribution of iron in the rat. *J. Nutr.*, 109, 129–37, 1979.
15. Semba, R.D., Vitamin A, immunity, and infection. *Clin. Infect. Dis.*, 19, 489–99, 1994.
16. Bloem, M.W., Interdependence of vitamin A and iron: an important association for programmes of anaemia control. *Proc. Nutr. Soc.*, 54, 501–8, 1995.
17. Garcia-Casal, M.N., Layrisse, M., Solano, L., Vitamin A and b-carotene can improve nonheme iron absorption from rice, wheat, and corn by humans. *J. Nutr.*, 128, 646–50, 1997.
18. Layrisse, M., Garcia-Casal, M.N., Solano, L., Vitamin A reduces the inhibition of iron absorption by phytates and polyphenols. *Food Nutr. Bull.*, 19, 3–5, 1998.
19. Baldwin, C. and Olarewaju, O., Hemolytic anemia, in: *StatPearls*, StatPearls Publishing, Treasure Island, FL, USA, 2020.
20. Phillips, J. and Henderson, A.C., Hemolytic anemia: Evaluation and differential diagnosis. *Am. Fam. Physician*, 98, 354–361, 2018.
21. Khan, I. and Shaikh, H., Cooley anemia, in: *StatPearls*, StatPearls Publishing, Treasure Island, FL, USA, 2020.
22. Mariani, R., Trombini, P., Pozzi, M., Piperno, A., Iron metabolism in thalassemia and sickle cell disease. *Mediterr. J. Hematol. Infect.*, 2, 9–6, 2009.
23. Fung, E.B., Harmatz, P., Milet, M., Ballas, S.K., Multi-center study of iron overload research group. Morbidity and mortality in chronically transfused subjects with thalassemia and sickle cell disease: A report from the multi-center study of iron overload. *Am. J. Hematol.*, 82, 255–265, 2007.
24. Svobodová, A., Walterova, D., Psotova, J., Influence of silymarin and its flavonolignans on H2O2-induced oxidative stress in human keratinocytes and mouse fibroblasts. *Burns*, 32, 973–979, 2006.
25. Alidoost, F., Gharagozloo, M., Bagherpour, B., Jafarian, A., Effects of silymarin on the proliferation and glutathione levels of peripheral blood mononuclear cells from beta-thalassemia major patients. *Int. Immunopharmacol.*, 6, 1305–1310, 2006.
26. Cunningham-Rundles, S., Giardina, P.J., Grady, R.W., Califano, C., Effect of transfusional iron overload on immune response. *J. Infect. Dis.*, 182, 115–121, 2000.

27. Ezer, U., Gulderen, F., Çulha, V.K., Akgul, N., Gurbuz, O., Immunological status of thalassemia syndrome. *Pediatr. Hematol. Oncol. J.*, 19, 51–58, 2002.
28. Loizzo, M.R., Tundis, R., Menichini, F., Pugliese, A., Bonesi, M., Chelating, antioxidant and hypoglycaemic potential of Muscari comosum (L.) mill. bulb extracts. *Int. J. Food Sci. Nutr.*, 61, 780–791, 2010.
29. Jomova, K. and Valko, M., Importance of iron chelation in free radical-induced oxidative stress and human disease. *Curr. Pharm. Des.*, 17, 3460–3473, 2011.
30. Hatcher, H.C., Singh, R.N., Torti, F.M., Torti, S.V., Synthetic and natural iron chelators: Therapeutic potential and clinical use. *Future Med. Chem.*, 1, 1643–1670, 2009.
31. Gazak, R., Walterova, D., Kren, V., Silybin and silymarin: New and emerging applications in medicine. *Curr. Med. Chem.*, 14, 315–338, 2007.
32. Darvishi, K.H., Salehifar, E., Kosaryan, M., Aliasgharian, A., Jalali, H., Potential effects of silymarin and its flavonolignan components in patients with β-thalassemia major: A comprehensive review in 2015. *Adv. Pharmacol. Sci.*, 304–307, 2015.
33. Gharagozloo, M., Karimi, M., Amirghofran, Z., Immunomodulatory effects of silymarin in patients with β-thalassemia major. *Int. Immunopharmacol.*, 16, 243–247, 2013.
34. Moayedi, B., Gharagozloo, M., Esmaeil, N., Maracy, M.R., Hoorfar, H., Jalaeikar, M., A randomized double-blind, placebocontrolled study of therapeutic effects of silymarin in β-thalassemia major patients receiving desferrioxamine. *Eur. J. Haematol.*, 90, 202–209.
35. Hagag, A., Elfaragy, M., Elrifaey, S., Abd El-Lateef, A., Therapeutic value of combined therapy with deferiprone and silymarin as iron chelators in Egyptian children with beta thalassemia major. *Infect. Disord. Drug Targets*, 15, 189–195, 2015.
36. Hagag, A.A., Elfrargy, M.S., Gazar, R.A., Abd El-Lateef, A., Therapeutic value of combined therapy with deferasirox and silymarin on iron overload in children with beta thalassemia. *Mediterr. J. Hematol. Infect. Dis.*, 5, 1–7, 2013.
37. Marks, P.W., Anemia: Clinical approach, in: *Concise Guide to Hematology*, H.M. Lazarus and A.H. Schmaier (Eds.), pp. 21–27, Springer, Cham, Switzerland, 2019.
38. Forget, B.G. and Bunn, H.F., Classification of the disorders of hemoglobin. *Cold Spring Harb. Perspect. Med.*, 3, 11684, 2013.
39. Imaga, N.A., Phytomedicines and nutraceuticals: Alternative therapeutics for sickle cell anemia. *Sci. World J.*, 269–659, 2013.
40. Ameh, S.J., Tarfa, F.D., Ebeshi, B.U., Traditional herbal management of sickle cell anemia: Lessons from Nigeria. *Anemia*, 60–74, 2012.
41. Oniyangi, O. and Cohall, D.H., Phytomedicines (medicines derived from plants) for sickle cell disease. *Cochrane Database Syst. Rev.*, 15–20, 2015.

42. Abraham, D.J., Mehanna, A.S., Wireko, F.C., Whitney, J., Thomas, R.P., Orringer, E.P., Vanillin, a potential agent for the treatment of sickle cell anemia. 77, 1334–1341, 1997.
43. Silva, D.G.H. and Belini, E., Oxidative stress in sickle cell disease: An overview of erythrocyte redox metabolism and current antioxidant therapeutic strategies. *Free Radic. Biol. Med.*, 65, 1101–1109, 2013.
44. Al Balushi, H., Hannemann, A., Rees, D., Brewin, J., Gibson, J.S., The effect of antioxidants on the properties of red blood cells from patients with sickle cell anemia. *Front. Physiol.*, 10, 976, 2019.
45. Cristina, M.J. and Ferreira, M.S., Investigation of cytotoxic, apoptosis-inducing, genotoxic and protective effects of the flavonoid rutin in HTC hepatic cells. *Exp. Toxicol. Pathol.*, 63, 459–465, 2011.
46. Nafees, S., Rashid, S., Ali, N., Hasan, S.K., Sultana, S., Rutin ameliorates cyclophosphamide induced oxidative stress and inflammation in wistar rats: Role of NFκB/MAPK pathway. *Chem. Biol. Interact.*, 231, 98–107, 2015.
47. Guo, R., Wei, P., Liu, W., Combined antioxidant effects of rutin and vitamin C in triton X-100 micelles. *J. Pharm. Biomed. Anal.*, 43, 1580–1586, 2007.
48. Muhammad, A., Waziri, A.D., Forcados, G.E., Sanusi, B., Sani, H., Sickling-preventive effects of rutin is associated with modulation of deoxygenated haemoglobin, 2,3- bisphosphoglycerate mutase, redox status and alteration of functional chemistry in sickle erythrocytes. *Heliyon*, 5, 1905, 2019.
49. Segel, G.B. and Lichtman, M.A., Aplastic anemia: Acquired and inherited, in: *Williams Hematology*, 8th ed, K. Kaushansky, and W.J. Williams, (Eds.), pp. 569–590, McGraw-Hill Medical, New York, NY, USA, 2010.
50. Scheinberg, P. and Chen, J., Aplastic anemia: What have we learned from animal models and from the clinic. *Semin. Hematol.*, 50, 156–164, 2013.
51. Ahire, E.D., Sonawane, V.N., Surana, K.R., Talele, G.S., Drug discovery, drug-likeness screening, and bioavailability: Development of drug-likeness rule for natural products, in: *Applied pharmaceutical Practice and Nutraceuticals*, pp. 191–208, Apple Academic Press, 2021.
52. Surana, K.R., Ahire, E.D., Sonawane, V.N., Talele, S.G., Talele, G.S., Molecular modeling: Novel techniques in food and nutrition development, in: *Natural Food Products and Waste Recovery*, pp. 17–31, Apple Academic Press, 2021.
53. Keservani, R.K., Kesharwani, R.K., Vyas, N., Jain, S., Raghuvanshi, R., Sharma, A.K., Nutraceutical and functional food as future food: A review. *Der Pharm. Lett.*, 2, 1, 106–116, 2010a.
54. Keservani, R.K., Kesharwani, R.K., Sharma, A.K., Vyas, N., Chadoker, A., Nutritional supplements: An overview. *Int. J. Curr. Pharm. Rev. Res.*, 1, 1, 59–75, 2010b.

55. Keservani, R.K., Sharma, A.K., Kesharwani, R.K., An overview and therapeutic applications of nutraceutical and functional foods, in: *Recent Advances in Drug Delivery Technology*, pp. 160–201, 2017.
56. Keservani, R.K., Sharma, A.K., Kesharwani, R.K. (Eds.), *Nutraceuticals and Dietary Supplements: Applications in Health Improvement and Disease Management*, CRC Press, 2020.

12
Vitamins as Nutraceuticals for Oral Health

Tushar N. Lokhande[1], Snehal D. Pawar[2]*, Snehal S. Kolpe[2], Khemchand R. Surana[3], Smita C. Bonde[4] and Sunil K. Mahajan[1]

[1]*Mahatma Gandhi Vidyamandir Pharmacy College, Panchavati, Nashik, India*
[2]*MGV's Samajshri Prashant Dada Hiray, College of Pharmacy, Malegaon, Nashik, India*
[3]*Shreeshakti Shaikshanik Sanstha, Divine College of Pharmacy, Satana, Nashik, India*
[4]*School of Pharmacy and Tech. Management, Mukesh Patel Technology Park, Babulde, Shirpur, Dist: Dhule, Maharashta, India*

Abstract

The vitamins are well known used according to medicinal perspective but there is no scientific clarification about use of vitamins for the purpose of oral health as nutraceuticals. Nutraceuticals are products which has various physiological benefits and it protect against different chronic diseases. They are nutrient that prevent diseases. They are different from pharmaceuticals where drugs are used in treatment of diseases. Though there is no scientific clarification in brief that clarifies vitamins as nutraceuticals for oral health. There are different types of vitamins which help in prevention of oral diseases and improving oral health. The present study helps us to understand nutraceuticals, vitamins and role of vitamins as nutraceutical for oral health.

Keywords: Vitamins, nutraceuticals, oral health, dental health

---

Corresponding author: snehal.pawar152295@gmail.com

Eknath D. Ahire, Raj K. Keservani, Khemchand R. Surana, Sippy Singh and Rajesh K. Kesharwani (eds.) *Vitamins as Nutraceuticals: Recent Advances and Applications*, (281–300) © 2023 Scrivener Publishing LLC

12.1 Introduction

The term "Nutraceutical" was termed by combination of two words "nutrition" and "pharmaceutical" by Stephen L. Defelice, MD, founder and chairman of the foundation for Innovation in Medicine (FIM), Cranford, NJ, in 1989 [1–3]. He also defined nutraceuticals as a "food or part of food which provides medicinal and health benefits which includes the prevention and treatment of various diseases and are made from botanical raw materials [4, 5]. As per AAFCO 1996, 'Nutrient' is a feed constituent which is in a form and at a level that will result in the sustain a life of human being or animal whereas 'Nutraceutical' means any of the non-toxic food constituent that has scientifically proven health benefits together with prevention as well as the treatment of diseases. Products are isolated or purified from food which is available in medicinal forms not usually related with food. A nutraceutical has benefit of providing protection against chronic diseases [6]. Nutraceuticals are the products that are other than nutrition which are also used as medicine [7]. The term nutraceutical is used commonly in marketing. It does not have regulatory definition [8]. Canada's health ministry additionally described nutraceuticals because the product that is isolated or that is purified from the food or food sources, this is commonly bought in medicinal form that isn't assisted with food and are verified to have a physiological advantage and which gives safety towards the persistent diseases [9]. Nutraceuticals are regulated through FDA that is beneathneath authority of the Federal Food Drug and Cosmetics Act [10]. The idea of Nutraceuticals drew back about 3000 years ago. Hippocrates (460–377 B.C) allows meals are thy medication and medication is thy meals. Early withinside the 1900s the us producers introduced the small amount of iodine into salt with a view to save you goiter [11]. The generally used opportunity remedy is nutritional dietary supplements which incorporates nutraceuticals and medicinal herbs as said through Merck Manual. 6.1 billion people which is nearly two third part of the total world's population simply rely on healing power of plant base materials for many reasons includes availability, affordability, safety, belief (Traditional affordability) or belief in traditional cures [12]. As medicinal benefits of food have been explored since for thousands of years, development of nutraceutical industry began during the 1980s [13].

The medical and health industries of these centuries have enclosed nutraceutical for different products and option for treatment of diseases. In countries like US, Europe and Japan the nutraceuticals have become a million dollars industry. They are the products that gives single or multiple ingredients together. They are available in the form of herbal products or are genetically engineered as food products. Process foods also contain nutraceutical with addition of nutrients [14]. Nutraceutical are products which are used to improve health, also help in delaying ageing process, prevent chronic diseases, it increases life expectancy or support function and structure of body [15]. Substances in nutraceuticals include natural diet, herbal products, biofortified crops, genetically engineered and process food products [16].

Nutraceuticals are already becoming part of dietary landscape in England, Japan and other countries. Germany, France, and UK were first to consider diet as it is a more important factor rather than exercise or hereditary factors for getting good health [17].

12.1.1 Nutraceuticals Categorized Based on Food Available in Market

1. Traditional nutraceuticals [18]
   a) Chemical constituents
      i. Nutrients: They include amino acids, fatty acids, minerals and vitamins with known nutritional functions.
      ii. Herbals: Herbal nutraceuticals are useful to enhance fitness and prevent chronic diseases. Most of those consist of analgesic, anti-inflammatory, astringent, antipyretic and antiarthritic.
      iii. Phytochemicals: Phytochemicals are plant nutrients which have a particular biological action thataid human health [19].
      iv. Polyunsaturated fatty acids (PUFAs).
   b) Probiotics and prebiotics: Probiotics mean 'for life' [20].
   c) Nutraceutical enzymes: Those Enzymes are enzymes which can be derived from plant, animal and microbial sources.
2. Non-traditional nutraceuticals
   a) Fortified nutraceuticals
   b) Recombinant nutraceuticals
3. Commercial Nutraceuticals
   a) Dietary supplements
   b) Functional food
   c) Medicinal food [21–23]

Difference between nutraceuticals and pharmaceuticals (Table 12.1):

Table 12.1 Difference between nutraceuticals and pharmaceuticals [24].

Sr. no.	Nutraceutical	Pharmaceutical
1	There is inhibition of the diseases.	There is treatment of the diseases.
2	Long term application or effects.	Short term application or effects.
3	Weak interaction with target.	Strong interaction with target.
4	Low potency.	High potency.

Difference between nutraceuticals and functional foods (Table 12.2):

Table 15.2 Difference between functional foods and nutraceuticals.

Sr. no.	Functional foods	Nutraceuticals
1	Natural.	Natural or synthetic and available as piils, capsules or liquids.
2	Naturally contains bioactive compounds found in foods.	The bioactive compounds from fortified food, dietary supplement/herbal products.
3	The bioactive component in them is different from traditional nutrients.	Include traditional nutrients.

The reason for shift towards nutraceuticals is [25–28]

1. The consumer concern about healthcare costs has been increase.
2. Nutraceuticals helps consumer by improving, sustaining the proper functioning of the body.
3. The healthcare providers found that fact that heavy process food of ours are coming from crops which are grown using chemical fertilizers, pesticides, herbicides and also genetically modified seed which has less sufficient nutrients present which are required for good health.
4. Now day's peoples focus on prevention of diseases rather than cure.

5. The people that may have chronic disease and they had not got any good results from allopathic medicines.
6. People with less economic conditions [25–28].

12.2 Vitamins

Vitamins are mainly classes of molecules that play a vital role in the metabolism in order to fulfill all the nutritional value of food and it is sometimes necessary to add those vitamins during processing [29]. The term diet became coined in 1912 by the polish biochemist Casimir Funk from "vitamine", a compound phrase even as operating on the Lister Institute of Preventive Medicine. They are institution of molecules wanted for everyday cell function, increase and development [30]. Vitamins are catalysts for metabolic reactions which uses proteins, fats as well as carbohydrates.

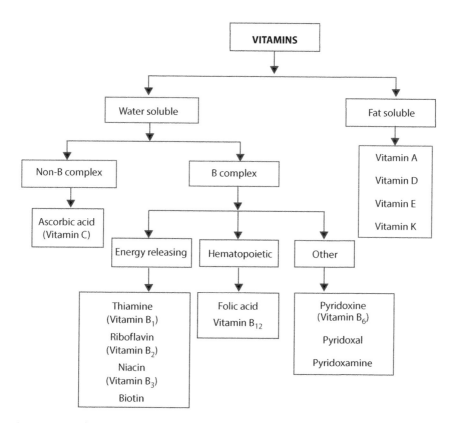

Figure 12.1 Classification of vitamin based on solubility.

For energy, growth and for the cell maintenance [31]. In total there are 13 essential vitamins which are required for body to work properly. Based on solubility vitamins are classified in below Figure 12.1.

Vitamin is classified into two categories based on how they are absorbed. Water soluble vitamins B and C dissolve in water upon entering the body. Vitamins A, C, D, E, and K which are fat soluble vitamins are stored in liver and fats tissues as reserved. Each vitamin play different role in the body and person requires a specific or different amount of each vitamin to stay fit and healthy [32, 33].

12.2.1 History of Vitamins

The year wise discovery of vitamins is listed below (Table 12.3) [34].

Table 12.3 List of vitamins with the year of discovery.

Sr. no.	Vitamin	Year of discovery
1	Vitamin A (Retinol)	1913
2	Vitamin B_1 (Thiamine)	1910
3	Vitamin C (Ascorbic acid)	1920
4	Vitamin D (Calciferol)	1920
5	Vitamin B_2 (Riboflavin)	1920
6	Vitamin E (Tocopherol)	1922
7	Vitamin K_1 (Phylloquinone)	1929
8	Vitamin B_5 (Pantothenic acid)	1931
9	Vitamin B_6 (Pyridoxine)	1934
10	Vitamin B_7 (Biotin)	1936
11	Vitamin B_3 (Niacin)	1936
12	Vitamin B_9 (Folic acid)	1941
13	Vitamin B_{12} (Cobalamins)	1948

12.2.2 Importance of Vitamins for Humans

Vitamins are very important substances necessary for humans who cannot be consolidate by them or only in limited quantities. They are obtained from human diet. The vitamin deficiency is not only caused due to insufficient food requirements but also because of poor absorption, inadequate utilization, people who are on diet or smokers. It helps to boost immune system [35].

12.3 Role of Vitamins as Nutraceutical for Oral Health

The root cause of gum diseases lies in poor nutritional support which is due to weakened immune system. As the result there is need to meet all the nutritional requirements of the oral cavity while recovering from the dental treatment. Now days tested dentists as well as hygienists have been recommending dental nutraceuticals to the patients to maintain good oral health. Dental nutraceutical consisting of nutrition and pharmaceuticals which is in the form of food it helps to build up the bones and the teeth [36].

The role of vitamin is very well known in a medical perspective but the scientific evidences in accordance to the oral health is not yet clarified properly [37]. It is general knowledge that the vitamins play a vital effect on oral as well as general health. Its imbalance leads to malnutrition. The chewing process allows one to extract more quantity of nutrients and number of distribution of teeth effect the chewing efficacy [38].

12.3.1 Vitamins Associated with the Oral Health as Nutraceuticals

12.3.3.1 Vitamin C (Ascorbic Acid)

Vitamin is water soluble. The bodily concentration is balance by the consumption of vitamin C because humans are not able to synthesized ascorbic acid de nova. This vitamin is very good antioxidant and it is free radical scavenger which helps to protect our tissues, cell membrane and DNA from oxidative damages. Vitamin C is an enzyme cofactor that refers to dehydroascorbic acid. Vitamin C is involved in biochemical reactions, which catalyzed by monooxygenases, dioxygenases [39, 40].

Vitamin C has multiple benefits out of which is keeping the connective tissues in the mouth healthy. If the body lacks the vitamin C, the teeth become fragile, loose and more susceptible to developing the gum diseases. As study done by Eydouetal shows that the vitamin C plays vital role in preventing the development of the dental caries [41]. The role of Vitamin C in oral health is not yet studied in depth and detail [42, 43].

Sources of Vitamin C: Most common sources of vitamin C include citrus fruits like lemons and limes, peppers (red and green), oranges, kale, berries, sweet potatoes vegetables, broccoli, tomato, Brussels sprouts, cauliflower, cabbage and raw and cooked leafy greens. Another fruit like strawberries, watermelon, papaya, grapes, kiwi, mango and pineapple contain higher concentrations of vitamin C. Meat organs (liver, kidney and heart) are also good sources of vitamin C Figure 12.2 [44, 45].

Vitamin C Deficiency in Oral Health: Role of vitamin C is stimulating collagen synthesis by increasing the transcription of procollagen genes. Collagen is a major component of the gingival connective tissue. Because of that, vitamin C leads to osteoblast differentiation and periodontal ligament differentiation. Severe vitamin C deficiency results in scurvy. Some of the clinical features include: petechiae, ecchymosis, coiled hairs, follicular hyperkeratosis, bleeding gums, perifollicular haemorrhages, joint effusions, arthralgia, and impaired wound healing [46].

(The Figure 12.2 shows vitamin C rich food, it includes citrous fruits like orange and lemons, banana, broccoli, peppers, potatoes, brussels sprout, amla).

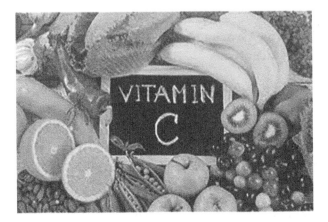

Figure 12.2 Vitamin C rich fruits.

12.3.3.2 Vitamin D

If the body has insufficient levels of vitamin D, it will prevent body from absorbing calcium as efficiently. Vitamin D plays significant role in keeping teeth healthy. Vitamin D is obtained through sunlight after siting in sun for at least 15 minutes a day, which is adequate for soaking vitamin D. Vitamin D is a hormone produced by the photolytic action of solar UVB light on the 7-dehydro-cholesterol present on the skin. It is also called as 1, 25-dihydroxyvitamin D or calcitriol and is found in the diet and supplements (Ergocalciferol and Cholecalciferol) [47].

Sources of Vitamin D: Natural sunlight organ meats (liver), fatty fish (salmon, sardines, herring, pilchards and tuna), egg yolks, fish oils and dairy products like milk and yogurt shown in Figure 12.3.

Vitamin D Deficiency in Oral Health: Vitamin D is responsible for the maintenance of calcium/phosphate homeostasis, regulation of bone remodelling, and modulation of cell proliferation and differentiation. Severe vitamin D deficiency has been associated with rickets, osteoporosis, osteomalacia, myopathy, severe hyperparathyroidism, impaired immune and cardiacfunctions, and death. Vitamin D deficiency is due to inadequate intake of vitamin D rich foods and sunlight exposure. Vitamin D deficiency causes liver, kidney and bowel diseases. In children vitamin D deficiency has been reported in with inflammatory bowel disease. Its deficiency effects on dental calcified tissues. Children who are affected with dental rickets have the risk of presenting with nonsyndromic

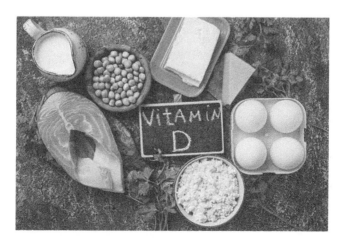

Figure 12.3 Sources of Vitamin D.

dentinogenesis and amelogenesis imperfecta. In some cases, vitamin D resistant rickets, the vitamin D receptor functions are affected and permanent teeth may develop enamel hypoplasia and hypomineralization defects giving them an abnormal shape [48]. The Figure 12.3 shows vitamin D rich food, it includes fish, eggs, fortifiedmilk, cheese, butter, cereal.

12.3.3.3 Vitamin E

Vitamin E is a group of organic compounds, which includes tocopherols and tocotrienols. Vitamin E exists in eight forms as a natural source like α, β, γ, and δ-tocopherols and α, β, γ, and δ-tocotrienols. The two common forms of vitamin E in the American diet are γ and β-tocopherol. α-Tocopherol is mostly found in wheat germ and sunflower oil. γ-Tocopherol is mostly found in corn, soybean oil and margarine. Because of vitamin E anti inflammatory properties scientists suspect a link between this essential vitamin and the prevention of gum diseases [49].

Sources of Vitamin E: Wheat germ, vegetable oil, seeds and nut, fish, and avocados shown in Figure 12.4.

Vitamin E Deficiency in Oral Health: In Vitamin E, α-tocopherol, act as antioxidant in the glutathione peroxidase pathway. It alsopreventscell membranes from oxidation by reacting it with radicals produced in the lipid peroxidation chain reaction. Its functions include serving as an antioxidant, a regulator for enzymatic activity and gene expression. It is involved

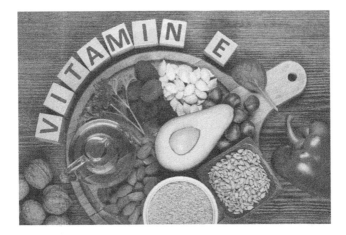

Figure 12.4 Vitamin E sources.

in supporting eye and neurological function, as well as in the inhibition of platelet coagulation. Vitamin E deficiency is due to inadequate supply of dietary fats and fat-soluble nutrients. Diseases include cystic fibrosis, pancreatitis, and cholestasis, loss of muscular mass, anaemia, delayed growth, and poor outcomes during pregnancy for both the infantand the mother. Its effects on oral health are not as clear as those of other vitamin [50]. The Figure 12.4 shows vitamin E rich food, it includes avocado, sunflower oils, wheat germ oil, almonds, spinach, and pumpkin.

12.3.3.4 Vitamin K (MKs)

Vitamin K is critical nutrient for oral and dental health. It helps oral microbiome in balance, prevents cavities and support remineralization Vitamin K is related to the γ-glutamyl carboxylase activity. These compounds existin two forms on the basis of synthesis, vitamin K1 (synthesized from green plants) and MKs (synthesized from anaerobic bacteria). MK series of vitamin or menaquinones are produced by anaerobic bacteria. Various forms of menaquinones or MKs have been identified, but only MK 7, 8 and 9 are produced by bacteria in the human colon. The other MK-4 menaquinone necessary for human metabolism and it is found in animal tissues such as the liver and blood vessels [51].

Sources of Vitamin K: Green, leafy vegetables like collards, spinach and broccoli. It can also be found in some fats and oils, like soybean oil and canola oil. MKs can be found in cheese and fermented soyabean products [51].

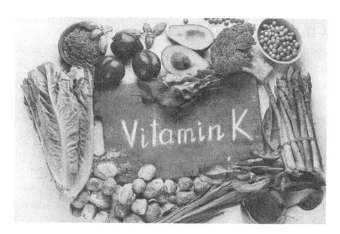

Figure 12.5 Vitamin K_2 sources.

Vitamin K Deficiency in Oral Health: Vitamin K has their roles in blood coagulation, bone metabolism and atherosclerosis prevention. Deficiency of vitamin K in adults produces occult bleeding and abnormal blood coagulation. In infant's vitamin K deficiency causes haemorrhagic disease of the new born, or bleeding. There are some oral complications due to vitamin K deficiency, except for haemorrhage after oral injury or surgery. This must be taken into consideration in patients on vitamin K antagonist medications [52]. The Figure 12.5 shows vitamin K_2 rich food, it includes broccoli, spinach, kale, Brussels sprouts, cabbage, lettuce, and blueberry.

12.3.3.5 Vitamin A

Vitamin A plays very crucial role in measles, oral leukoplakia, oral submucous fibrosis, growth promotion and wound healing in oral cavity. It is important for maintaining oral cavity lining, bone growth, normal cell development and permits normal tooth spacing. It also plays an important role in stimulating salivary glands that helps to prevent tooth decay by washing away bacteria inside the mouth. As a result, we should ensure that the mouth is moist that is best line for defense [53].

Vitamin A includes retinal, retinol, retinoic acid and provitamin A carotenoids. Retinoic acid mostly found in animal tissues and is derived from the oxidation of retinol. Retinal is a polyene chromophore, and is bound to a set of proteins called as opsins. Carotenoids are organic pigments produced by plants, algae, fungi, and bacteria [54, 55].

Sources of Vitamin A: Vitamin A found in sweet potatoes, yams, peppers, kale, eggs yolk and fish as shown in Figure 12.6.
Vitamin A Deficiency in Oral Health: A decrease consumption of vitamin A reasons reduced oral epithelial tissue development, impaired teeth formation, teeth hypoplasia and the presence of periodontitis. Vitamin A is needed to assist cell differentiation, hold epithelial integrity, red blood cell production, and duplicate additionally increase resistance in opposition to infections. Vitamin A deficiency constitutes a major health problem, which mostly seen in developing countries. Severe vitamin A deficiency causes vision problems (xeroph thalmia). Some time observed that even moderate vitamin A deficiency may impair vaccine elicited immunity for certain types of vaccines. Vitamin A deficiency is due to lack of vitamin A rich foods. It is often present among populations whose diets do not include sufficient animal products. It may be

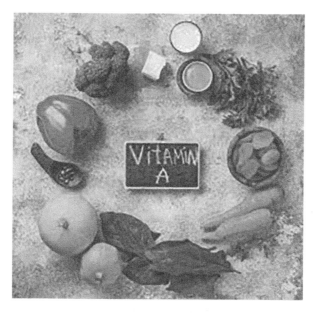

Figure 12.6 Vitamin A source.

further problem like measles, diarrhoea and respiratory infections [56]. The Figure 12.6 shows vitamin A rich food, it includes broccoli, carrots, curly kale, cheese, yogurt, egg yolks.

12.3.3.6 Vitamin B-Complex

Vitamin B complex includes thiamine (vitamin B1), riboflavin (vitamin B2), niacin (vitamin B3), pantothenic acid (vitamin B5), pyridoxine (vitamin B6), biotin (vitamin B7 or B8), and folic acid (vitamin B9) andcobalamin (vitamin B12). Vitamin B complex is necessary for cell growthand metabolism but each member of the B-complex has a different structureand performs different functions. Vitamins B1, B2, B3, and biotin involved energy production, vitamin B6 is essential for amino acidmetabolism, and vitamin B12 and folic acid facilitate steps required forcellular division. The relationship between vitamin B12 deficiency and oral health still remains unclear. Vitamin B12 is one of the most important micronutrients for brain developmentand their function. Vitamins prevent sores and oral inflammation including canker sores inflammed gums and other injuries inside mouth [57].

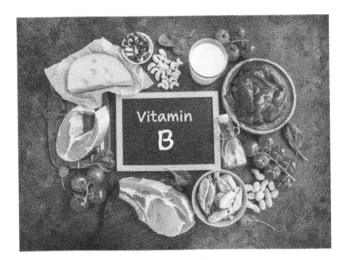

Figure 12.7 Vitamin B sources.

Sources of Vitamin B-Complex: Some most common food sources of vitamin B-Complex are fresh fruits like bananas and orange, nuts, almonds, spinach, legumes, red meats, mushrooms, egg and dairy products as shown in Figure 12.7.

Vitamin B-Complex Deficiency in Oral Health: Vitamin B12 deficiency may cause an increase in dental caries andgingival diseases in children. Inadequate intakes of (riboflavin, vitamin D, and vitamin B12) were associated with increased caries experience and low adequate intakes vs inadequate or high adequate intakes) of nutrients (vitamin B12 and vitamin C) were related with decreased caries experience. It also causes glossitis, angular cheilitis, recurrent oral ulcer, oral candidiasis, diffuseerythematous mucositis, and pale oral mucosa. Folic acid is required for essential biochemical reactions for the synthesis of amino acids, purines, and DNA. Insufficient intake of folic acidduring the pregnancy includes increase the risk for cleft palate. The Figure 12.7 shows vitamin B rich food, it includes fish, cheese, cashew, milk, salmon, cereal, chicken, spinach [58].

12.4 Before Nutraceuticals

Before nutraceutical the only systemetic care a patient should be given would antibiotics which target the released of enzyme collagenase but scope of antibiotics is now less as usage of antibiotics, damages the immune system and the nutraceuticals inhibit the release of multiple enzymes which include collagenase which effectively prevent further plaque build-up and that strengthens immune system of the person and it enhance soft tissue healing [59].

Advantages of nutraceuticals

- It improves overall health.
- It boosts the energy.
- It prevents chronic diseases.
- Improves sleeping pattern.
- Relieves anxiety.

12.5 Conclusion

This chapter helps us to know in detail about vitamins, what actually it means. They are classified based on solubility as fat soluble and water soluble. Nutraceuticals were studied in detail. The role of vitamins as nutraceutical for oral health was described and it is reported that vitamins have its different role in dental treatment. The sources of different vitamins are varried. The chapter helps us in getting idea about vitamins and its role in oral health.

Acknowledgement

The authors wish to thank M.G.V'S Samajshri Prashant Dada Hiray, College of Pharmacy, Malegaon Nashik, India.

References

1. Onyeka, K.N. and Kingsley, I.U., Nutraceuticals: History, classification and market demand, in: *Functional Foods and Nutraceuticals*, Egbuna, C. and Tupas, G.D. (eds.), pp. 13–22, Springer International Publishing, New York, 2020.
2. Jian, W., Sanjay, G., Mattheos, A.G.K., Yajun, Y., Microbial production of value-added nutraceuticals. *Current Opinion in Biotechnology,* United States, 37, 97–104, 2016.
3. Avrelija, C. and Walter, C., The role of functional foods, Nutraceuticals and food supplements in intestinal health. *Nutrients*, 2, 611–625, 2010.

4. Defelice, S.L., The nutraceutical evolution: Its impact on food industry R and D. *Trends Food Sci. Technol.*, 6, 59–61, 1995.
5. Hamid, N., Azar., B., Mahmoud, R.K., New concept in nutraceuticals as alternative for pharmaceuticals. *Int. J. Prev. Med.*, 5, 12, 1487–1499, 2014.
6. Zeisel, S.H., Regulation of nutraceuticals. *Science*, 285, 185–186, 1999.
7. Brower, V., Nutraceuticals: Poised for a healthy slice of the healthcare market? *Nat. Biotechol.*, 16, 728–731, 1998.
8. Bieselskl, H.K., Chapter 3: Nutraceuticals: The link between nutriton and medicine, in: *Nutraceuticals in Health and Disease Prevention*, vol. 2, pp. 1-26, Marcel Deckker, New York, 2001.
9. Raman, D., Nutraceuticals for healthy life. *Indian J. Pharm. Educ. Res.*, 51, 3, 148–151, 2017.
10. Alamgir, N.M., Vitamins, nutraceuticals, food additives, enzymes, anesthetic aids and cosmetics, in: *Progress in Drug Research*, pp. 407–534, 2018.
11. Nutraceutical: New era's. *Pharmaceutical's J. Pharm. Res.*, 3, 1243–1247, 2010.
12. Namdeo, S., Bhaskar, B., Sunil, D., Pratik, K., Nutraceuticals: A review on current status. *Res. J. Pharm. Technol.*, 7, 1, 110–113, 2014.
13. Kharb, S. and Singh, V., Nutraceuticals in health and disease prevention. *Indian J. Clin. Biochem.*, 19, 1, 50–53, 2004.
14. Shilpa, P.C., Priyatam, V.P., Mahesh, N.P., Nutraceuticals: Review. *World J. Pharm. Pharm. Sci.*, 6, 8, 681–739, 2017.
15. Dighe, S.A., Nalkar, R.S., Kakad, S.B., A review on nutraceuticals and its role in treatment of disease. *World J. Pharm. Res.*, 9, 12, 1285–1297, 2020.
16. Rajasekavan, A., General perspective, in: *The Future of Drug Discovery*, p. 108, 2017.
17. Chauhan, B., Kumar, G., Kalam, N., Ansari, S.H., Current concepts and prospects of herbal nutraceutical: A review. *J. Adv. Pharm. Technol. Res.*, 4, 1, 4–8, 2013.
18. Zhao, J., Nutraceuticals, nutritional therapy, phytonutrients, and phytotherapy for improvement of human health: A perspective on plant biotechnology application, Bentham Science Publishers, Pubmed.org vol. 1, pp. 75–97, USA, 2007.
19. Michail, S., Sylvester, F., Fuchs, G., Issenma, R., Clinical efficacy of probiotics: Review of the evidence with focus on children, clinical practice guideline. *J. Pediatr. Gastroenterol. Nutr.*, 43, 4, 15–20, 2006.
20. Holzapfel, W.H., Haberer, P., Geisen, R., Bjorkroth, J., Schillinger, U., Taxonomy and important features of probiotic microorganisms in food and nutrition. *Am. J. Clin. Nutr.*, 73, 365–373, 2001.
21. Sascha, S. and Annabell, P., Health-beneficial nutraceuticals—Myth or reality? *Eur. J. Appl. Microbiol. Biotechnol.*, 101, 3, 951–961, 2016.
22. Maria, G.C., Thomas, G.W., Guglielmo, C., The role of vitamins in oral health. A systematic review and meta analysis. *Int. J. Environ. Res. Public Health*, 17, 3, 938, 2020.

23. Dickinson, A. and Mackay, D., Health habits and other characteristics of dietry supplement users: A review. *J. Nutr.*, 13, 14, 2014.
24. Parveen, S.S. and Srinivas, P., The role of vitamins and trace elements an oral health: A systematic review. *Int. J. Med. Rev.*, 4, 1, 22–31, 2017.
25. Kogl, and Tonnis, Uber das bios problem. Drastellung von kvy stallisertem biotin aur eigel 6.20. Mitteilung uber pflanzliche wachstumss toffee. *Hoppe Seylers Z. Physiol. Chem.*, 242, 1-2, 43–73, 1936.
26. Sona, S., Seaweed vitamins as nutraceuticals. *Adv. Food Nutr. Res.*, 64, 357–369, 2011.
27. Varela-Lopez, A., Navarro-Hortal, M.D., Giampierif, F., Bullon, P., Battino, M., Quius, J.L., Nutraceuticals in periodontal health maintainance. *Molecules*, 20, 23–26, 2018.
28. Eydou, Z., Jad, B.N., Elsayed, Z., Ismail, A., Magaogao, M., Hossain, A., Investigation on the effect of vitamin C on growth & biofilm-forming potential of Streptococcus mutans isolated from patients with dental caries. *BMC Microbiol.*, 20, 231–235, 2020.
29. Cagetti, M.G., Wolf, T.G., Tennert, C., Comoni, N., Lingstrom, P., Campus, G., The role of vitamins in oral health. A systematic review and meta-analysis. *Int. J. Environ. Res. Public Health*, 17, 938–405, 2020.
30. Murererehe, J., Uwitonze, A.M., Nikuze, P., Patel, J., Razzaque, M.S., Beneficial effects of vitamin C in maintaining optimal oral health. *Front. Nutr.*, 8, 1–5 2022.
31. Botelho, J., Machado, V., Mendes, J.J., Proenca, L., Delgado., A.S., Vitamin D-deficiency and oral health: A comprehensive review. *BMC*, 12, 5, 147–154, 2020.
32. Perez, A., What are vitamins and how do they work. *Med. News Today*, 1–2, 2020.
33. Souyoul, S.A., Saussy., K.P., Lupo, M.P., Nutraceuticals: A review. *Dermatol. Ther.*, 8, 5–16, 2018.
34. Subrrramni, T., Yeap, S.K., Omar, A.R., Aziz, S.A., Rahman, N.M., Vitamin suppresses cell death in MCF-7 human breast cancer cells indused by jall MoL. *Int. J. Environ. Res. Public Health*, 18, 305–313, 2014.
35. Taqa, A.A., Vitamins and their relation to oral health: A review study. *IJRP*, 22, 1, 510–522, 2019.
36. Wilson, M., *Food Constituents and Oral Health: Current Status and Future Prospects*, pp. 168–174, CRC Press, Boca Raton, 2009.
37. Ross, A.C., Caballero, B., Cousins, R.J., Tucker, K., Ziegler, T., *Modern Nutrition in Health and Disease Philadelphia*, vol. 11, pp. 260–398, Wolters Kluwer Health/Lippincott Williams & Wilkins, United States, 2014.
38. Kau, A.L., Ahern, P.P., Griffin, N.W., Goodman, A.L., Gordon, J.I., Human nutrition, the gut microbiome, and immune system: Envisioning the future. *Nature*, 474, 327–336, 2011.

39. Akhtar, S., Ahmed, A., Randhawa, M.A. et al., Prevalence of vitamin A deficiency in South Asia: Causes, outcomes, and possible remedies. *J. Health Popul. Nutr.*, 31, 413–423, 2013.
40. Kaufman, D.R., Calisto, J., Simmons, N.L. et al., Vitamin A deficiency impairs vaccine-elicited gastrointestinal immunity. *J. Immunol.*, 187, 1877–1883, 2011.
41. Park, J.A., Lee, J.H., Lee, H.J., Association of some vitamins and minerals with periodontitis in a nationally representative sample of Korean young adults. *Biol. Trace Elem. Res.*, 178, 171–179, 2017.
42. Sheetal, A., Hiremath, V.K., Patil, A.G., Sajjansetty, S., Kumar, S.R., Malnutrition and its oral outcome–a review. *J. Clin. Diagn. Res.*, 7, 178–180, 2013.
43. Chaitanya, N.C., Muthukrishnan, A., Babu, D.B.G., , Role of and vitamin A in oral mucositis induced by cancer chemo/radiotherapy–a meta-analysis. *J. Clin. Diagn. Res.*, 11, 06–09, 2017.
44. Yan, Y., Zeng, W., Song, S. et al., Vitamin C induces periodontal ligament progenitor cell differentiation via activation of ERK pathway mediated by PELP1. Protein cell. *J. Clin. Diagn. Res.*, 4, 620–627, 2013.
45. Alagl, A.S. and Bhat, S.G., Ascorbic acid: New role of an age-old micronutrient in the management of periodontal disease in older adults. *Geriatr. Gerontol. Int.*, 15, 241–254, 2015.
46. Herrmann, W. and Obeid, R., *Vitamins in the Prevention of Human Diseases*, pp. 41–61, De Gruyter, Berlin, 2011.
47. Lerner, V. and Miodownik, C., *Vitamin D Deficiency*, pp. 23–33, Hauppaege, Nova Science, Sultan Qaboos University, 2011.
48. Combs, G.F., *The Vitamins: Fundamental Aspects in Nutrition and Health Amsterdam*, vol. 3, pp. 3–177, 345–354, Elsevier, Academic Press, Ithaca, 2008.
49. Freedman, J.E. and Keaney Jr., J.F., Vitamin E inhibition of platelet aggregation is independent of antioxidant activity. *J. Nutr.*, 131, 374–377, 2001.
50. Garrow, J.S., Ralph, A., James, W.P.T., *Human Nutrition and Dietetics*, pp. 211–282, Churchill Livingstone, Edinburgh, 2000.
51. Weingartner, J., Lotz, K., Fanghänel, J., Gedrange, T., Bienengräber, V., Proff, P., Induction and prevention of cleft lip, alveolus and palate and neural tube defects with special consideration of B vitamins and the methylation cycle. *J. Orofac. Orthop.*, 68, 4, 266–277, 2007.
52. Wang, H., Li, L., Qin, L.L., Song, Y., Vidal-Alaball, J., Liu, T.H., Oral vitamin B12 versus intramuscular vitamin B12 for vitaminB12 deficiency. *Cochrane Database Syst. Rev.*, 15, 3, 4655, 2018.
53. Ahire, E.D., Sonawane, V.N., Surana, K.R., Talele, G.S., Drug discovery, drug-likeness screening, and bioavailability: Development of drug-likeness rule for natural products, in: *Applied Pharmaceutical Practice and Nutraceuticals*, pp. 191–208, Taylor and Francis, 2021.

54. Surana, K.R., Ahire, E.D., Sonawane, V.N., Talele, S.G., Talele, G.S., Molecular modeling: Novel techniques in food and nutrition development, in: *Natural Food Products and Waste Recovery*, pp. 17–31, Taylor and Francis, 2021.
55. Gupta, M., Aggarwal, R., Raina, N., Khan, A., Vitamin-loaded nanocarriers as nutraceuticals in healthcare applications, in: *Nanomedicine for Bioactives*, pp. 451–470, Springer, Singapore, 2020.
56. Isola, G., The impact of diet, nutrition and nutraceuticals on oral and periodontal health. *Nutrients*, 12, 9, 2724, 2020.
57. Ahire, E.D., Sonawane, V.N., Surana, K.R., Role of drug repurposing in current treatment strategies against COVID-19; Systemic review. *Pharm. Reson.*, 24–9, 2020.
58. Sachdeva, V., Roy, A., Bharadvaja, N., Current prospects of nutraceuticals: A review. *Curr. Pharm. Biotechnol.*, 21, 10, 884–896, 2020.
59. Gupta, S., Parvez, N., Sharma, P.K., Nutraceuticals as functional foods. *J. Nutr. Ther.*, 4, 2, 64–72, 2015.

Index

Advantages of nutraceuticals, 295
Anti-cancer, 176
Anti-infective vitamins, 117
Anti-inflammatory, 116, 118, 173, 175, 177
Antioxidants, 63, 64, 66, 70–72, 110, 112–113, 115, 117–120, 123, 173
Apoptosis, 118
Arachidonic acid, 10
Ariboflavinosis, 15
Arthritis, 88
Ascorbic acid lead to cancer, 228
Attenuating virus, 119
Autoimmune diseases, 88
Autoimmune inflammatory disorder, 97
Avitaminosis, 3

Before nutraceuticals, 294
Beneficial effects, 68, 70, 73, 76
Bioactive compounds, 129–130, 153, 167, 169–170, 175, 178–179
Biochemical functions, 168, 174
Biosynthesis, 242, 245
Biotin, 237, 242, 244–246

Cancer, 217
Carbohydrate, 240
Cardiac, 61, 65–67, 70
Cardiovascular disease, 61–70, 215, 218
Cardiovascular health, 62, 73
Causes of anemia, 258

Chitin, 129, 131–133, 135–136, 138, 155
Chitosan, 129, 131–136, 138, 154–155
Chlorophytes, 169
Cholecalciferol, 40
Chronic diseases, 179
Chronic kidney disease, 220
Classification of vitamins, 36
Clinical research, 67, 70
Clotting factors, 116, 121
Coagulation-vitamins, 120
Complex vitamin, 173
COVID-19, 116–117, 119

Defensive system, 117
Deficiency, 61, 63, 64, 235–237, 240, 244–246
Diabetes mellitus, 122, 167, 175
Diet and nourishment in pregnancy, 186
Dietary, 235, 236, 244, 249
Dietary fibers, 170–171, 175
Difference between nutraceuticals and functional foods, 284
Difference between nutraceuticals and pharmaceuticals, 284
Disease management, 175, 178

EAAs, 129, 131, 142
Ectopic mineralization, 221
Ergocalciferol, 40
Essential, 235, 236, 239, 240, 244, 245, 249

Fat-soluble vitamins, 92, 107–108, 110–113, 116–117, 123, 169, 196, 208
Folacin, 20
Folic acid, 62, 63, 66, 67
Functional foods, 129–130, 155–156, 169, 175, 178–179
Fundamental food, 109

Health, 61–76, 236, 238, 241, 243, 245–247, 249
Hematopoiesis, 117–118
Hepatic steatosis, 216
Herbals, 107–110
Hippocrates, 168
Huntington's disease, 223
Hydrosoluble vitamins, 62, 63, 76
Hypertension, 176, 179
Hypervitaminosis, 3, 9
Hypovitaminosis, 3, 236

Immune system, 89, 108, 116, 118–119
Immunity, 87
Immunological, 115–117, 119–120
Inflammation, 216
Insulin secretion, 215
Insulin sensitivity, 216
Intervention, 61

Liposoluble vitamins, 61, 62, 64–66

Macular degeneration, 213
Marine algae, 168, 177
Marine-derived, 130, 155
Measles, 213
Menadione, 42
Menaquinone, 42
Metabolic diseases, 205, 207, 210, 211, 213, 215, 218
Micronutrients, 235, 244
Mineral bone disorder, 220
Minerals, 129, 131, 143–144, 149, 150, 153, 155
Multivitamins, 4

Niacin, 2, 237, 241, 244–246
Nicotinamide, 17
Nicotinic acid, 16, 17
Non–insulin-dependent diabetes mellitus, 227
Nutraceuticals, 3, 107–124, 129–131, 136, 167–171, 175, 179–180, 194
  non-traditional, 255
  traditional, 255
Nutraceuticals categorized based on food available in market,
  commercial nutraceuticals, 283
  non-traditional nutraceuticals, 283
  traditional nutraceuticals, 283
Nutrients, 107–110, 112, 118, 123
Nutrition, 236, 244, 247
Nutritional, 129–131, 135, 140, 150, 153–155

Obesity, 175–176, 179, 221
Omega-3 fatty acids, 129, 145
Osteromalacia, 7

Pantothenic acid, 237, 242, 244, 246
Peptides, 129–131, 142, 150–151, 154–155
Phenolic compounds, 129, 140, 153
Pheophytes, 169
Phylloquinone, 42
Phytochemicals, 169, 171
Polysaccharides, 129–131, 133, 138, 140, 155, 168–176
Prohormones, 115
Proteins, 129, 136–137, 140, 142, 150–151, 153
Psoriasis, 88
Pyridoxine, 2

Retinoic acid, 39
Retinoids, 37
Rhodophytes, 168–169
Riboflavin, 237, 240, 241, 244, 246
Role of vitamins, 73, 205

Role of vitamins in nutraceuticals for anemia,
  folate, 262–263
  riboflavin, 263–264
  role of iron in anemia as nutraceutical, 258–259, 265
  vitamin A, 259–260
  vitamin B12, 263–264
  vitamin C, 260–261, 269
  vitamin E, 261–262, 271–273

Seafood, 129, 131–132, 135, 141, 143–144, 147–149
Seaweeds, 167–180
Stroke, 226
Structure of vitamin,
  vitamin B-complex, 266–269
  vitamin D, 270
  vitamin K, 273–274
Sunshine vitamin, 111
Superfood, 172
Supplement, 68–76

Targeted nutrition foods for pregnancy, 195
Thiamine, 237–241, 244, 246
Thiamine diphosphate, 14
Tocopherol, 8, 41
Tocotrienol, 41
Type 2 diabetes, 213, 214
Types of anemia,
  based on etiology, 257
  based on physiological abnormality, 257
  based on the category, 257
  based on the Hb level, 256
  based on the RBC morphology, 256

Vegetables, 240
Vitamin A, 4, 37, 92, 211–214
Vitamin A/retinol, 188
Vitamin B1, 12, 13, 95
Vitamin B1/thiamine, 191
Vitamin B12, 22, 48, 99, 225

Vitamin B12/cobalamin/cyanocobalamin, 192
Vitamin B2, 15, 44, 96, 224
Vitamin B3, 16, 45, 97, 222
Vitamin B5, 17, 223
Vitamin B6, 19, 98
Vitamin B7/biotin, 191
Vitamin B7/H, 46
Vitamin B9, 20, 98, 225
Vitamin B9/folic acid, 47, 191
Vitamin C, 2, 24, 49, 99
Vitamin C/ascorbic acid, 192
Vitamin D, 3, 6, 39, 64, 65, 68, 69, 73–75, 93
Vitamin D/calciferol, 189
Vitamin deficiency, 61–63
Vitamin E, 8, 41, 94, 219
Vitamin E/tocopherol, 189
Vitamin F, 9
Vitamin K, 2, 10, 42, 219
Vitamin M, 20
Vitamin supplementation, 63, 72
Vitaminoids, 2
Vitamins, 1, 2, 36, 61–77, 107–123, 129–131, 140, 144, 149, 150, 153–155, 167–175, 178, 207–229, 235–249
  history of vitamins, 285–286
  importance of vitamins for humans, 287
Vitamins associated with the oral health as nutraceuticals,
  vitamin A, 292–293
  vitamin B-complex, 293–294
  vitamin C, 287–288
  vitamin D, 289–290
  vitamin E, 290–291
  vitamin K, 291–292
Vitamins in CVP, 71, 73

Water-soluble, 235–240, 245, 247–249
Water-soluble vitamins, 95, 107–108, 110, 167, 171, 196, 208

Printed and bound by CPI Group (UK) Ltd, Croydon, CR0 4YY
25/06/2023

03230097-0003